The Specialty Practice of Rehabilitation Nursing

A Core Curriculum

Third Edition

(formerly published as *Rehabilitation Nursing: Concepts and Practice—A Core Curriculum*)

Editor

Ann E. McCourt, MS RN
Consultant
Ormond Beach, FL
formerly Coordinator of Rehabilitation
New England Sinai Hospital and Rehabilitation Center
Stoughton, MA

Associate Editors

Brenda Emick-Herring, MSN RN CRRN
Staff Development Specialist
Iowa Methodist Medical Center
Des Moines, IA

Maureen Habel, MA RN CRRN CNA
Director, Nursing Staff Development
Rancho Los Amigos Medical Center
Downey, CA

Nancy Davis Kipnis, MS RN CRRN
Unit Leader
Rush-Presbyterian-St. Luke's Medical Center
Chicago, IL

Terri Patterson, MSN RN CRRN
President/Consultant
Nursing Consultation Services, Ltd.
Norristown, PA

The Rehabilitation Nursing Foundation of the Association of Rehabilitation Nurses
5700 Old Orchard Road, First Floor
Skokie, IL 60077-1057

3rd Edition
Formerly published as *Rehabilitation Nursing: Concepts and Practice—A Core Curriculum*

Library of Congress Catalog Card Number: 93-86096
ISBN 1-884278-00-0 (hardcover)
1-884278-01-9 (softcover)

NOTE: As new scientific information becomes available through basic and clinical research, recommended treatments and drug therapies undergo changes. The authors, editors, and publisher have done everything possible to make this book accurate, up-to-date, and in accord with standards accepted at the time of publication. The authors, editors, and publisher are not responsible for errors or omissions or for consequences from application of the book, and make no warranty, expressed or implied, in regard to the contents of the book. Any practice described in this book should be applied by the healthcare practitioner in accordance with professional standards of care used in regard to the unique circumstances that may apply in each situation. The reader is advised always to check product information (package inserts) for changes and new information regarding dose and contraindications before administering any drug. Caution is especially urged when using new or infrequently ordered drugs or treatments.

To those
who have made
rehabilitation nursing
a specialty practice

The Rehabilitation Nursing Foundation extends its thanks
to **Hollister Incorporated** of Libertyville, IL
for its generous support
of the publication of
The Specialty Practice of Rehabilitation Nursing:
A Core Curriculum

The Specialty Practice of Rehabilitation Nursing: A Core Curriculum
was developed in part through grants from these contributors:

New England Chapter of the Paralyzed Veterans of America
Walpole, MA

Teresa Cervantez Thompson, PhD RN CRRN
in memory of Malcom Maloof, MS RN CRRN

Medical Marketing Group, Inc.
Decatur, GA

Table of Contents

PREFACE

The Specialty Practice of Rehabilitation Nursing: A Core Curriculum reflects the evolution of a distinct specialty in nursing and provides information necessary to practice within the specialty. This third edition is a comprehensive, state-of-the-art guide to the practice of rehabilitation nursing, designed to meet the needs of both those just entering the specialty and those experienced in it. It also is an excellent reference for the rehabilitation component of nursing practice in general. Written and edited by rehabilitation nurses with wide-ranging experience in all areas of the specialty, the text is an authoritative resource for those providing nursing care for rehabilitation clients, those preparing for the Certified Rehabilitation Registered Nurse (CRRN) certification examination, and those providing instruction in rehabilitation nursing.

As the book evolved, the editors saw the need for including several new features. A major portion of this edition is devoted to integrating theory and assessment with functional health patterns and nursing diagnoses. This new approach should help rehabilitation nurses identify the relationship between scientific concepts and the nursing process. To meet the need expressed by ARN members for a concise, convenient reference on the most common disorders found among rehabilitation clients, the editors focused a section on stroke, prevalent musculoskeletal disorders, traumatic brain injury, and spinal cord injury. Topics new to this edition include ethical issues in rehabilitation nursing and the role of the rehabilitation nurse case manager. We also have added a glossary of terms frequently used in rehabilitation and have highlighted research-based works in the reference lists, in keeping with the specialty's growing emphasis on research.

The book is divided into eight sections that employ both narrative and outline formats. The narrative format was used to enhance the readability of broad general topics and historical data, as well as to summarize each section and chapter. The outline format is used extensively to present scientific data and to show the hierarchy of information under each topic, as well as to aid in teaching and learning.

To introduce the reader to the specialty, **Section I** furnishes a broad overview of the philosophy, objectives, and process of rehabilitation and rehabilitation nursing. A timeline chronicles the history of rehabilitation from the late 19th century to the present, and there are brief glimpses of a representative group of rehabilitation nursing pioneers. Historical information may not be seen as essential for entering the specialty, but it provides a very helpful perspective on accomplishments of the past and goals to be set for the future.

Section II contains new material that will improve and update knowledge relating to stroke, traumatic brain injury, spinal cord injury, and musculoskeletal disorders—osteoporosis, arthritis, and conditions associated with amputation. Understanding the anatomical, physiological, and pathophysiological changes and residual deficits associated with each disorder enables the nurse to teach clients and families about the processes and outcomes of injury and disease. Knowledge about the resulting sequelae also helps the nurse comprehend the etiology of possible nursing diagnoses that are listed for each disorder. Another innovation, the book's discussion of the impact of the aging process on rehabilitation, reflects the growing number of aging people in the rehabilitation population. Concepts related to the pediatric population are integrated throughout the text.

Section III focuses on the clinical practice of rehabilitation nursing. Functional health patterns serve as the unifying framework here, because using functional health patterns permits nurses to focus on the alteration in functional ability and life style that is seen in rehabilitation patients. A separate chapter for each pattern enhances the integration of scientific theory, appropriate nursing assessment, related nursing diagnoses, and interventions and outcomes. This design permits the reader to learn new material sequentially as a comprehensive unit or to focus on areas of particular interest. The listing of nursing diagnoses with interventions and outcomes will assist rehabilitation nurses in developing nursing care plans and guidelines for care.

Both managers and practitioners will find **Section IV** a helpful guide to fostering the team approach to care, as well as to understanding and meeting the challenges of accreditation. Accreditation standards require nursing staff to be involved in quality improvement activities; thus, the inclusion of this information. Portions of several pertinent patient evaluation systems are reproduced as well.

Section V is an overview of the community reentry of people with disabilities, with a focus on required life skills and obtaining access to health care. In keeping with the current trend in nursing practice, the role of the nurse case manager and issues associated with this role are highlighted.

Section VI and **Section VII** include legislative and economic issues and an overview of basic ethical principles with examples of current ethical dilemmas. To help consolidate this difficult topic for the reader, we have included in Section VII documents such as the American Hospital Association's 1992 revision of "A Patient's Bill of Rights" and the ANA Position Statement on Nursing and the Patient Self-Determination Act.

Section VIII discusses the future of rehabilitation nursing, citing the potential impact of the growing population of people with disabilities and of healthcare reform, alternate methods of care delivery, new legislation, and emerging technology.

There are two appendices. The first is a client and family guide to choosing a rehabilitation facility, designed to assist the nurse in helping families with the transition to rehabilitation. The second is a listing of community resources and healthcare-related organizations for rehabilitation nurses who need additional information on specific problems or who have clients with specific needs not covered in the text.

Throughout the book, the terms *patient* and *client* are used interchangeably, and the term *family* includes significant others.

The development of the third edition of this core curriculum was a complete team effort, accomplished through the combined knowledge and total commitment of the four associate editors: Brenda Emick-Herring, Maureen Habel, Nancy Davis Kipnis, and Terri Patterson. Without their perseverance and selfless support, the production of this text would not have been possible. Thanks also accrue to our many ARN colleagues who contributed their expertise as authors and reviewers.

—*Ann E. McCourt*
Editor

CONTRIBUTORS

Section I. Introduction to Rehabilitation and Rehabilitation Nursing

Chapter 1

Maureen Habel, MA RN CRRN CNA
Director, Nursing Staff Development
Rancho Los Amigos Medical Center
Downey, CA

Chapter 2

Helen Cioschi, MSN RN CRRN CRNP
Vice President of Nursing
Magee Rehabilitation Hospital
Philadelphia, PA

Chapter 3

Maureen Habel, MA RN CRRN CNA

Chapter 4

Dagny Engle, RN CAE
Executive Director
Association of Rehabilitation Nurses
Skokie, IL

Susan S. Novak, MS RN CRRN
Director of Nursing
Memorial Regional Rehabilitation Center
Jacksonville, FL

Section II. Common Disorders Among Rehabilitation Clients

Chapter 5

Brenda Emick-Herring, MSN RN CRRN
Staff Development Specialist
Iowa Methodist Medical Center
Des Moines, IA

Maureen Habel, MA RN CRRN CNA

Chapter 6

Brenda Emick-Herring, MSN RN CRRN

Chapter 7

Karen Gabrielson, MSN RN CRRN
Staff Nurse
Alta Bates-Herrick Hospital
Berkeley, CA

Pam Semanik, MSN RN
Clinical Specialist, Orthopedics
Rehabilitation Institute of Chicago
Chicago, IL

Nancy Davis Kipnis, MS RN CRRN
Unit Leader
Rush-Presbyterian-St. Luke's Medical Center
Chicago, IL

Chapter 8

Terri Patterson, MSN RN CRRN
President/Consultant
Nursing Consultation Services, Ltd.
Norristown, PA

Chapter 9

Karen Fried, MSN RN CRRN
Rehabilitation Clinical Specialist
Thomas Jefferson University Hospital
Philadelphia, PA

Chapter 10

Pamela Duchene, DNSc RN CRRN
Vice President, Nursing & Clinical Services
New England Rehabilitation Hospital
Woburn, MA

Section III. Functional Health Patterns and Nursing Diagnoses

Chapter 11

Karen Preston, MS PHN CRRN
Nurse Consultant
Rehabilitation Nursing Services, Inc.
Sacramento, CA

Bonnie Parker, MSN RN CRRN
Case Manager
NeuroCare of Texas
Irving, TX

Chapter 12

Brenda Emick-Herring, MSN RN CRRN

Karen Patton, MSN RN CRRN
Clinical Nurse Specialist
University of Missouri Hospitals-Rusk Rehabilitation Center
Columbia, MO

Randy Temple, RN CRRN
Research Data Manager
Rehabilitation Institute of Chicago
Chicago, IL

Peggy Matthews Kirk, BSN RN CRRN
Staff Nurse, Spinal Cord Injury Program
Rehabilitation Institute of Chicago
Chicago, IL

Kelly Johnson, MSN RN CRRN CFNP
Spinal Cord Injury Clinical Educator
Craig Hospital
Englewood, CO

Chapter 13

Helen Cioschi, MSN RN CRRN CRNP

Mary Mulrow, BSN RN CRRN
Rehabilitation Clinician
Charleston Area Medical Center
Charleston, WV

Chapter 14

Marion Phipps, MS RN CRRN
Clinical Nurse Specialist
Beth Israel Hospital
Boston, MA

Nancy Davis Kipnis, MS RN CRRN

Daniel Kopanke, MS RN CRRN
Unit Leader
Rush-Presbyterian-St. Luke's Medical Center
Chicago, IL

Ann McCourt, MS RN
Consultant
Ormond Beach, FL

Catherine Tracey, MS RN CRRN
Vice President, Patient Care Services
Northeast Rehabilitation Hospital
Salem, NH

Marie Femino Esposito, MS RN C
Director of Professional Services
Primary Health Service, Inc.
Brockton, MA

Lisa Cyr Buchanan, MS RN C CRRN
Director/Owner
Lisa B. Cyr & Associates
Charleston, ME

Michelle Young Stevenson, MS RN CRRN
Associate Vice President of Patient Care
Mt. Sinai Hospital
Philadelphia, PA

Margaret Reddy Daly, MN RN CRRN
Nurse Consultant
Nursing Consultation Services, Ltd.
Norristown, PA

Pamela Duchene, DNSc RN CRRN

Terri Patterson, MSN RN CRRN

Susanne Hays, MS RN CRRN
Nurse Specialist/Owner
Adaptations/Family Centered Pediatric Rehabilitation
Albuquerque, NM

Chapter 15

Maureen Habel, MA RN CRRN CNA

Chapter 16

Cindy Gatens, MN RN CRRN
Clinical Nurse Specialist
The Ohio State University Hospital
Columbus, OH

René Hébert, MS RN CRRN
Clinical Nurse Specialist
The Ohio State University Hospital
Columbus, OH

Pamela Duchene, DNSc RN CRRN

Carol Gleason, RN CRRN
Senior Marketing Representative
Greenery Rehabilitation Group
Newton, MA

Susanne Hays, MS RN CRRN

Chapter 17

Judy Popovich, DNSc RN CRRN
Assistant Professor
University of Kentucky College of Nursing
Lexington, KY

Chapter 18

Barbara Brillhart, PhD RN CRRN
Associate Professor
University of Colorado Health Sciences Center
School of Nursing
Denver, CO

Chapter 19

Laura Daly Williams, MN RN CS CRRN
Rehabilitation Clinical Nurse Specialist
Sexual Medicine Center
Lafayette, LA

Chapter 20

Shirley Hoeman, PhD RN CRRN CNAA
Consultant
Health Systems Consultations
Long Valley, NJ

Chapter 21

Melinda Hagee, RN CRRN
Nurse Manager
Chambersburg Hospital
Chambersburg, PA

Section IV. The Rehabilitation Team

Chapter 22

Kathryn Smart, MS RN CRRN
Rehabilitation Clinical Nurse Specialist
Rush-Presbyterian-St. Luke's Medical Center
Chicago, IL

Nancy Davis Kipnis, MS RN CRRN

Chapter 23

Nancy Davis Kipnis, MS RN CRRN

Chapter 24

Margaret Kelly-Hayes, EdD RN CRRN
Associate Clinical Professor
Boston University School of Medicine
Boston, MA

Bernadette Pohlmann, MS RN CRRN CPHQ
Quality Assurance Coordinator/Clinical Nurse Educator
Spinal Cord Injury and Rehabilitation Nursing Service
Edward Hines Jr. Department of Veterans Affairs Hospital
Hines, IL

Daniel Kopanke, MS RN CRRN

Nancy Davis Kipnis, MS RN CRRN

Section V. Community Reentry

Chapter 25

Janice Rook, MS RN CRRN
Rehabilitation Manager
Gates McDonald
Columbus, OH

Chapter 26

Lisa Cyr Buchanan, MS RN C CRRN

Chapter 27

Lisa Cyr Buchanan, MS RN C CRRN

Carol Gleason, RN CRRN

Section VI. Legislative and Economic Issues

Chapter 28

Gloria Craven, MS RN CRRN
Clinical Specialist
Beth Israel Hospital
Boston, MA

Carol Gleason, RN CRRN

Chapter 29

Lorraine Priestley, MSN RN CRRN
Senior Health Services Representative
ITT Hartford
Greenbelt, MO

Section VII. Ethics in Rehabilitation Nursing

Chapter 30

Terri Patterson, MSN RN CRRN

Margaret Reddy Daly, MN RN CRRN

Section VIII. The Future of Rehabilitation Nursing

Chapter 31

Aloma (Cookie) Gender, MSN RN CRRN
Director of Nursing
San Diego Rehabilitation Institute
San Diego, CA

Other contributors

Jan Brewer, PhD RN
Director, Nursing Research/Community Outreach
Rancho Los Amigos Medical Center
Downey, CA

Patricia Edwards, MA RN C
Nursing Practice Coordinator
Spaulding Rehabilitation Hospital
Boston, MA

Judith Stanton, MS RN
Yorba Linda, CA

REVIEWERS

Reviewers of the Entire Book

Christina Mumma, PhD RN CRRN
Assistant Professor
College of Nursing & Health Sciences
University of Alaska Anchorage
Anchorage, AK

Teresa L. Cervantez Thompson, PhD RN CRRN
Vice President for Hospital Services
Rehabilitation Institute of Michigan
Detroit, MI

Marilyn Pires, MS RN CRRN
Rehabilitation Clinical Nurse Specialist
Rancho Los Amigos Medical Center
Downey, CA

Jill Derstine, EdD RN
Chair, Division of Nursing
Neuman College
Aston, PA

Judy Siefke, BSN RN CRRN
Charge Nurse
Poudre Valley Hospital
Fort Collins, CO

Section Reviewers

Section I. Introduction to Rehabilitation and Rehabilitation Nursing

Beth Budny, MS RN CRRN CNA
Head Nurse
Veterans Administration Medical Center
West Roxbury, MA

Diane Burgher, MPA RN CRRN
Administrative Director, Rehabilitation
Providence Medical Center
Seattle, WA

Section II. Common Disorders Among Rehabilitation Clients

Joanne Baggerly, MSN RN CRRN
Clinical Nurse Specialist
Massachusetts General Hospital
Boston, MA

Karma Klauber, MS RN CRRN
Clinical Nurse
Sharp Memorial Hospital Rehabilitation Center
San Diego, CA

Section III. Functional Health Patterns and Nursing Diagnoses

Catherine A. Tracey, MS RN CRRN
Vice President, Patient Care Services
Northeast Rehabilitation Hospital
Salem, NH

Susan Greco, MSN RN CRRN
Clinical Specialist in Nursing/Director of Education
North Alabama Rehabilitation Hospital
Huntsville, AL

Jean M. Benjamin, MSN RN CRRN
Assistant Administrator-SRRC
Cape Fear Valley Medical Center
Fayetteville, NC

Section IV. The Rehabilitation Team

Charles Cumiskey, RN CRRN
Nurse Manager
St. Peter Hospital
Olympia, WA

Barbara H. Warner, MS RN
Director, Neuroscience-Rehabilitation Nursing
The Ohio State University Hospitals
Columbus, OH

Section V. Community Reentry

Carol Ann Balch, MN RN
Director, Clinical Operations-West Division
National Medical Enterprises
Santa Monica, CA

Rose Butler, MS RN CRRN
Clinical Specialist
Memorial Regional Rehabilitation Center
Jacksonville, FL

Section VI. Legislative and Economic Issues

Carol Ann Balch, MN RN

Judy A. Harris, MS RN CRRN CRC
Rehabilitation Consultant
Grimsley Rehabilitation Associates
Tallahassee, FL

Section VII. Ethics in Rehabilitation Nursing

Marilyn Ter Maat, MSN RN C CRRN CNAA
House Supervisor Coordinator
Memorial Hospital
Manhattan, KS

Judy A. Harris, MS RN CRRN CRC

RNF BOARD AND STAFF

RNF Board of Trustees

RNF Staff

The Specialty Practice of Rehabilitation Nursing

A Core Curriculum

Third Edition

Section I
Introduction to Rehabilitation and Rehabilitation Nursing

The purpose of this section is to provide the reader with a theoretical and historical perspective on rehabilitation and the specialty practice of rehabilitation nursing.

Chapter 1 addresses the philosophical beliefs and values held by rehabilitation professionals. These belief systems drive rehabilitation professionals to achieve clients' goals through the process of rehabilitation. Understanding the relationships among rehabilitation's philosophy, goals, and process will help rehabilitation nurses continue to influence the evolution of rehabilitation as a professional healthcare specialty.

Chapter 2 provides an overview of the recent history of rehabilitation. Factors that led to the development of rehabilitation as a specialty are included to help the nurse appreciate the origins of rehabilitation practice. This chapter also recognizes the rehabilitation nursing pioneers whose vision and contributions continue to influence our practice today.

Chapter 3 defines rehabilitation nursing practice, outlines its scope, and describes the settings in which rehabilitation nursing practice occurs. Theoretical nursing models useful for guiding rehabilitation nursing practice are summarized.

Chapter 4 traces the origins and development of the specialty's professional organization. The mission, philosophy, and major accomplishments of the Association of Rehabilitation Nurses are highlighted.

CHAPTER 1

Rehabilitation: Philosophy, Goals, and Process

Understanding the dynamics among a field's philosophy, goals, and process helps professionals in that field to understand and to value their contributions within a broad context. A philosophy essentially is a belief system; goals are outcomes, or ends, to be achieved. A process is a method of operating or proceeding in order to accomplish a goal. In rehabilitation, these three entities are closely intertwined. For example, the basic philosophical belief in rehabilitation is that the disabled individual has the right to become expert in his or her own healthcare management; therefore, the goal becomes the transfer of accountability for self-care from the healthcare professional to the client. Education of the client and the development of self-care skills are the operations, or the process, carried out by the rehabilitation team to support the person with a disability in achieving this goal.

The philosophy of rehabilitation

Understanding the philosophical bases of rehabilitation helps nurses to develop an awareness of how rehabilitation developed in terms of goals and processes, how it continues to evolve, and how nursing will participate in shaping its future.

Dittmar (1989) wrote that "a philosophy is a composite of personal feelings and beliefs about individuals, their interactions with social groups, and the effects of environmental influences and professional beliefs" (p. 4). Kemp, Brummel-Smith, and Ramsdell (1990) stated that rehabilitation includes a philosophy about how health care should be provided, includes principles that shape healthcare delivery, and focuses on a long-term commitment to providing services.

Rehabilitation is a unique and complex process whose outcome is to restore an individual to optimal functional status and to ensure use of all of the individual's resources to maintain that status at home and within a community. Thus, successful rehabilitation aims at helping each individual to strive for independence in order to achieve the highest quality of life possible (Kottke & Lehman, 1990). Figure 1.1 shows factors contributing to the quality of life within a rehabilitation context.

Some of the major philosophical tenets inherent in rehabilitation include the following:

- Rehabilitation recognizes the uniqueness and wholeness of each individual and views each person and his or her own environment as interdependent systems (Sayles, 1981).
- Despite the severity of an injury or illness, each individual has the potential to maintain or regain self-esteem and dignity and to transcend disability. Individuals can obtain optimal independence within the limits of disability when they participate fully in making decisions about their rehabilitation (Dittmar, 1989).
- Through rehabilitation, people with disabilities are enabled to mobilize their own resources, decide what they wish and are able to be, and achieve goals through their own efforts and in their own way (Wright, 1983).
- Each individual is a social organism motivated to work and contribute as a member of society; this contribution begins with self-support and extends to a commitment to family, community, nation, and the world (Wright, 1983). This philosophy holds that persons are part of a much larger interdependent system.

A systems approach recognizes that changes in any part of the system have an impact on all other parts of the system. In a systems approach, a problem at the organ level, such as a right-hemisphere CVA or a fracture dislocation of spinal segment C6, is viewed not only as affecting the individual involved, but also as having an impact on the family, society, and ultimately the nation and the world.

Two widely used conceptual frameworks within the field of rehabilitation are the International Classification of Impairments, Disabilities, and Handicaps (ICIDH) developed by the World Health Organization (WHO) (Storck & Thompson-Hoffman, 1991), and the Functional Limitations System devised by Saad Nagi (Pope & Tarlov, 1991).

The World Health Organization describes an impairment as occurring at the organ level, a disability as an experience occurring at the personal level, and a handicap as a phenomenon occurring at the societal level (Storck & Thompson-Hoffman, 1991). According to the WHO model, the following distinctions should be made among an impairment, a disability, and a handicap:

1. An *impairment* is defined as "a loss or abnormality of a psychological, physiological, or anatomical structure and function" (Storck & Thompson-Hoffman, 1991, p. 6). An impairment at the organ level does not itself result in a disability.
2. A *disability* occurs when there is a "restriction or lack (resulting from an impairment) of ability to perform an activity in the manner or within the range considered normal for a human being" (Storck & Thompson-Hoffman, 1991, p. 6).
3. A *handicap* occurs when there is "a disadvantage for a given individual resulting from impairment or disability that limits or prevents fulfillment of a role that is normal

for that individual" (Storck & Thompson-Hoffman, 1991, p. 7).

People with disabilities face societal barriers in the pursuit of independence. These obstacles may range from architectural barriers to policies and attitudes that hinder their potential to function as members of society. In this context, "there are no handicapped persons, only handicapping societies" (Brummel-Smith, 1990, p. 5).

The Nagi, or functional limitations, framework consists of four concepts: pathology, impairment, functional limitation, and disability. *Pathology* refers to cellular and tissue alterations occurring from disease, trauma, infection, or congenital problems. *Impairment* describes specific abnormalities of physical, mental, and biochemical functioning. A *functional limitation* exists when there is a decrease in an individual's actual or potential performance. Pathology, impairment, and functional limitations are all characteristics that apply to an individual (Nagi, 1965).

In Nagi's model, *disability* occurs when there are conditions that interfere with the performance of individuals in personal, social, and culturally expected roles (Pope & Tarlov, 1991). It is the interface with a person's physical and/or mental limitations within the setting and context of his or her environment and culture that potentially results in disability.

A proposed model of disability combining both the WHO and the Nagi models was published in 1991 by the Committee on a National Agenda for the Prevention of Disabilities, Division of Health Promotion, Institute of Medicine (Pope & Tarlov, 1991). The newly proposed framework builds on the WHO classification, including deletion of the term *handicap*, and the Nagi framework and adds the concepts of risk factors and quality of life to a model describing the disabling process.

Definitions of rehabilitation: The terms that have been used to define rehabilitation provide insight about belief systems held by rehabilitation professionals. Figure 1.2 provides definitions of rehabilitation as they have evolved over the past 50 years, from a definition in 1944 by the National Council on Rehabilitation to the present. These definitions illustrate the philosophical influences shaping the meaning of disability and the place of disabled persons in society. The beliefs underlying these definitions about individuals, disability, human potential, and the interdependence of people in society provide the philosophical structural supports for the goals and processes of rehabilitation.

Figure 1.1. Factors Contributing to the Quality of Life*

Highest Level of Attainment

Aspiration for personal achievement and creativity
Vocational performance and capability
Social interaction
Communicative abilities
- Writing
- Reading
- Speaking

Activities of daily living
Mobility
- Ambulation and transfers
- Manipulative skills
- Posture

Sensory perception
- Hearing
- Vision
- Touch
- Spatial orientation

Moderate Level of Attainment

Enjoyment and satisfaction
Sense of self-worth
Comfort versus pain
Awareness and cognition
Survival of essential organs
Supportive environment
Food, shelter, clothing, personal safety

Lowest Level of Attainment

*The factors underlying quality of life are arrayed from the bottom of the figure to the top, in ascending order of their attainment during rehabilitation. Restoration to each level requires the prior attainment of the functional capabilities of subordinate levels.

Reprinted with permission of W.B. Saunders Company from Kottke, F.J., & Lehman, J.F. (1990). *Krusen's handbook of physical medicine and rehabilitation* (4th ed.) (p. xx). Philadelphia: W.B. Saunders Company.

The goals of rehabilitation

Rehabilitation goals are the desired outcomes for each rehabilitation client. In 1949, rehabilitation nursing pioneer Alice Morrissey (1949) stated that "the great goal of rehabilitation is to return the patient to the community as a useful citizen capable of using whatever ability he has left and independent of the support of others. Although this high objective cannot always be achieved, a certain amount of independence can be restored to every patient through the wise guidance and expert teaching of nurses qualified in the field of rehabilitation" (p. 545).

According to Brummel-Smith (1990), the major goals of rehabilitation are improving function, promoting independence and life satisfaction, and preserving self-esteem. "These goals are not, however, simply a matter of increasing cardiovascular reserves, stabilizing gait, increasing muscular strength, improving activities of daily living, or improving range of motion in a joint. Improving function means maximizing the person's ability to live in the least restrictive and most desirable environment" (Brummel-Smith, 1990, p. 42). The goal of promoting independence is accomplished through the promotion of life satisfaction and the preservation of the disabled person's self-esteem. The consensus among healthcare professionals is that people who can value and enjoy themselves in spite of a disability are minimally handicapped by it.

The major goal of rehabilitation as described in *Rehabilitation Nursing: Concepts and Practice—A Core Curriculum* (Sayles, 1981) is to enable an individual to achieve his or her highest level of function by preventing complications, modifying the effects of disability, and increasing independence.

The 1987 edition of *Rehabilitation Nursing: Concepts and Practice—A Core Curriculum* (Mumma, 1987, pp. 2-4) outlined the goals of rehabilitation as the following:

1. achieving maximal functional potential and self-sufficiency,
2. achieving and maintaining an acceptable quality of life,

Figure 1.2. Definitions of Rehabilitation

- "Rehabilitation is the restoration of the handicapped to the fullest physical, mental, social, vocational, and economic usefulness of which they are capable" (National Council on Rehabilitation, 1944, cited in Wright, 1983, p. 3).
- "Rehabilitation is the process of maximizing the use of an individual's capabilities or resources to foster optimal growth and functioning. It recognizes the uniqueness and wholeness of each individual and views each person and his [or her] environment as interdependent systems" (Sayles, 1981, p. 3).
- "Rehabilitation is a dynamic process in which a disabled person is aided in achieving optimum physical, emotional, psychological, social or vocational potential in order to maintain dignity and self-respect in a life that is as independent and self-fulfilling as possible" (Hickey, 1986, p. 179).
- "Rehabilitation is the physical restoration of a sick or disabled person by therapeutic measures and reeducation to participation in the activities of a normal life within the limitation of his/her physical disability" (Mumma, 1987, p. 2).
- "Rehabilitation is an approach, an attitude, and a process involving the specialized techniques and interactions of members of the rehabilitation team. The individualized rehabilitation plan is developed by all rehabilitation team members, including the client and family" (Dittmar, 1989, p. 2).
- "Rehabilitation assists disabled persons in recovering lost physical, psychologic, or social skills so that they may be more independent, live in personally satisfying environments, and maintain meaningful social interactions" (Brummel-Smith, 1990, p. 3).
- "Rehabilitation is a creative procedure which includes the cooperative efforts of various medical specialists and their associates in other health fields to improve the mental, physical, social, and vocational aptitudes of persons who are handicapped, with the objective of preserving their ability to live happily and productively on the same level and with the same opportunities as their neighbors" (Kottke & Lehman, 1990, p. xxii).
- Rehabilitation is "the process of providing, in a coordinated manner, those comprehensive services deemed appropriate to the needs of a person with a disability in a program designed to achieve objectives of improved health, welfare, and the realization of the person's maximal physical, social, psychological, and vocational potential for useful and productive activity" (Commission on Accreditation of Rehabilitation Facilities, 1991, p. 138).

Figure 1.3. Basic Guidelines for Interdisciplinary Rehabilitation Teams

- Treat the underlying disease.
- Prevent a secondary disability.
- Treat the primary disabilities.
- Set realistic goals.
- Emphasize functional independence.
- Enhance residual function.
- Provide adaptive tools.
- Alter the environment.
- Use a team approach.
- Be aware of motivational and other psychological factors (of both the patients and the caregivers).

Reprinted with permission of PRO-ED, Inc., from Kemp, B., Brummel-Smith, K., & Ramsdell, J.W. (Eds.) (1990). *Geriatric rehabilitation* (p. 348). Austin, TX: PRO-ED, Inc.

Figure 1.4. Steps to Be Taken by the Rehabilitation Team to Achieve Optimal Outcomes

1. Stabilize the primary problem(s).
2. Prevent secondary complications.
3. Restore lost functional abilities.
4. Promote adaptation of the person to his or her environment.
5. Adapt the environment to the person.
6. Promote family adaptation.

Reprinted with permission of PRO-ED, Inc., from Kemp, B., Brummel-Smith, K., & Ramsdell, J.W. (Eds.) (1990). *Geriatric rehabilitation* (p. 6). Austin, TX: PRO-ED, Inc.

3. ensuring that the client's specific needs are addressed,
4. promoting adaptation and adjustment of the client and family to a changed life,
5. preventing complications and promoting optimal wellness, and
6. returning to successful function within the community.

The process of rehabilitation

The rehabilitation process consists of a planned and orderly sequence of individualized services designed to meet the unique needs of each disabled person. To achieve the complex goals of rehabilitation, an interdisciplinary approach that maximizes the specific contributions of members of a variety of professional healthcare disciplines is required. The collaborative interactive efforts of interdisciplinary teams distinguish rehabilitation as a healthcare specialty (see Chapter 22). Within the team setting, highly effective performance occurs when team members pursue excellence within each specialty, while understanding that the contribution of each discipline is an integral part of holistic patient care (American Congress of Rehabilitation Medicine, 1992). Figure 1.3 lists the basic guidelines that members of interdisciplinary rehabilitation teams should follow as they strive to achieve successful rehabilitation outcomes.

Each member of the treatment team is accountable for supporting and enhancing the treatment program being implemented by other members of the rehabilitation team (CARF, 1991). Regardless of the setting or client population, the rehabilitation team uses a problem-solving approach that includes the following components:

1. an interdisciplinary patient evaluation,
2. a listing of all patient problems,
3. a determination of treatment goals,
4. implementation of an individual treatment plan, and
5. an evaluation of the success of the treatment plan in achieving goals.

Elements taken into consideration by the rehabilitation team during this complex process are a recognition of the unique impact of the disability for each individual, a consideration of the need for overall rehabilitation rather than a concentration on a particular aspect of the process, and an awareness of the role that societal attitudes about disability may play in allowing a disability to become a handicap. Suggested steps to be followed by the rehabilitation team to achieve optimal outcomes are found in Figure 1.4.

References

American Congress of Rehabilitation Medicine. (1992). *Guide to interdisciplinary practice in rehabilitation settings.* Skokie, IL: Author.

Brummel-Smith, K. (1990). In B. Kemp, K. Brummel-Smith, & J.W. Ramsdell (Eds.), *Geriatric rehabilitation* (pp. 3-12). Austin, TX: PRO-ED, Inc.

Commission on Accreditation of Rehabilitation Facilities (CARF). (1991). *Standards manual for organizations serving people with disabilities.* Tucson, AZ: Author.

Dittmar, S. (Ed.). (1989). *Rehabilitation nursing: Process and application.* St. Louis: The C.V. Mosby Company.

Hickey, J.V. (1986). *The clinical practice of neurological and neurosurgical nursing* (2nd ed.). Philadelphia: J.B. Lippincott Company.

Kemp, B., Brummel-Smith, K., & Ramsdell, J.W. (Eds.). (1990). *Geriatric rehabilitation.* Austin, TX: PRO-ED, Inc.

Kottke, F.J., & Lehman, J.F. (1990). *Krusen's handbook of physical medicine and rehabilitation* (4th ed.). Philadelphia: W.B. Saunders Company.

Morrissey, A.B. (1949). The nursing technics in rehabilitation. *American Journal of Nursing, 49*, 545-555.

Mumma, C.M. (Ed.) (1987). *Rehabilitation nursing: Concepts and practice—A core curriculum* (2nd ed.). Evanston, IL: Rehabilitation Nursing Foundation.

Nagi, S.Z. (1965). Some conceptual issues in disability and rehabilitation. In M.B. Sussman (Ed.), *Sociology & rehabilitation* (pp. 100-113). Washington, DC: American Sociological Association.

Pope, A.M., & Tarlov, A.R. (Eds.). (1991). *Disability in America: Toward a national agenda for prevention.* Washington, DC: National Academy Press.

Sayles, S.M. (Ed.). (1981). *Rehabilitation nursing: Concepts and practice—A core curriculum.* Evanston, IL: Rehabilitation Nursing Institute.

Storck, I.F., & Thompson-Hoffman, S. (1991). Demographic characteristics of the disabled population. In S. Thompson-Hoffman & I.F. Storck (Eds.), *Disability in the United States: A portrait from national data* (pp. 1-12). New York: Springer Publishing Company.

Wright, B. (1983). *Physical disability: A psychological approach.* New York: Harper & Row Publishers, Inc.

CHAPTER 2

The History of Rehabilitation and Rehabilitation Nursing in the 20th Century

The 20th century has been characterized by an explosion of change, growth, turmoil, creativity, and scientific and technological advances. Many of these changes have been stimulated by societal needs resulting from entering or recovering from war, enjoying the creativity and prosperity of peacetime, and attempting to treat and cure disease and its sequelae.

Thomas McKeown (1979) pointed out that in the late 19th and early 20th centuries, improvements in hygiene and nutritional status, the development of immunization programs, and the introduction of new medications (especially sulfonamides and other chemotherapeutics) resulted in a decrease in mortality and a significant increase in the health status of modern societies. During this same period, an explosion of specialties occurred in the medical field in Europe and North America. The development of rehabilitation as a phenomenon of the 20th century has been a challenging process, including the emerging specialty role of the physiatrist and the evolution of a variety of roles in professional rehabilitation health care.

Many technological advances in the 20th century have influenced the need for rehabilitation. The introduction of the automobile and other industrial achievements created a potential for injury that had not existed prior to the Industrial Revolution. At the beginning of the century, a workweek as short as 5 days was unknown. As the concept of respite from work evolved for the first time in history, leisure-time activities—some of which involved physical risk—began to account for an increasing incidence of traumatic disability. Significant increases in life expectancy also have changed the demographics in the United States and Canada dramatically, resulting in large numbers of individuals who can expect to have at least one disabling condition over the course of an extended life span.

Experience in trauma care gained from the century's two world wars, the Korean War, and the Vietnam War has increased the survival rate for traumatically injured persons in the civilian population. Evolving side by side with the scientific and technological advances that have supported physical rehabilitation has been the human rights movement that emerged in mid-century and has had far-reaching effects for all minority groups. Persons with disabilities, a large minority group in America, have begun to receive national support for their rights to lead normal, high-quality lives despite physical disabilities. These factors are the major ones that shaped the healthcare specialty known as rehabilitation.

1900-1917: The state of rehabilitation at the turn of the century

During the first decade of the 20th century, society began to focus on the needs of individuals with disabilities by providing a therapeutic environment for the treatment of specific disabilities while beginning to address individuals' educational and vocational needs. Initial signs of change in attitudes toward the disabled had become evident when the first schools for crippled children were developed in Norway (1892), the United States (1893), and Belgium (1908). Individuals such as Susan Tracy, a nurse and author; George Barton, an architect recovering from tuberculosis; and Eleanor Slagle, a social worker, laid the foundation for the promotion of occupational and vocational training for individuals recovering from illness or trauma or for those living with a disabling condition.

During this same period, the foundation for rehabilitation

Rehabilitation in the Late 19th and 20th Centuries: A Timeline

1892: First handicraft school for crippled children was established in Norway.
1893: First vocational training school for crippled children was established in the United States.
1904: First clinic in North America for crippled children was opened.
1908: The first vocational school for disabled adults was established in Belgium.
1917: The federal Division of Special Hospitals and Physical Reconstruction was developed at Massachusetts General Hospital.

was laid. In 1904, the first clinic for crippled children in North America was established. The use of electrotherapy as a therapeutic modality required a controlled scientific approach that led to the development of the American Electrotherapeutic Association in 1917 through the American Medical Association (AMA). Joel Goldthwait, MD, and Elliott Brackett, MD, developed the medicomechanical department at Massachusetts General Hospital, where physical therapy modalities were instituted for the treatment of certain diseases. These modalities included chemotherapy, dietetics, exercise, hydrotherapy, mechanical vibration therapy, psychotherapy, and thermotherapy.

From the beginning of the 20th century until the 1920s, competition between physician and nonphysician groups working in disability treatment stimulated the need for licensure and a definition of the specialty. At the same time, social reformers became concerned with the increasing number of persons who were unemployed as a result of work-related injuries. During this period, 500,000 people of working age were affected by occupational injuries.

1917-1918: The impact of World War I on physical medicine

In 1917, America joined the Allied forces that were fighting World War I. The war ended a year and a half later in November 1918—but despite the brevity of America's involvement in the war, the conflict had an enormous impact on the American practice of physical medicine. In 1917, under the direction of the surgeon general of the United States, the federal Division of Special Hospitals and Physical Reconstruction was developed at Massachusetts General Hospital to treat wounded soldiers and others requiring rehabilitation. Also recognized was the need to bring disabled veterans beyond surgery—to provide educational and vocational rehabilitation that would restore a sense of meaning to their wounded lives.

In 1917, Frank Granger, MD, was named president of the American Association of Electrotherapeutics and Radiology and the director of the physiotherapy program of Massachusetts General Hospital. Granger was also the first to train physical reconstruction aides, who were sent to France by the U.S. government to treat war casualties. These individuals were later described as experts in military massage and muscle reeducation. Many of the reconstruction aides were nurses or had a background in physical education.

By 1921, 123,000 disabled American veterans had returned to America to be treated under the Division of Physical Reconstruction and the Federal Board for Vocational Education, which were established by the federal government. During this period, other physician's groups—such as orthopedic surgeons—claimed the right to treat orthopedic injuries and traumatic injuries, which included war-related amputations. During this period, the AMA attempted to broaden its power by demanding control of the Federal Board for Vocational Education. However, these efforts were thwarted in 1920 when the passage of the Vocational Rehabilitation Law provided for federal control of vocational rehabilitation, separate from the jurisdiction of the Surgeon General of the United States.

On the European front, particularly in England, the need to care for wounded veterans resulted in a proposal to establish the first spinal centers, which would incorporate the concepts of aseptic intermittent catheterization and functional reeducation. These centers later served as a model for the future development and expansion of regional spinal injury centers in the United States after World War II.

1920-1943: The post-World War I period

In 1920, the first Rehabilitation Act was passed by the U.S. Congress. This act was to be monitored by the League of Red Cross Societies. The passage of this law and other events set in motion by World War I led to the development of the American Women's Physical Therapy Association in 1921 by Harold Corbusier, MD; Frank Granger, MD; and physical therapist Mary McMillan. The American Occupational Therapy Association was established in 1923 by occupational therapist T.B. Kinder and others. Throughout this period, the role, placement, and governance of these therapies became a focus for the emerging specialty of rehabilitation.

Attempts were made during this period to organize, define, and implement the role of therapists to take them beyond the military arena into the mainstream of society's hospitals. The need for registries was met by the establishment of the first federal occupational therapy registry in 1926 and the first federal physical therapy registry in 1934. In 1933, the AMA established guidelines to accredit physical therapy schools. A year later, in 1934, a formal alliance was established between the AMA Council on Medical Education and Hospitals and the American Physical Therapy Association.

The Social Security Act of 1935 first defined rehabilitation as a process that helped a disabled person become capable of engaging in a remunerative occupation. At this time, the government began to provide rehabilitation services beyond the needs of the military and outside hospital walls.

In a 1938 address to members of the American Congress of Physical Therapy Physicians, Frank Krusen, MD, urged them to establish their practice based on the use of physical therapy modalities and, at the same time, encouraged the group to support the use of simple modalities by all physicians. Krusen's address established the hallmarks of physical medicine as controlling disease, relieving suffering, and shortening the period of disability.

The influence of poliomyelitis and the development of spinal cord injury centers: Physical medicine was being established in Europe as well, as evidenced by the growth of spinal cord centers and the development of specialty hospitals and clinics for the treatment of poliomyelitis. From 1923 through

1917: Frank Granger, MD, was named president of the American Association of Electrotherapeutics and Radiology.
1920: The first Rehabilitation Act was passed by the U.S. Congress and was monitored by the League of Red Cross Societies; the Vocational Rehabilitation Law was passed.
1921: The American Women's Physical Therapy Association was formed.
1923: The American Occupational Therapy Association was formed.
1933: The American Medical Association (AMA) established guidelines to accredit physical therapy schools.

1939, Sister Elizabeth Kenny, a nurse who used muscle manipulation and eliminated the use of rigid orthoses, developed numerous centers throughout Australia for the treatment of polio. These centers provided muscle reeducation therapy, attendant services, and community support.

Throughout the 1940s, numerous articles on Sister Kenny's methodologies and results were published in America, while Australian physicians attempted to squelch the efforts of the Sister Kenny Institute. However, in the United States in 1943, the National Foundation for Infantile Paralysis provided funding for research and training in Sister Kenny's techniques. Research grants were awarded to study her treatment techniques and the resulting patient outcomes. A few centers for the treatment of polio were established in the United States; one of the most prominent of these was the Sister Kenny Institute in Minneapolis, which later became affiliated with the University of Minnesota Medical School. The impact of polio stimulated many advances in rehabilitation, including the development of the iron lung, positive pressure ventilation, pneumobelts, wrist-driven hand splints, and prototypes for other orthoses and mobility devices (Raymond, 1986).

Needs of children: As the 19th century came to an end, the needs of children with physical disabilities became a societal concern; this was demonstrated by the establishment of private and public rehabilitation programs and hospitals. The primary mission of these programs and facilities was to promote the rehabilitation of individuals whose disabilities resulted from congenital defects, disease, or trauma and whose age ranged from birth to 21 years.

The development of these early pediatric hospitals was in response to the standard "asylum" care offered to children with birth or acquired disabilities, which offered little more than group shelter. In contrast, rehabilitation or curative programs typically included restorative procedures, exercise, and the application of physical modalities in a hospital environment. Hallmark programs were developed at the Hospital for Sick Children in Washington, DC (1883), the Cleveland Rehabilitation Center (1889), the Children's Country Home in Westfield, NJ (1892), the Blythedale Children's Hospital in Valhalla, NY (1892), the Boston Institute School for Crippled and Deformed Children (1893), Cleveland's Health Hill Hospital (1895), and the Curative Workshop of Milwaukee (1919).

Pediatric rehabilitation programs grew in number in the first half of the century (see Figure 2.1) and this growth continues today, as programs focus on a continuum of care within a developmental, educational, and family systems framework. The impact of technological advances; heroic lifesaving measures taken at life stages from intrauterine life to early adolescence; and the success and sequelae of survival from transplants, cancer, and near-fatal neurological traumas require demanding restorative and preventive care for the pediatric client with rehabilitation needs.

1941-1945: The impact of World War II

Prior to World War II, relatively little attention was paid to the field of rehabilitation. The inability to manage shock and to prevent life-threatening infection resulted in high casualty rates from traditional injuries. During the early 1940s, new methods of handling shock and treating infection as well as an increasing sophistication in trauma care resulted in longer survival rates.

The many problems that soon appeared with increased survival posed a tremendous challenge to the Veterans Administration (VA) when large numbers of the war-injured were transferred from military to VA hospitals. The VA responded with clinical programs, research, and education that has benefited the rehabilitation population at large.

By the 1940s, the United States had begun again to prepare for the return of war casualties. Howard Rusk, MD, established the Army Air Corps Convalescent Training Program and recommended the establishment of separate convalescent centers capable of providing numerous services to meet the needs of disabled veterans. In 1942, the U.S. government established a 3-month program to train physicians in physical therapy techniques.

In 1943, Bernard Baruch, an industrialist, financier, and government adviser, made appeals to President Franklin D. Roosevelt, who was disabled, to develop comprehensive rehabilitation programs that would provide for the physical, psychological, and vocational needs of disabled veterans and facilitate the resocialization of these individuals. Also in 1943, Public Law 113 was passed, defining bureaucratic responsibility for the treatment of soldiers; thus, war once again provided the catalyst for the growth of rehabilitation practice.

Significant events occurred in the 1940s that reinforced a comprehensive rehabilitation philosophy. In 1943, the U.S. Congress passed the Vocational Rehabilitation Act, which further broadened the scope of rehabilitation to include vocational rehabilitation. The same year saw the establishment of the National Foundation for Infantile Paralysis. In 1944, the Stoke Mandeville Center for the treatment of spinal cord injury was founded in England. Fundamental to this center's success was its management by experienced rehabilitation physicians, its employment of a sufficient number of specialist allied health professionals, and its vocational placement and social reintegration. By 1945, the American Paraplegia Association had been founded, as had eight spinal cord injury units within the United States.

1946-1960: The post-World War II period

By 1946, the term *physiatrist* began to be used to describe physician specialists who were trained in rehabilitation medicine. This period further established rehabilitation as a medical specialty and differentiated it as a distinct hospital mission for a few institutions. Practice acts were developed to foster legal recognition and authority for the growing number of rehabilita-

1934: A formal alliance was established between the AMA Council on Medical Education and the Hospitals and the American Physical Therapy Association.
1935: The Social Security Act defined rehabilitation.
1938: In an address to the American Congress of Physical Therapy Physicians, Frank Krusen, MD, established the hallmarks of physical medicine.
1939: Sister Elizabeth Kenny implemented new treatment techniques for patients with polio in Australia.

Figure 2.1. Early Pediatric Rehabilitation Facilities in the United States

1883
The Hospital for Sick Children, Washington, DC

1889
The Cleveland Rehabilitation Center, Cleveland, OH

1892
The Children's Country Home, Westfield, NJ
The Blythedale Children's Hospital, Valhalla, NY

1893
The Boston Institute School for Crippled and Deformed Children

1895
Health Hill Hospital in Cleveland

1902
The Home for Crippled Children (now The Rehabilitation Institute), Pittsburgh, PA

1919
The Curative Workshop of Milwaukee

1922
Happy Hills Convalescent Center (now Mt. Washington Pediatric Hospital), Baltimore, MD

1930
Elizabethtown Hospital and Rehabilitation Center (now University Hospital Rehabilitation Center for Children and Adults), Elizabethtown, PA

1937
Children's Rehabilitation Institute (now the Kennedy Institute) Baltimore, MD

1940
Alfred I. duPont Institute, Wilmington, DE (as a hospital for crippled children)

1949
Kennedy Memorial Hospital (now Franciscan Children's Hospital and Rehabilitation Center), Boston, MA

1950
Children's Orthopedic Hospital (now Cardinal Hill Rehabilitation Hospital), Lexington, KY

Source Consulted
Edwards, P.A. (1992). The evolution of rehabilitation facilities for children. *Rehabilitation Nursing, 17,* 191-192.

tion professionals, including physical therapists, occupational therapists, communication disorders specialists, and vocational counselors. Physical therapy technicians, who had been known as *corrective therapists* during the war, attempted to achieve status as physical therapists in the civilian healthcare arena. However, a united force consisting of the AMA, the American Congress of Physical Medicine and Rehabilitation, and the American Physical Therapy Association blocked their efforts, based on the belief that the growth of corrective therapists would impede the development of physical therapy as a profession.

The appearance and importance of nurses in a rehabilitation role was recognized by the insurance industry when Liberty Mutual Insurance Company hired the first insurance rehabilitation nurse. This came about because Medicare legislation created a demand for the employment of rehabilitation nurses by insurance companies. Later, the American Nurses' Association (ANA) published *Guidelines for the Practice of Nursing on the Rehabilitation Team: An Answer to a Growing Need* (ANA, 1965).

Throughout the post-World War II era, technological advancements in medical and surgical care and chemotherapeutics, including antibiotics, resulted in a lowered morbidity and mortality rate.

1960-1990: A new society, a new beginning for rehabilitation

Throughout the 1960s, the specialty practices of physical and occupational therapy continued to evolve. Specialty practice in these areas was defined either through licensing laws as created by the Board of Physical Therapy Examiners or through voluntary certification offered to occupational therapists. The movement of rehabilitation into nontraditional treatment settings also occurred during this period.

The emphasis on the workplace and a focus on improving reentry for the individual with a disability was supported by legislation during this period, including the Workmen's Compensation and Rehabilitation Law, passed in 1965, and the Vocational Rehabilitation Act amendments of 1967. These acts authorized funding and described the need to provide programmatic support to all disabled individuals with vocational needs. The federal Medicaid program (primarily for the poor) and the Medicare program (primarily for the elderly) broadened access to health care. The intent of these programs was to increase

1942: War readiness programs were developed and physicians were trained in physical therapy techniques.
1943: The National Foundation for Infantile Paralysis was established in the United States.
1943: Public Law 113 defined bureaucratic responsibility for the treatment of soldiers.
1943: The Vocational Rehabilitation Act broadened the scope of rehabilitation.
1945: The American Paraplegia Association was formed.
1946: *Physiatrist* was accepted as a term for physician specialists who were trained in rehabilitation medicine.

comprehensive care and improve the quality of outcomes.

By 1966, the issue of quality control for rehabilitation services was addressed through the establishment of the Commission on Accreditation of Rehabilitation Facilities (CARF). This body continues to serve as the intermediary for quality control in the rehabilitation industry. CARF seeks the establishment of guidelines and standards through the input of sponsoring and associate members that include the major associations of the professional team and the rehabilitation industry.

When the Vocational Rehabilitation Act was amended, services were offered to the families of persons with disabilities. Further progress was made during this period, when a focus on access and architectural barriers resulted in the passage of the Architectural Barriers Act of 1968. This act established standards for buildings whose construction is funded by the federal government.

In 1970, the Developmental Disabilities Services and Construction Act was passed and provided extended programming not only for individuals with mental retardation, but also for those with congenital and other developmental disabilities.

By the early 1970s, regional health care became a focal point in rehabilitation services. Medicare legislation forced healthcare providers to focus on quality outcomes while defining and controlling costs. The successful development of the regional concept of care for individuals with spinal cord injury, modeled by John Young, MD, and others, provided a framework to measure the outcome of regionalization of rehabilitative care.

In 1973, the Rehabilitation Act of 1973 was passed. This act increased societal awareness of the needs of persons with disabilities by developing guidelines for nondiscriminatory employment and promoting community access through the reduction and elimination of physical barriers.

At the same time, many attitudinal barriers regarding putting the person with a disability back into the workplace and into the community at large remained in place. By the late 1960s, the independent living movement, initiated in Berkeley, CA, established the groundwork for a more self-directed social and healthcare environment. Its focus was on self-determination, legislative support, community awareness, and community access.

In 1974, the Association of Rehabilitation Nurses was founded in Illinois with an initial nationwide membership of more than 200 (see Chapter 4). Ten years later, the association established the first certification program for rehabilitation nurses, which gave successful participants the Certified Rehabilitation Registered Nurse (CRRN) credential.

Throughout the 1970s and 1980s, the needs of the disabled population became more prominent as a social issue. The special needs of disabled persons were recognized in 1981, which was declared the International Year of the Disabled Person. Tertiary medical centers established rehabilitation units to meet growing demands for services. Fortunately, at the same time, the development of rehabilitation units and hospitals provided healthcare institutions an attractive reimbursement alternative to the prospective payment system affecting acute care. Many freestanding rehabilitation centers also were created to address the diverse needs of people with disabilities, which included the development of programs that focused on aftercare and community reintegration.

Traumatic injuries related to sports and motor vehicle accidents influenced the passage of important legislation covering the use of seat belts and the integration of disability prevention programs in educational and occupational areas. Although seat belts had been standard equipment in passenger vehicles since 1966, consumer resistance to being restrained needed to be overcome. Aggressive educational efforts, media campaigns, and state police monitoring have reduced this behavioral problem to some degree. In 1984, New York became the first state in the country to mandate safety-belt use for drivers and front-seat passengers based on successes with similar programs in Canada, West Germany (now the Federal Republic of Germany), and the United Kingdom. The use of seat belts has led to the development of consumer and industry demands for more safety measures. Supplemental restraint systems, including driver's-side and front-seat passenger air bags, may reduce the incidence and/or severity of head, neck, and abdominal trauma.

In addition to concerns about vehicular safety, concerns related to sports and motorcycle safety have influenced local and federal legislative activity in the areas of safe sport practices and the use of helmets for cyclists and motorcyclists. These developments are crucial, as injuries to the brain that are often the result of motor vehicle injuries require a significantly more intense and expensive trauma management and rehabilitation program, as well as incur long-term costs of care management and alternative life plans.

Head injuries were identified in the 1980s as a major cause of morbidity and mortality. According to Max, MacKenzie, and Rice (1991), 39,000 people died of head injuries between 1979 and 1986. The development of regional training centers and head injury centers has fostered early intervention, aggressive rehabilitation, and resocialization of this typically young patient group through the continuum of rehabilitative care.

1990 to the present: Toward the 21st century

With the trend toward survival increasing for patients with severe trauma, rehabilitation has found a niche across the entire life span. In the 1990s, geriatric rehabilitation demands greater attention, as at least 11% of Americans who turned 65 in 1990 will spend 5% of their remaining years in a nursing home or rehabilitation program.

Deaths from traumatic injury and once-life-threatening cardiovascular disease have declined; therefore, the demand for continued rehabilitative efforts has not only increased, but also intensified. The increased number of early interventions and

1965: The American Nurses' Association (ANA) published *Guidelines for the Practice of Nursing on the Rehabilitation Team: An Answer to a Growing Need.*
1965: Workmen's Compensation and Rehabilitation Law was passed.
1965: The initial Medicaid legislation, which defined the need for access to health care for the poor and the disabled, was passed.
1966: Medicare legislation stimulated a demand for employment of rehabilitation nurses by insurance companies.
1966: The Commission on Accreditation of Rehabilitation Facilities was established.

aggressive technological treatment has shifted the intensity of care to all points on the continuum. This shift requires high technology, which formerly was placed only in the hands of the intensive-care team, but now resides in rehabilitation hospitals and life care communities as well as in the individual's home.

The Americans with Disabilities Act, passed in 1990, is expected to have lasting effects across all segments of society, from the government to the community, in providing access and opportunities for individuals with disabilities to the community, employment, education, and health care.

As of 1991, the Centers for Disease Control (through the U.S. Department of Health and Human Services) continues to recognize the need for the prevention of physical and mental disabilities. The national financial impact to date of both mental and physical disabilities is enormous.

The future of rehabilitation is in the hands of scientists, technologists, researchers, educators, employers, healthcare professionals, individuals with disabilities, and the community—all of whom must remain open to challenge, growth, and the ability of the individual to succeed beyond the limits of physical constraints.

Rehabilitation nursing pioneers

The emergence of rehabilitation nursing can be attributed to a relatively small group of pioneers, now deceased or retired, whose contribution and foresight established the foundation for the specialty. Unfortunately, there is little in the way of biographical information about or printed material relating to the early and rich history of the founders of rehabilitation nursing. The following individuals were responsible for many of the major early accomplishments and contributions to the practice. As specialists, rehabilitation nurses need to begin to systematically and scientifically collect data on today's leaders for the present and future generations of rehabilitation nurses.

Alice Morrissey, BS RN

- During the 1940s, served as nursing supervisor of the department of physical medicine and rehabilitation at Bellevue Hospital, NY, the site of the country's first medical rehabilitation program for people with disabilities
- Gave the specialty of rehabilitation nursing its name
- In 1951, wrote *Rehabilitation Nursing*, the first textbook in the field

Lena Plaisted, MS RN PT

- In 1956, founded the first graduate program in rehabilitation nursing at Boston University
- Served as director of the Boston University program and prepared nurses at the master's level with the theory and clinical expertise needed to function as teachers and managers of rehabilitation nursing
- Testified before congressional committees and the Vocational Rehabilitation Administration to obtain federal funding for both graduate fellowships and short-term continuing education
- In 1969, wrote *The Clinical Specialist in Rehabilitation*, one of the first publications to describe this new role

Barbara Madden, MA RN

- During the 1950s, contributed significantly to the development of nursing programs for acute and postpolio patients
- Assisted in establishing 13 regional respiratory centers for the National Foundation for Infantile Paralysis (NFIP)
- Established the first rehabilitation nursing residency program for graduate students in rehabilitation nursing in 1965, while serving as director of nursing at Rancho Los Amigos Medical Center

Harriet Lane, MA RN

- In 1951, became the first nurse to be hired by the Liberty Mutual Insurance Company to coordinate patient rehabilitation programs at the company's rehabilitation center in Boston
- In the 1960s, pioneered gerontological rehabilitation nursing as a specialty at Boston University
- In 1972, became the first nurse to establish an independent practice in rehabilitation and gerontological nursing

Mary Ann Mikulic, MS RN

- Was one of the first rehabilitation nursing clinical specialists appointed by the Veterans Administration
- Was the first ARN member to serve as editor of *ARN Journal* (now *Rehabilitation Nursing*)
- Received the Olin Teague Award from the Veterans Administration, which is given in recognition of achievement that has been extraordinarily beneficial to the rehabilitation of war-injured veterans

References

American Nurses' Association (ANA). (1965). *Guidelines for the practice of nursing on the rehabilitation team: An answer to a growing need.* Kansas City, MO: Author.

Edwards, P.A. (1992). The evolution of rehabilitation facilities for children. *Rehabilitation Nursing, 17*, 191-192, 195.

Max, W., MacKenzie, E., & Rice, D. (1991). Head injuries: Costs and consequences. *Journal of Head Trauma Rehabilitation, 6*(2), 76-91.

McKeown, T. (1979). *The role of medicine: Dream, mirage or nemesis.* Princeton, NJ: Princeton University Press.

Raymond, C. (1986). Polio survivors spurred rehabilitation advances. *Journal of the American Medical Association, 255*, 1403-1404.

1967:	The Vocational Rehabilitation Act was amended to offer services to families of people with disabilities.
Late 1960s:	The independent living movement was initiated in Berkeley, CA.
1968:	The Architectural Barriers Act was passed.
1970:	Developmental Disabilities Services and Construction Act was passed.
1973:	The Rehabilitation Act of 1973 was passed.
1974:	The Association of Rehabilitation Nurses was founded.

Suggested Readings

Affeldt, J. (1988, February). The 1987 Mary E. Switzer Lecture: The tapestry of rehabilitation, its weaves and threads. *Journal of Allied Health, 17*(1), 53-58.

Barker, J.T. (1982). Women as leaders in the field of rehabilitation. *Journal of Rehabilitation, 48*(1), 9-18, 68-70.

Bedbrook, G.M. (1987). The development and care of spinal cord paralysis (1918 to 1986). *Paraplegia, 25*(3), 172-184.

Colman, W. (1990). Evolving educational practices in occupational therapy: The War Emergency Courses, 1936-1954. *The American Journal of Occupational Therapy, 44*, 1028-1036.

Devereaux, E. (1990). American Occupational Therapy Foundation: Milestones of a quarter century. *The American Journal of Occupational Therapy, 44*, 295-297.

Gritzer, G., & Arluke, A. (1985). *The making of rehabilitation: A political economy of medical specialization, 1890-1980.* Berkeley, CA: University of California Press.

Harvey, R. (1991, Summer). Rehabilitation's best of times/worst of times. *Physiacare: Marianjoy Rehabilitation Center*, p. 2.

Harvey-Kreftig, L. (1985). The concept of work in occupational therapy: A historical review. *The American Journal of Occupational Therapy, 39*, 301-307.

Herbison, G. (1984). The Walter J. Zeitzer Lectures: Research—Ends, setting, environment, activities, resources, creativity, health. *Archives of Physical Medicine and Rehabilitation, 65*, 112-114.

Jamieson, E.N., & Sewall, M.F. (1960). *Trends in nursing history.* New York: W.B. Saunders Company.

Johnson, J.H. (1980). Symposium on rehabilitation nursing: Foreword. *The Nursing Clinics of North America, 15*, 221-223.

Jones, F. (1948). The nurse's responsibility in rehabilitation. *American Journal of Nursing, 48*(2), 76-79.

King, R.B., & Dudas, S., (1980). Rehabilitation of the patient with a spinal cord injury. *The Nursing Clinics of North America*, 15(2), 221-223.

Lipson, M. (1977). Medical legislation: Its effect on rehabilitation programs. *Archives of Physical Medicine and Rehabilitation, 58*, 386-392.

Marshall, E. (1985). Looking back. *The American Journal of Occupational Therapy, 39*, 297-300.

Martin, N., Holt, N., & Hicks, D. (Eds.). (1981). *Comprehensive rehabilitation nursing.* New York: McGraw-Hill Book Company.

Morrissey, A. (1949). Rehabilitation care for patients. *American Journal of Nursing, 49*, 453-454.

Morrissey, A. (1951). *Rehabilitative nursing.* New York: G.P. Putnam's Sons.

Mumma, C.M. (Ed.). (1987). *Rehabilitation nursing: Concepts and practice—A core curriculum* (2nd ed.). Evanston, IL: Rehabilitation Nursing Foundation.

National Association of Rehabilitation Facilities (NARF). (1985). *Exclusion of rehabilitation units from the Medicare prospective payment system for inpatient medical rehabilitation services.* Washington, DC: Author.

Petrucelli, E. (1987). Seat belt laws: The New York experience—Preliminary data and some observations. *The Journal of Trauma, 27*, 706-710.

Plaisted, L.M. (1969). The clinical specialist in rehabilitation nursing. *American Journal of Nursing, 69*, 562-564.

Riffle, K. (1973). Rehabilitation: The evolution of a social concept. *The Nursing Clinics of North America, 8*, 665-671.

Romano, P., & McLaughlin, E. (1991). Helmet use and fatal motorcycle injuries in California, 1987-1988. *Journal of Head Trauma Rehabilitation, 6*(2), 21-37.

Rusk, H. (1981). An equal chance. *Journal of the American Medical Association, 246*, 1503-1505, 1509-1510.

Rusk, H.A. (1977). *Rehabilitation medicine* (4th ed.). St. Louis: The C.V. Mosby Company.

Singer, C. (1962). *A short history of medicine* (2nd ed.). New York: Oxford University Press.

Smoyak, S. (1976). Specialization in nursing: From then to now. *Nursing Outlook, 27*, 676-681.

Sorenson, S., & Krass, J. (1991). Occurrence, severity and outcomes of brain injury. *Journal of Head Trauma Rehabilitation, 6*(2), 11-20.

Stryker, R. (1972). *Rehabilitation aspects of acute and chronic nursing care* (2nd ed.). Philadelphia: W.B. Saunders Company.

Whitten, E.B. (1974). Editorial: The Rehabilitation Act of 1973 and the severely disabled. *Journal of Rehabilitation, 40*(4), 29-40.

Wilson, J. (1986). The Sister Kenny clinics: What endures? *The Australian Journal of Advanced Nursing, 3*(2), 13-21.

1980s: Traumatic head injuries were identified as a major cause of morbidity and mortality.
1981: The International Year of the Disabled Person was celebrated.
1984: New York was the first state to pass a law making seat belts mandatory.
1984: The first Certified Rehabilitation Registered Nurse (CRRN) certification examination was held.
1990: The Americans with Disabilities Act was passed.
1991: The Centers for Disease Control acknowledged the need for a focus on prevention of disability.

CHAPTER 3

Rehabilitation Nursing Practice

It has been estimated that approximately 25% of the world's population is affected by disabilities (Acton, 1982). People with disabilities, their families, and their significant others rarely are prepared for the physical, psychosocial, and economic consequences of disability. The sequelae of disability—including functional loss, frustration, potential rejection, stigma, social barriers, and feelings of lowered self-esteem—can be overwhelming. Rehabilitation nurses, in conjunction with other members of the interdisciplinary rehabilitation team, help people with disability to manage those sequelae and to lead fulfilling and productive lives (Fraley, 1992).

Although professional nurses use rehabilitation nursing techniques in many practice settings, rehabilitation nursing is a unique nursing specialty whose practitioners operate with a common body of knowledge, skills, and attitudes about nursing and about disability. The purpose of this chapter is to define rehabilitation nursing as a specialty practice; to describe how it differs from other areas of professional nursing practice in terms of philosophy, goals, and processes; to describe nursing models related to rehabilitation nursing practice; to address the necessary educational preparation for rehabilitation nursing; to describe rehabilitation nursing certification; and to outline roles and settings in which rehabilitation nursing is practiced.

Rehabilitation nursing as a specialty practice

The American Nurses Association (ANA) and the Association of Rehabilitation Nurses (ARN) stated that rehabilitation nursing is a specialty practice area within the scope of professional nursing practice (ANA & ARN, 1988). They defined rehabilitation nursing as "the diagnosis and treatment of human responses of individuals and groups to actual or potential health problems stemming from altered functional ability and altered life style" (p. 4).

Descriptions of rehabilitation nursing written in the 1981 and 1987 editions of *Rehabilitation Nursing: Concepts and Practice—A Core Curriculum* (Mumma, 1987; Sayles, 1981) have stood the test of time. In the 1981 edition, a description of rehabilitation formulated by Lena M. Plaisted stated that "rehabilitation nursing is nursing with an awareness of the patient's tomorrow and the relationship between what does and what does not happen today and the tomorrow that follows" (Goldenson, 1978). In the 1987 edition, Willis-Sukosky (1987) listed the following characteristics of rehabilitation nursing as an area of nursing specialization:

- Rehabilitation nursing is practiced within a dynamic, therapeutic, and supportive relationship that is constantly changing, progressing, or regressing as clients and nurses influence one another.
- The rehabilitation nurse interacts therapeutically with clients and their support systems over long periods of time.
- Rehabilitation nursing is practiced within many types of healthcare and community settings.
- Rehabilitation nursing demands specialized knowledge, skills, and attitudes.
- Rehabilitation nurses use the nursing process to achieve individual quality outcomes for each client based on standards delineated in *Standards of Rehabilitation Nursing Practice* (ANA & ARN, 1986).
- Rehabilitation nursing is practiced in collaboration with other members of the interdisciplinary team to achieve the goals of rehabilitation for individual clients.
- Rehabilitation nurses practice a high level of independent nursing functions.

The philosophy, goals, and process of rehabilitation nursing

The philosophical basis of rehabilitation nursing: As with the specialty of rehabilitation (see Chapter 1), rehabilitation nursing can be described in terms of the values and beliefs, the goals formulated with clients to achieve successful rehabilitation outcomes, and the processes used by rehabilitation nursing professionals to achieve those goals. Rehabilitation nurses share a belief system about disability and the rights of individuals with disabling conditions and chronic illness. Rehabilitation nurses believe that a person with a disability has intrinsic worth that transcends the disability, and that each person is a unique holistic being who has both the right and the responsibility to make informed personal choices regarding health and lifestyle (ANA & ARN, 1988).

The ANA and ARN (1988) document *Rehabilitation Nursing: Scope of Practice; Process and Outcome Criteria for Selected Diagnoses* describes the foundations, definitions and goals, specialized practice characteristics, and ethical aspects of rehabilitation nursing. This document also delineates the characteristics of generalists and advanced practitioners in rehabilitation nursing.

The goals of rehabilitation nursing: The major goal of rehabilitation nursing is to assist persons with disability and chronic illness in attaining maximum functional ability, maintaining optimal health, and adapting to an altered lifestyle. Professional rehabilitation nurses assist clients in formulating goals that are realistic and attainable and that consider the clients' continuing accountability for optimal wellness. Dittmar (1989) stated that the goal of rehabilitation is to "facilitate the movement of individuals toward independence while helping them satisfy their needs. Therefore, the approach is holistic, caring, and optimistic" (p. 6).

The process of rehabilitation nursing: The process of rehabilitation nursing involves a problem-solving approach that is based on the nursing process. Using assessment data, rehabilitation nurses formulate nursing diagnoses. They identify actual or potential responses to alterations in functional ability and lifestyle and identify relevant etiologies or risk factors associated with physical and mental status, self-care abilities, emotional responses to disability, pain, alterations in self-concept, and individual and family coping issues. Based on the client's nursing diagnoses, rehabilitation nurses design and implement treatment strategies that promote quality of life for their clients. They communicate nursing diagnoses and planned interventions to other members of the rehabilitation interdisciplinary team. Lastly, they evaluate the effectiveness of nursing interventions in achieving clients' goals and revise nursing diagnoses, as necessary, to achieve desired outcomes (ANA & ARN, 1988).

Rehabilitation nurses have the responsibility to try to raise the public's awareness about preventing disability and chronic illness and to promote the quality of life for persons with disabilities. Rehabilitation nurses should influence communities to take steps to prevent disability and to adopt positive attitudes toward people with disabilities. Rehabilitation nurses use their skills as educators, advisers, consultants, and advocates to break down societal barriers and to promote meaningful and effective public policies that support the needs of individuals with disabilities (ANA & ARN, 1988).

Nursing models related to rehabilitation nursing practice

Fundamental to every professional discipline is the ability to develop and refine a body of knowledge that can be applied to its practice (Huckabay, 1991; Torres, 1990). This body of evolving knowledge is expressed in terms of concepts and theories; formulating theory is the goal of scientific work (McLeis, 1991). Haughey and Dittmar (1989) stressed that the nursing profession has only started to recognize the relevance and significance of theory as the basis for nursing practice, research, and education.

McLeis (1991) used the term *nursing conceptualizations* to characterize theories used to both describe and prescribe aspects of nursing care. One way to look at a conceptual model of nursing is to describe it as the overall picture of how something is or should be. ANA and ARN (1986) defined a theory as "the coherent set of hypothetical, conceptual, and pragmatic principles developed in association with practice in a field of activity and forming its content as an intellectual discipline" (p. 14). From the time of the nursing pioneers described in Chapter 2 to the present, all rehabilitation nurses have practiced from a theoretical basis.

Each encounter with a client, assessment of that client's needs, development of a plan of treatment, and evaluation of outcomes is derived from the nurse's belief system about human beings, the environment that surrounds them, the meaning of health, and the discipline of nursing.

The incorporation of theoretical models into rehabilitation nursing practice allows for testing, expansion, and refinement of nursing theories and models. Derstine and Mandzak-McCarron (1990) stressed that theories provide the framework for nurses to examine what they do and emphasize the criticality of theory development to the science of nursing. According to Huckabay (1991), the significance of nursing theory lies in the extent to which it is able to explain and shape nursing practice. Sorrentino (1991) viewed theories as mechanisms that facilitate nursing practice and as "guiding lights" that illuminate the path to nursing empowerment and the achievement of desired outcomes in clients, practice, and healthcare systems (p. 54).

As a basis for practice, conceptual models and the theories that drive them allow rehabilitation nurses to do the following:

- *assess*, guide, and give focus and perspective;
- *explain* phenomena and behaviors observed in practice;
- *diagnose* by providing a framework for the development of nursing interventions and client goals;
- *establish* goals based on assessed needs;
- *predict* outcomes based on interventions;
- *direct* nursing interventions toward meeting clients' needs and goals; and
- *evaluate* outcomes in a systematic manner.

The key to the effective use of a conceptual model in rehabilitation nursing practice is to choose a model that is compatible with the scientific basis of rehabilitation nursing as practiced (or as desired) in the individual setting. A framework compatible with the organization's philosophy enables nursing and team practice to function at its most efficient level for the achievement of the highest level of client outcomes possible.

Nursing theories developed by King (1981), Neuman (1982), Orem (1985), and Roy (1984) will be described below in terms of their major concepts and their applicability to rehabilitation nursing practice. (See Table 3.1 for a brief comparison of these theorists' work.) Although there are several nursing models and theories, those of King, Neuman, Orem, and Roy were chosen because of their applicability to and widespread use in rehabilitation.

Imogene King—Theory of Goal Attainment

Definitive works: *Toward a Theory for Nursing: General Concepts of Human Behavior,* 1971; *A Theory for Nursing: Systems, Concepts, Process,* 1981

Major focus: King identified the conceptual framework of her theory as an open-systems framework and the theory as one of goal attainment (George, 1990).

Summary of concepts: The client is a personal system within the environment that coexists with other personal systems. Individuals form groups that compose interpersonal systems, and interpersonal systems combine to form social systems. These three systems interact continuously and dynamically with the environment.

Concepts relevant to the personal system include perception, self, body image, growth and development, time, and space. The interpersonal system includes the concepts of role, interaction, communication, transaction, and stress. Concepts relevant to the social system are power, organization, authority, status, and decision making. From these three interacting systems and the concepts of person, health, environment, and nursing, King derived a theory of goal attainment (George, 1990).

The theory of goal attainment describes interactions between the client and the nurse. King described this interaction as occurring between two people, usually strangers, coming together in a healthcare organization to help and to be helped in

Table 3.1. Comparison of Four Nursing Models

	King Open Systems Model	Neuman Health-Care Systems Model	Orem Self-Care Model	Roy Adaptation Model
Major Focus	Goal attainment through interaction	Relationship and reaction to stressors and regenerative factors	Self-care • dependence • independence	Holistic, biopsychosocial adaptation
Pragmatic Use for Rehabilitation Nursing	Strong interactive basis with a goal-setting emphasis	Strong intervention based on primary, secondary, and tertiary prevention activities	Individual and/or family self-care abilities; emphasizes independence	Strong nursing process base with heavy assessment
Client Involvement	Unique open system (personal, interpersonal, social) interacting with the environment	Unique, holistic open system composed of physiological, sociocultural, psychological, developmental, and spiritual variables	System that involves the client when self-care needs exceed capabilities	Holistic level-of-adaptation system (regulator and cognator mechanisms function as internal control processes)
Nursing Involvement	Process of action, reaction, and interaction with the client	Concern for the total person and all the variables affecting the response to stressors	Helping the client and/or family to become capable of meeting self-care needs	Managing stimuli to promote adaptation
Goals for Health and Well-being	Attain, maintain, or restore health to function in life roles	Maintain adaptation after reconstitution and stability occur	A whole, sound state of being	Promote integrity and positive adaptation
Environment	Personal set of systems interacting with other personal systems in the environment	Reciprocal: Prevention-limitation of stressors and effects (flexible, internal, and adaptive lines of defense)	External surroundings, including biological and psychosocial	Internal and external stimuli (focal, contextual, and residual)
Limitations	Interaction of clients with cognitive and/or communication deficits may be limited Implies compliance as a result of interaction Minimal guidelines for assessment, diagnosis, and intervention	Can apply to all healthcare disciplines (a two-edged sword, as it can be challenging and problematic to define each discipline's unique contribution)	Focus is on individual self-care deficits rather than biopsychosocial aspects; illness/acute care focus of philosophy may be a barrier to rehabilitation nursing practice Assumes that independence is of value in self-care	Boundaries between psychosocial modes are blurred Assessment and diagnoses focus on nursing, which may interfere with an interdisciplinary approach

maintaining a state of health that permits optimum role functioning. Interactions between the client and the nurse focus on the interventions necessary to achieve goals. "In King's perspective, the goal of nursing action is to interact purposefully with clients to mutually establish goals and [the] means for achieving them. The focus of nursing action is the patient who is potentially stressed and unable to cope with changes in daily activities" (Haughey & Dittmar, 1989, p. 25).

King proposed a holistic open-systems view of clients that is compatible with a rehabilitative philosophy, including the concepts of body image; growth and development; stress; time; space; and functioning in the roles of a disabled person, family member, and member of a community.

Limitations: Mumma (1987b) cited limitations in King's theory in several areas that have an impact on rehabilitation nursing. According to Mumma, the theory's focus on interaction has limited applicability to clients who have cognitive or communication deficits, and the transactions described assume that the client shares the goal of being an active participant in his or her own care.

Betty Neuman—Health-Care Systems Model

Definitive works: *The Betty Neuman Health-Care Systems Model: A Total Person Approach to Patient Problems,* 1974; *The Neuman Systems Model,* 1982

Major focus: The major focus of Neuman's model is the individual's relationship to stress, his or her reaction to stress, and his or her reaction to regenerative factors that are dynamic in nature.

Summary of concepts: Each person is a unique holistic system composed of physiological, sociocultural, and developmental variables. As an open system, the person interacts with and adjusts to the environment. Each individual has a normal line of defense, or unique steady state, that is composed of a normal range of response to stressors. Flexible lines of defense protect individuals from stressors. Lines of resistance are internal factors that help each individual mount a stress response. Lines of resistance protect the core of the person and stabilize and return individuals to normal lines of defense when they are overwhelmed by stressors.

According to Cross (1990), Neuman described nursing as a unique profession that concerns itself with all the variables affecting human responses to stressors, with primary concerns for the total person (p. 267). Nurses act at levels of primary, secondary, and tertiary prevention. *Primary prevention* identifies and alleviates risk factors associated with stressors; this level of intervention strengthens the flexible lines of defense. *Secondary prevention* bolsters the internal lines of defense by focusing on symptoms, interventions, and treatment modalities. The goal of *tertiary prevention* is to maintain a degree of adaptation after reconstitution and stability have occurred.

Applicability to rehabilitation nursing: A basic strength of this model is the clear direction it provides for interventions through primary, secondary, and tertiary prevention activities. According to Cross (1990), Neuman's model also has applicability to many disciplines.

Limitations: A unique potential limitation of Neuman's model is its applicability to all healthcare professional disciplines. Using a model for nursing that can describe the functions of other disciplines as well can present a challenging problem and could interfere with the ability of each discipline to articulate its unique contribution to health care.

Dorothea E. Orem—Theory of Self-Care Deficit

Definitive works: *Nursing: Concepts of Practice,* 1971; *Nursing: Concepts of Practice* (2nd ed.), 1980; *Nursing: Concepts of Practice* (3rd ed.), 1985

Major focus: The major focus of Orem's theory is self-care, defined as "the practice of activities that individuals initiate and perform on their own behalf in maintaining life, health, and well-being" (Orem, 1985, p. 31).

Summary of concepts: Orem described three categories of self-care: universal, developmental, and health deviation healthcare requisites or requirements.

Universal self-care requisites are the basic physiological and psychological needs shared by all human beings. *Developmental self-care requisites* are the activities that promote developmental processes across the life span. *Health deviation self-care requisites* come into play when there are changes in health status. Orem (1985) saw the nurse's role as one of helping clients to "maintain continuously that amount and quality of self-care which is therapeutic in maintaining life and health, in recovering from disease or injury or in coping with their effects" (p. 18). Orem described three levels of nursing interventions, depending on the potential involvement of the client. A *wholly compensatory nursing system* occurs when the client has no active role in performing self-care. A *partially compensatory system* exists when the nurse helps the client perform self-care. A *supportive-educative system* exists when the client requires support, guidance, a developmental environment, and education to acquire the knowledge and skills necessary to meet self-care needs independently.

Applicability to rehabilitation nursing: Orem's theory of self-care deficit has been popular in rehabilitation nursing due to its focus on client autonomy for self-care, family involvement as agents of self-care, and the inclusion of the client's perspective (Mumma, 1987b). Orem (1985) proposed that persons engaged in the rehabilitation process require nursing whenever their ability to provide self-care is inadequate to meet healthcare needs. Orem believed that a rehabilitation client's potential to manage his or her own self-care is not related to a particular dysfunction but, rather, to his or her overall capability of maintaining self-care—what Orem (1985) called *self-care agency* (p. 97).

In describing the role of rehabilitation nurses, Orem stated, "Nurses can help persons [with disabilities] to remain competent in their relationships with others, to be in touch with cultural changes and trends, to be effective community members, and to know how they fit within the healthcare system. Serious attention by nurses to both the self-care requisites and the self-care capabilities of their clients will facilitate this movement.

"If persons are to attain and maintain their social positions and roles, they must be able to maintain their health and well-being by the continuous meeting of their universal, developmental, and health deviation self-care requisites; surmount existing or emerging interferences; live with dysfunctional conditions that in themselves may be hazards to continued health and well-being and to life itself; and to identify, adapt, and operate within their own functional norms" (Orem, 1985, p. 36).

Limitations: Knust and Quarn (1983) viewed Orem's theory as having some limitations for rehabilitation in terms of its focus on physical disability at the expense of psychosocial abilities in clients who would be seen in Orem's model as requiring a wholly compensatory approach by the nurse to meet self-care needs. They stated that "while a severely disabled person might be wholly dependent on others to perform universal self-care requisites, the person might be wholly independent in directing and taking responsibility for his own care" (p. 27).

The strong acute care foundations of Orem's theory and its implication that a whole or sound state of being is necessary to achieve health could be an intrinsic barrier in the model's philosophical foundation to its use in rehabilitation nursing.

Sister Callista Roy—Theory of Adaptation

Definitive works: *Introduction to Nursing: An Adaptation Model,* 1976; *The Roy Adaptation Model,* 1980; *Introduction to Nursing: An Adaptation Model* (2nd ed.), 1984

Major focus: The major focus of Roy's theory is that humans, as biopsychosocial beings, are interacting constantly with their environment (Roy, 1984). To cope with change, individuals use genetically determined and learned biological, psychological, and social mechanisms to achieve positive adaptation.

Summary of concepts: In Roy's model, the person is an adaptive system. Roy has identified four models of adaptation: physiological needs, self-concept, role mastery, and interdependence. *Physiological needs* include basic biological needs such as circulation, regulation of temperature, oxygenation, fluid balance, sleep, activity, digestion, and elimination. The *self-concept* mode of adaptation refers to "conscious and unconscious thoughts, beliefs, attitudes, and values that an individual has regarding himself [or herself] and his [or her] world" (Roy, 1984, p. 300). In the *role mastery* mode of adaptation, the individual regulates the performance of roles based on changes in his or her position in society. In the *interdependence* adaptation mode, "the self-concept of a person and his [or her] role mastery interact with other persons in the environment in an inter-dependent way" (Roy, 1984, p. 300). Two adaptive mechanisms are used by the individual. The *regulator* mechanism describes an automatic neuroendocrine response; the *cognator* mechanism represents perception, information processing, and judgments influenced by learning.

The nurse, through the nursing process, promotes adaptive responses. System responses in each mode are assessed using objective and subjective data. As a result of this first-level assessment, the nurse makes a preliminary judgment on whether the behavior is adaptive or ineffective. In the second-level assessment, focal, contextual, and residual stimuli influencing the adaptive system are identified. A nursing diagnosis is formulated, mutually agreed-upon goals are established, and interventions are designed. Factors precipitating ineffective behaviors are modified and adaptive coping behaviors are strengthened.

Applicability to rehabilitation nursing: According to Haughey and Dittmar (1989), "Roy's adaptation theory can be used as a framework for rehabilitation nursing practice. The disabled person experiences both overt and covert physiological changes that may affect self-concept negatively and hinder successful adaptation to a disability. Roy views the role of the nurse as assisting the client and family in achieving a positive response and, thus, adaptation to environmental stimuli—a role that is often enacted by rehabilitation nurses" (p. 26).

Piazza and Foote (1990) viewed Roy's model as an appropriate framework for rehabilitation nursing. "Roy's model provides a holistic, biopsychosocial view of persons through the identification of four modes of adaptation that provide structure for the nursing process" (p. 257). They also related it to other important aspects of care: "Use of a nursing model, such as Roy's, could promote continuity of care through identification of not only the physiological but also the psychological and sociological aspects of care that have an impact on patients during their stay in a rehabilitation nursing unit and following discharge" (p. 254).

Limitations: A potential limitation of Roy's model is its strong emphasis on assessment and diagnosis from a nursing perspective. This emphasis may interfere with an optimal interdisciplinary approach.

Educational preparation for rehabilitation nursing

The practice of rehabilitation nursing demands specialized knowledge and skills for responding therapeutically to the significant impact that disability has on clients, on their support systems, and on the community at large. It is uncommon for nursing students in undergraduate programs to have exposure to specialized course work in rehabilitation nursing principles and practices. Overall exposure to general concepts of healthcare restoration more often is achieved within an integrated curriculum and within the context of clinical nursing rotations that focus on the care of adult clients.

According to ANA and ARN (1988), the knowledge base required for rehabilitation nursing in all practice settings includes the concepts of optimum wellness, socialization, sexuality, adaptation, the process of change, learning, growth and development, and role theory. Rehabilitation nursing experts also recommend development of a sound knowledge base in the areas of anatomy and physiology—with a special emphasis on the neurological, musculoskeletal, gastrointestinal, and urological systems—as well as an understanding of functional assessment and kinesiology.

The ability to function effectively within an interdisciplinary team requires knowledge of group dynamics and effective team functioning. Rehabilitation nurses must acquire excellent manual skills in therapeutic positioning, range of joint motion, transfers, ambulation, and activities of daily living (ADL) tasks that often include the use of many types of adaptive equipment. The Association of Rehabilitation Nurses provides opportunities for ongoing education in this specialized field through publications, national educational conferences, and a variety of learning opportunities sponsored at both the national and chapter levels. Community-based programs, self-directed learning, and other educational opportunities are vehicles used by rehabilitation nurses to develop professionally.

Because of the expertise they derive from education, experience, and professional growth, rehabilitation nurses focus on clients as holistic beings. Hanlon and Sharkey (1989) stated that rehabilitation nurses "implement a rehabilitation philosophy, incorporate rehabilitation principles in practice, and apply rehabilitation knowledge and skills within the framework of the nursing process" (p. 76).

Certification in rehabilitation nursing

Healthcare certification validates that the individual holding the certification credential has demonstrated a certain level of skill within a specialty. The goal of the ARN certification examination is to recognize nurses who, through an examination process, are able to demonstrate an agreed-upon level of expertise in rehabilitation nursing. The certification process represents a synthesis of a unique body of knowledge and skill that promotes effective resolution of the clinical challenges confronting rehabilitation nurses (Pierce, Gibbons, & Cullen, 1991).

The first certification examination for the specialty practice of rehabilitation nursing—which, if passed, results in attaining the credential of Certified Rehabilitation Registered Nurse (CRRN)—was given in December 1984 under the auspices of ARN's Rehabilitation Nursing Certification Board. As of 1993, there are more than 7,000 registered nurses certified in rehabilitation nursing in the United States and Canada. Drew (1985) stated that certification is a form of self-regulation by rehabilitation nursing professionals. In her view, certification "implies ethically responsible behavior in the course of nursing practice and is a form of public protection and an aid to the professional by encouraging and recognizing high professional achievement" (p. 20).

Nurses acquiring rehabilitation nursing specialty certification are entitled to use the CRRN credential in their interactions with clients and other healthcare professionals. The ARN certification examination certifies nurses who have concentrated their practice in the area of rehabilitation for at least 2 years. By the year 2000, eligibility requirements will include a baccalaureate degree in nursing. In addition, candidates will be asked to demonstrate successful completion of a continuing education course that includes the concepts contained in the core curriculum of rehabilitation nursing published by ARN. Those nurses already certified as CRRNs at that point will be exempt from revised criteria, provided they maintain their certification status.

Many rehabilitation nurses also have achieved certification

in the area of insurance rehabilitation. The certified insurance rehabilitation specialist (CIRS) designation is available to all professionals within the insurance rehabilitation field who complete certification requirements. The CIRS designation evolved from the need to regulate practitioners within the insurance industry. The intent of the CIRS credential is to demonstrate a minimum acceptable level of knowledge regarding disability compensation (Drew, 1985).

Roles and settings in rehabilitation nursing practice

Rehabilitation nurses serve in a variety of roles with clients across the life span in settings that include acute care and rehabilitation facilities, skilled nursing facilities, residential facilities, day-care agencies, and private homes. The *Report on the Rehabilitation Nurses Job Analysis* published by the Association of Rehabilitation Nurses and the Rehabilitation Nursing Certification Board (Dungan & McCourt, 1991) described many settings in which rehabilitation nursing is practiced. Primary practice rehabilitation nursing settings as reported in this survey appear in Table 3.2.

Table 3.2. Primary Practice Settings of Rehabilitation Nurses in 1991

Setting	%
General hospital with a rehabilitation unit	55.9%
General hospital without a rehabilitation unit	1.4%
Freestanding rehabilitation facility	23.1%
Outpatient rehabilitation facility	0.9%
Long-term care facility	2.4%
Veterans Administration hospital	1.3%
Community health/home health/hospice	6.0%
State/regional health agency	0.1%
Insurance company	4.6%
Private company/private practice	0.6%
Educational institution	2.0%
Other	1.7%

Reprinted with permission of the Association of Rehabilitation Nurses and the Rehabilitation Nursing Certification Board from Dungan, L., & McCourt, A. (1991). *Report on the Rehabilitation Nurses Job Analysis* (p. 39). Skokie, IL: Association of Rehabilitation Nurses and Rehabilitation Nursing Certification Board.

Role overview: The rehabilitation nurse engages in roles ranging from educator to expert witness.

The primary role of a rehabilitation nurse is as a *client educator*. In this role, the nurse shares information and helps clients develop the skills needed to move on an illness-wellness continuum toward wellness by promoting independence and by rewarding achievement (Berni, 1980; Willis-Sukosky, 1987). In the role of *caregiver*, the rehabilitation nurse provides direct personal care services to clients until accountability for care and role performance can be transferred effectively to the clients, the family, and/or significant others. Caregiving activities are focused on restoring and maintaining function, preventing complications, and avoiding further functional loss (Willis-Sukosky, 1987).

Serving as a *counselor*, the rehabilitation nurse helps clients and families anticipate and practice responses to the challenges of community reintegration.

As a *coordinator of care*, the rehabilitation nurse helps clients transfer and apply skills learned in other areas of the broad rehabilitation program. Throughout the therapeutic relationship, the nurse aids clients in acquiring effective problem-solving skills and becoming their own healthcare experts.

As a *client advocate*, the nurse provides information and insight to others about the rehabilitation process and clients' responses, reactions, needs, and progress.

In the role of *researcher*, the rehabilitation nurse may participate in data collection for research studies, use the findings of nursing research to improve practice, or may design and conduct original research studies.

As a *legal consultant and expert witness* in litigation proceedings, the rehabilitation nurse provides knowledge and skills that are essential in the areas of personal injury, workers' compensation, and malpractice litigation (Faherty, 1991). As the life span increases for persons with disabling catastrophic injuries, rehabilitation nurses may become involved in life care planning as a service to clients, families, and medical and legal professionals who have responsibilities for persons with disabilities. Life care plans devised by rehabilitation nurse consultants can project current and future healthcare needs and predict the costs that will be involved in meeting clients' needs over time.

Generalist and advanced practice roles in rehabilitation nursing: Rehabilitation nurses function in both generalist and advanced practice roles. Rehabilitation nurse *generalists* practice in a variety of healthcare and community settings. The role of rehabilitation nurse generalists is influenced by basic nursing educational preparation, continuing education, and experience in meeting the needs of disabled individuals and their support systems. Certification in rehabilitation nursing helps to validate the basic knowledge and skill level of rehabilitation nurse generalists.

Rehabilitation nurses practicing at a generalist level are educationally prepared with a diploma or an associate's degree and have acquired their knowledge about and skills in rehabilitation nursing through a combination of on-the-job training and both formal and informal continuing education. Nurses prepared at the baccalaureate level may demonstrate intermediate-to-advanced skills through formal education, self-directed learning, and ongoing job experience (Dittmar, 1989).

For *advanced practice* roles in rehabilitation nursing, graduate preparation at a master's-degree level or higher is needed. Rehabilitation nurse specialists bring to their practice special expertise in the areas of clinical practice, education, research, and consultation.

Rehabilitation nurse specialists, as a result of their graduate preparation in rehabilitation nursing, demonstrate the application of advanced knowledge and skill, design and/or use nursing research as a basis for their practice, and serve as change agents for staff, clients, families, and other interdisciplinary team members. Five graduate programs prepare rehabilitation nurses as clinical specialists. These programs are sponsored by the University of Alabama in Birmingham, AL; Rush-Presbyterian-St. Luke's Medical Center in Chicago; State University of New York in Buffalo, NY; Thomas Jefferson University in Philadelphia; and the University of Texas in Arlington, TX.

A description of roles at both the generalist and advanced practice levels is contained in the publication *Rehabilitation Nursing: Scope of Practice; Process and Outcome Criteria for Selected Diagnoses* (ANA & ARN, 1988).

Subspecialty and advanced practice

Many subspecialty roles have been formalized by ARN into categories of special interest groups (SIGs). Current ARN SIGs include groups for rehabilitation staff nurses, gerontological rehabilitation nurses, pain management rehabilitation nurses, pediatric rehabilitation nurses, rehabilitation clinical nurse specialists, rehabilitation nurse case managers, rehabilitation nurse educators, rehabilitation nursing administrators, and rehabilitation nurse researchers.

The rehabilitation staff nurse: The major role of the rehabilitation nurse is to act as the *primary educator* for clients and their families. In this capacity, rehabilitation staff nurses teach clients to help themselves toward the goal of self-management. The staff nurse's teaching agenda includes, but is not limited to, helping clients and their families learn to maintain skin integrity, to become independent in self-care and mobility, to manage an effective bowel-and-bladder management program, to manage safety, and to use problem solving and creativity as a means of adapting and coping.

Rehabilitation staff nurses are the *primary caregivers* within the rehabilitation team. In this role, nurses use the nursing process to intervene therapeutically on behalf of clients. Rehabilitation staff nurses perform and/or delegate to ancillary caregivers tasks that restore and maintain function, prevent complications, and avoid further functional loss.

Rehabilitation staff nurses provide a therapeutic environment for clients and their families. They assertively communicate clients' needs and desires to others and share the clients' successes and struggles during the rehabilitation process. As team facilitators, rehabilitation staff nurses collaborate and consult with other healthcare disciplines. As client advocates and counselors, rehabilitation staff nurses work with clients on a 24-hour basis, encouraging clients to use their remaining abilities, helping to prepare them for a return to successful functioning, and referring them to other healthcare professionals, as appropriate, to meet complex current and future care needs.

Rehabilitation staff nurses transmit their specialized clinical practice knowledge to nursing students and experienced nurses entering rehabilitation nursing through both formal and informal teaching. In addition, they promote the development of research-based practice in rehabilitation nursing through research utilization and through direct participation in nursing research studies.

The gerontological rehabilitation nurse: Gerontological rehabilitation nursing practice provides care and expertise to promote health, maintain and restore function, and provide education and counseling to older clients and their families. Gerontological rehabilitation nurses combine the knowledge of and skills associated with rehabilitation and gerontological principles to focus on individuals who are 65 years of age and older.

Persons 80 years of age and older now represent the fastest growing segment of the population in the United States and in many other countries. Due to its advancing age and lengthening life span, this heterogeneous group is one of the largest consumers of healthcare services, regardless of setting.

The incorporation of rehabilitation practices and skills is essential for maintaining or restoring functional ability for elderly clients who have a multitude of medical and psychosocial problems. Using an interdisciplinary approach, gerontological rehabilitation nurses focus on prevention, safety strategies, client-family education, discharge planning, and a knowledge of community resources that enhances the care of elderly clients.

The pain management rehabilitation nurse: Rehabilitation nurses who practice in the area of pain management use a specialized scientific knowledge base to facilitate self-management plans for clients with pain.

Pain management rehabilitation nurses develop and initiate an individualized self-management plan that emphasizes biopsychosocial factors. Appropriate self-management through the use of learned skills and mutual goal setting becomes the client's responsibility. These strategies promote compliance and increase clients' coping mechanisms, thus minimizing pain behaviors. Pain management rehabilitation nurses provide staff development education and consultation to practitioners, clients, and members of the community.

The pediatric rehabilitation nurse: Pediatric rehabilitation nursing is the specialty practice committed to improving the quality of life for children, adolescents, and their families. The mission of this subspecialty is to provide a continuum of nursing care from injury and diagnosis to productive adulthood in collaboration with the interdisciplinary team.

Pediatric rehabilitation nursing is both specialized and diverse—a combination clearly reflected in the populations served. Infants, children, and adolescents with a variety of disabling conditions receive specialized care from pediatric rehabilitation nurses in a variety of settings—hospital, clinic, home, and school.

Developmental theory is a cornerstone of pediatric rehabilitation nursing, because a major interruption of normal life experiences can jeopardize a child's growth and development. Pediatric rehabilitation nurses recognize the importance of family involvement in the young person's development and are child/family advocates. Each child and family form the core of the rehabilitation team.

The publication *Pediatric Rehabilitation Nursing: Role Description* (ARN, 1992) provides further information regarding the roles of the pediatric rehabilitation nurse and the components of pediatric rehabilitation nursing practice.

The rehabilitation clinical nurse specialist: Rehabilitation clinical nurse specialists provide clinical expertise in rehabilitation nursing. Clinical nurse specialists educate clients, families, and staff and serve as consultants and liaisons within the organization and within the community. They use research findings in their practice and often design and conduct research studies. Variations on how this role is implemented depend on the needs of particular client populations and the settings in which the clinical nurse specialist practices. *The Rehabilitation Clinical Nurse Specialist: Role Description* (ARN, 1991a) describes role components in the areas of practitioner, educator, consultant, and researcher. The expertise needed for this role requires graduate-level preparation in rehabilitation nursing.

The rehabilitation nurse case manager: Rehabilitation nurse case managers provide comprehensive and cost-effective healthcare services by effectively planning, organizing, coordinating, and monitoring the services and resources needed to meet the individual client's healthcare needs.

The Rehabilitation Nurse Case Manager: Role Description (ARN, 1991b) includes the goals of case management, describes the roles of the rehabilitation nurse case manager and the settings in which the nurse case manager operates, and outlines the functions of practitioners in this role. It also addresses the qualifications for rehabilitation nurse case managers.

The rehabilitation nurse educator: Rehabilitation nurse educators function in both academic and institutional settings. In formal academic settings they serve as faculty for both undergraduate and graduate programs. Educators in institutional settings provide staff development and continuing education activities to ensure competent and up-to-date practice in the specialty of rehabilitation nursing. The rehabilitation staff development educator assists in assessing the proficiency of practitioners, develops and implements appropriate educational interventions, evaluates the effectiveness of training, and maintains documentation of the educational process. Programs such as orientation, demonstrations of safe use of products for patient care, updates on policies and procedures, and continuing education sessions for specialty practice are core components of the rehabilitation nursing educational process.

As role models for rehabilitation nurse clinicians, rehabilitation staff development educators participate in patient education activities, help to apply applicable research findings to rehabilitation nursing practice, and involve themselves in quality improvement projects. As advocates for rehabilitation nursing specialty practice and for people with disabilities, rehabilitation nurse educators promote and interpret rehabilitation nursing concepts to and for the professional nursing community and to the lay community at large.

The rehabilitation nursing administrator: Rehabilitation nursing administrators provide leadership in an organization to influence others toward the achievement of desired goals for nursing and patient care and to obtain the necessary resources to provide care.

The rehabilitation nursing administrator participates in strategic management by defining, implementing, and controlling the direction of an organization and is accountable for the quality of patient care and for the effective use of human resources.

The duties of this role include planning and implementing resource allocation and utilization within organizations. The rehabilitation nursing administrator influences professional rehabilitation nursing by supporting and engaging in educational and research activities and participating at the executive level with colleagues from other disciplines to provide leadership for rehabilitative services. Graduate preparation in nursing administration assists the rehabilitation nursing administrator in performing the many role requirements of his or her position.

The rehabilitation nurse researcher: Professional nurses contribute to the scientific base of nursing practice and the development of rehabilitation nursing through participation in research activities. As generalists at an undergraduate level, rehabilitation nurses participate in the research process at levels appropriate to their experience and education. They ensure the protection of human subjects involved in research, apply research findings in practice decisions, and may participate in the dissemination of research results. The practice of rehabilitation nurse generalists should reflect the use of current, validated research findings. At an advanced-practice level, rehabilitation nurses are prepared at the master's or doctoral level; this preparation involves active participation in research.

As researchers, rehabilitation nurses develop research programs within an interdisciplinary framework. Research utilization, theory development, and the development of research programs are primary responsibilities of nurse researchers.

References

Acton, N. (1982). The world's response to disability: Evolution of a philosophy. *Archives of Physical Medicine and Rehabilitation, 63*, 145-149.

American Nurses' Association (ANA) & the Association of Rehabilitation Nurses (ARN). (1986). *Standards of rehabilitation nursing practice* (rev. ed.). Kansas City, MO: American Nurses' Association.

American Nurses' Association & the Association of Rehabilitation Nurses. (1988). *Rehabilitation nursing: Scope of practice; process and outcome criteria for selected diagnoses.* Kansas City, MO: American Nurses' Association.

Association of Rehabilitation Nurses. (1991a). *The rehabilitation clinical nurse specialist: Role description.* Skokie, IL: Author.

Association of Rehabilitation Nurses. (1991b). *The rehabilitation nurse case manager: Role description.* Skokie, IL: Author.

Association of Rehabilitation Nurses. (1992). *Pediatric rehabilitation nursing: Role description.* Skokie, IL: Author.

Berni, R. (1980). Changing trends in rehabilitation nursing. In A. Walsh (Ed.), *The expanded role of the rehabilitation nurse.* Thorofare, NJ: Charles B. Slack.

Cross, J.R. (1990). Betty Neuman. In J.G. George (Ed.), *Nursing theories: The base for professional nursing practice* (3rd ed.) (pp. 258-286). Norwalk, CT: Appleton & Lange.

Derstine, J., & Mandzak-McCarron, K. (1990). Theory-based practice in the workplace: The next step. *Rehabilitation Nursing, 15*, 138-139.

Dittmar, S. (Ed.). (1989). *Rehabilitation nursing: Process and application.* St. Louis: The C.V. Mosby Company.

Drew, J. (1985). Certification in rehabilitation nursing. *Rehabilitation Nursing, 10*(2), 20-24.

Dungan, L., & McCourt, A. (1991). *Report on the Rehabilitation Nurses Job Analysis.* Skokie, IL: Association of Rehabilitation Nurses and Rehabilitation Nursing Certification Board.

Faherty, B.L. (1991). The nurse legal consultant and disabling injuries. *Rehabilitation Nursing, 16*, 30-33.

Fraley, A. (1992). *Nursing and the disabled across the life span.* Boston: Jones & Bartlett Publishers, Inc.

George, J.B. (Ed.). (1990). *Nursing theories: The base for professional nursing practice* (3rd ed.). Norwalk, CT: Appleton & Lange.

Goldenson, R.M. (Ed.) (1978). *Disability and rehabilitation handbook.* New York: McGraw-Hill Book Company.

Hanlon, D., & Sharkey, E.L. (1989). The professional practice of rehabilitation nursing. In S. Dittmar (Ed.), *Rehabilitation nursing: Process and application* (pp. 73-79). St. Louis: The C.V. Mosby Company.

Haughey, B., & Dittmar, S. (1989). Theoretical bases of rehabilitation nursing. In S. Dittmar (Ed.), *Rehabilitation nursing: Process and application* (pp. 16-29). St. Louis: The C.V. Mosby Company.

Huckabay, L. (1991). The role of conceptual frameworks in nursing practice, administration, education, and research. *Nursing Administration Quarterly, 15*(3), 17-28.

King, I. (1981). *A theory for nursing: Systems, concepts, process.* New York: John Wiley & Sons, Inc.

Knust, S.J., & Quarn, J.M. (1983). Integration of self-care theory with rehabilitation nursing. *Rehabilitation Nursing, 8*(4), 26-28.

McLeis, A. (1991). *Theoretical nursing: Development and progress* (2nd ed.). Philadelphia: J.B. Lippincott Company.

Mumma, C.M. (Ed). (1987a). *Rehabilitation nursing: Concepts and practice—A core curriculum* (2nd ed.) (pp. 27-101). Evanston, IL: Rehabilitation Nursing Foundation.

Mumma, C.M. (1987b). Theoretical background. In C.M. Mumma (Ed.), *Rehabilitation nursing: Concepts and practice—A core curriculum* (2nd ed.) (pp. 27-101). Evanston, IL: Rehabilitation Nursing Foundation.

Neuman, B. (1982). *The Neuman systems model.* New York: Appleton-Century-Crofts.

Orem, D. (1985). *Nursing: Concepts of practice* (3rd ed.). New York: McGraw-Hill Book Company.

Piazza, D., & Foote, A. (1990). Roy's adaptation model: A guide for rehabilitation nursing practice. *Rehabilitation Nursing, 15*, 254-259.

Pierce, L.L., Gibbons, K.B., & Cullen, J.M. (1991). The CRRN examination: Preparation and strategies. *Rehabilitation Nursing, 16*, 148-152.

Roy, C. (1984). *Introduction to nursing: An adaptation model* (2nd ed.). Englewood Cliffs, NJ: Prentice-Hall, Inc.

Sayles, S.M. (Ed.). (1981). *Rehabilitation nursing: Concepts and practice—A core curriculum.* Evanston, IL: Rehabilitation Nursing Institute.

Sorrentino, E.A. (1991). Making theories work for you. *Nursing Administration Quarterly, 15*(3), 54-59.

Torres, G. (1990). The place of concepts and theories within nursing. In J.B. George (Ed.), *Nursing theories: The base for professional nursing practice* (3rd ed.) (pp. 1-12). Norwalk, CT: Appleton & Lange.

Willis-Sukosky, N. (1987). Introduction to the field of rehabilitation and rehabilitation nursing. In C.M. Mumma (Ed.), *Rehabilitation nursing: Concepts and practice—A core curriculum* (2nd ed.) (pp. 1-25). Evanston, IL: Rehabilitation Nursing Foundation.

Suggested Readings

Ackerman, M.L., Brink, S.A., Jones, C.G., Moody, S.L., Perlich, G.L., & Prusinski, B.B. (1986). Imogene King: Theory of goal attainment. In A. Marriner (Ed.), *Nursing theorists and their work* (pp. 231-245). St. Louis: The C.V. Mosby Company.

American Congress of Rehabilitation Medicine. (1992). *Guide to interdisciplinary practice in rehabilitation settings.* Skokie, IL: Author.

Andrews, H.A., & Roy, C. (1986). *Essentials of the Roy Adaptation Model.* Norwalk, CT: Appleton-Century-Crofts.

Blue, C.L., Brubaker, K.M., Papazian, K.R., & Riser, C.M. (1986). Sister Callista Roy: An adaptation model. In A. Marriner (Ed.), *Nursing theorists and their work* (pp. 297-307). St. Louis: The C.V. Mosby Company.

Brody, S.K., & Pawlson, L.G. (Eds.). (1990). *Aging and rehabilitation: The state of the practice.* New York: Springer Publishing Company.

Brummel-Smith, K. (1990). In B. Kemp, K. Brummel-Smith, & J.W. Ramsdell (Eds.), *Geriatric rehabilitation.* Boston: Little, Brown and Company-College Hill Press.

Butler, M. (1991). Geriatric rehabilitation nursing. *Rehabilitation Nursing, 16*, 318-320.

Chinn, P.L., & Jacobs, M.K. (1987). *Theory and nursing: A systematic approach* (2nd ed.). St. Louis: The C.V. Mosby Company.

Commission on Accreditation of Rehabilitation Facilities (CARF). (1991). *1991 standards manual for organizations serving people with disabilities.* Tucson, AZ.

Davidhizar, R., & Cosgray, R. (1990.) The use of Orem's model in psychiatric rehabilitation assessment. *Rehabilitation Nursing, 15*, 39-41.

Dimond, M., & Jones, S.L. (1983). *Chronic illness across the life span.* Norwalk, CT: Appleton-Century-Crofts.

Eisenberg, M.G., Griggens, C., & Duvall, R.J. (1982). *Disabled persons as second-class citizens.* New York: Springer Publishing Company.

Eisenberg, M.G., & Marazarro, R.G. (1982). *Behavioral approaches to rehabilitation.* Springer Publishing Company.

Eisenberg, M.G., Sutkin, L.C., & Jansen, M.A. (Eds.). (1984). *Chronic illness and disability through the life-span.* New York: Springer Publishing Company.

Fawcett, J. (1989). *Analysis and evaluation of conceptual models of nursing* (2nd ed.). Philadelphia: F.A. Davis Company.

Foster, P.C., & Janssens, N.P. (1990). Dorothea E. Orem. In J.B. George (Ed.), *Nursing theories: The base for professional nursing practice* (3rd ed.) (pp. 91-112). Norwalk, CT: Appleton & Lange.

Galbreath, J.G. (1990). Sister Callista Roy. In J.B. George (Ed.), *Nursing theories: The base for professional nursing practice* (3rd ed.) (pp. 231-258). Norwalk, CT: Appleton & Lange.

George, J.B. (1990). Imogene M. King. In J.B. George (Ed.), *Nursing theories: The base for professional nursing practice* (3rd ed.) (pp. 193-210). Norwalk, CT: Appleton & Lange.

Gillies, D.A. (1987). Family assessment and counseling by the rehabilitation nurse. *Rehabilitation Nursing, 12*, 65-69.

Gillies, D.A. (1989). *Nursing management: A systems approach* (2nd ed.). Philadelphia: W.B. Saunders Company.

Halstead, L.S., & Grabois, M. (1985). *Medical rehabilitation.* New York: Raven Press.

Hermiz, M.E., & Meininger, M. (1986). Betty Neuman: Systems model. In A. Marriner (Ed.), *Nursing theorists and their work* (pp. 313-334). St. Louis: The C.V. Mosby Company.

Hiltz, D. (1989). The Neuman systems model: An analysis of a clinical situation. *Rehabilitation Nursing, 15*, 330-332.

Jones, F.T. (1948). The nurse's responsibility in rehabilitation. *American Journal of Nursing, 48*, 76-79.

King, I.M. (1971). *Toward a theory for nursing: General concepts of human behavior.* New York: John M. Wiley & Sons, Inc.

Latus, M.J. (1982). The role of the insurance rehabilitation nurse. *Rehabilitation Nursing, 7*(5), 26-29.

Marriner, A. (Ed). (1986). *Nursing theorists and their work.* St. Louis: The C.V. Mosby Company.

Martin, N., Holt, N., & Hicks, D. (1981). *Comprehensive rehabilitation nursing.* New York: McGraw-Hill Book Company.

Morrissey, A.B. (1949). The nursing technics in rehabilitation. *American Journal of Nursing, 49*, 545-555.

Morrissey, A.B. (1949). Rehabilitation care for patients. *American Journal of Nursing, 49*, 453-454.

Nelson, N. (1989). The certification process. *Nursing Clinics of North America, 24*(1), 151-159.

Oliver, N.R. (1991). True believers: A case for model-based nursing practice. *Nursing Administration Quarterly, 15*(3), 37-43.

Orem, D.E. (1971). *Nursing: Concepts of practice.* New York: McGraw-Hill.

Orem, D.E. (1980). *Nursing: Concepts of practice* (2nd ed.). New York: McGraw-Hill.

Orem, D. (1985). A concept of self-care for the rehabilitation client. *Rehabilitation Nursing, 10*(3), 33-36.

Power, P., Dell Orto, A., & Gibbons, M. (1988). *Family interventions through chronic illness and disability.* New York: Springer Publishing Company.

Rigger, T.F., Maki, D.R., & Wolf, A. (Eds.). (1988). *Applied rehabilitation counseling.* New York: Springer Publishing Company.

Roy, C. (1976). *Introduction to nursing: An adaptation model.* Englewood Cliffs, NJ: Prentice-Hall, Inc.

Roy, C. (1980). The Roy adaptation model. In J.P. Riehl & C. Roy (Eds.), *Conceptual models for nursing practice* (2nd ed.) (pp. 119-134). New York: Appleton-Century-Crofts.

Steel, J.E. (1985). The impact of certification on specialty practice.

Rehabilitation Nursing, 10(2), 16-19.

Styles, M.M. (1983). The anatomy of a profession. *Rehabilitation Nursing, 8*(5), 10-13, 35.

Stryker, R.P. (1977). *Rehabilitative aspects of acute and chronic care* (2nd ed.). Philadelphia: W.B. Saunders Company.

Taylor, L.J., Colter, M., Golter, G., & Backer, T.E. (Eds.). (1985). *Handbook of private sector rehabilitation.* New York: Springer Publishing Company.

Ter Maat, M. (1990). Tales of a new rehabilitation director of nursing. *Rehabilitation Nursing, 15*, 329-330.

Thompson-Hoffman, S., & Storck, I. (Eds.). (1991). *Disability in the United States: A review of the state of knowledge.* New York: Springer Publishing Company.

Trieschmann, R. (1987). *Aging with a disability.* New York: Demos Publishing Company.

Vash, C.C. (1981). *The psychology of disability.* New York: Springer Publishing Company.

Watson, P.G. (1985). Components of rehabilitation nursing practice advancement. *Rehabilitation Nursing, 10*(5), 28-31.

Weiner, S.M. (1983). Rehabilitation nursing in the private sector. *Rehabilitation Nursing, 8*(2), 31-32.

Wright, B. (1983). *Physical disability: A psychological approach.* New York: Harper & Row Publishers, Inc.

CHAPTER 4

The Association of Rehabilitation Nurses

The Association of Rehabilitation Nurses (ARN) was founded in 1974. The purpose of the organization is to advance the quality of rehabilitation nursing services by promoting educational programs and the exchange of ideas among rehabilitation nurses.

In the beginning

When the organizers of the Association of Rehabilitation Nurses (ARN) began their work in 1974 in the northern suburbs of Chicago, they identified two major challenges: obtaining funding for their endeavor and locating rehabilitation nurses who might be interested in joining ARN. Initial funding was obtained from Lutheran General Hospital, in Park Ridge, IL, which supplied a start-up grant. Association Management Center, a management firm in Glenview, IL, agreed to provide management and administrative services. Fees would be collected as money became available. Susan Novak, MS RN CRRN, spearheaded the organization's growth efforts in her position as ARN's first president.

To locate potential members, surveys were sent to the American Hospital Association's list of rehabilitation facilities and units. More than 200 nurses responded to the survey. They became the first members and leaders of ARN.

Structure and growth of ARN

Regions and chapters: For organizational purposes, ARN leaders divided the United States into seven geographic regions when the association was formed. Regions are not structural components of the organization, but ARN members from each region elect one director to the ARN Board of Directors every 2 years.

State chapters began to form simultaneously with the national organization; by 1977, 10 chapters were chartered and others were forming in many states across the country. In 1986, the board decided to allow chapters to be formed in local areas, rather than just on a statewide basis. The result was a rapidly growing number of chapters that reached more than 75 by 1992. Some chapters still cover an entire state, others simply a metropolitan area; some have only the required minimum of 16 members and others have dozens.

The chapter structure made it possible for rehabilitation nurses to network and take advantage of educational opportunities on a local level, while it also provided a means for organizational growth and leadership development. The ARN Board of Directors recognized the need to nurture chapter leadership and in May 1988 inaugurated an annual Leadership Institute to help train and develop current and future chapter leaders.

Planning activities: Thc basis for ARN was its purpose statement and bylaws. But early on, leaders recognized the need to provide structure and to plan for the future.

The ARN board held its first long-range planning session in 1982; subsequent sessions took place in 1985, 1987, and 1992. These sessions provided the basis for orderly growth and the ability to create opportunities. The plan is reviewed annually by the board and committees, and every new challenge and existing program are evaluated according to the plan.

Throughout the formal and informal planning activities, attention has been given to the documents that form the core of the organization: the definition of rehabilitation nursing; ARN's mission statement, philosophy, and conceptual framework; and ARN's goals and objectives.

Professional activities

Educational conferences: One hundred forty-three nurses and six exhibitors attended the first ARN educational conference in Minneapolis in August 1975. Thereafter, the annual conference was held in various cities around the country and grew steadily in size and sophistication. The fifth anniversary conference was held in Chicago in 1979, the 10th in Cincinnati in 1984, and the 15th in Nashville in 1989.

Publications: *ARN Journal* was launched in November 1975. The journal was designed not only as an educational publication, but also as a membership recruitment tool. It replaced the original newsletter, *Rehab RN News*, which was published from June 1974 through the end of 1975. In 1980, the journal's name was changed to *Rehabilitation Nursing*. Over the years, the editorial content of the journal has evolved. Authors looked increasingly toward *Rehabilitation Nursing* as the vehicle in which to publish, so the journal's editorial board could be more selective. More research was published, and in 1991, the journal began to offer continuing education credit for several articles in each issue.

At its 1992 conference, ARN launched a new publication, *Rehabilitation Nursing Research*. Although begun as an annual issue, the publication was planned to become a quarterly journal, one of the first specialty journals devoted to research in nursing.

In 1984, *ARN News* was published for the first time. This newsletter was issued in months that alternated with publication of the journal and provided another source of organizational communication. By 1988, all organizational news was published in the newsletter rather than in the journal.

Standards of practice: ARN published the first edition of *Standards of Rehabilitation Nursing Practice* in 1977 with the American Nurses Association (ANA) (ANA & ARN, 1977). As with most of its other projects, ARN accomplished this project far earlier in its history than have other specialty nursing organizations. The standards were revised in 1986, again with ANA (ANA & ARN, 1986), and another publication, *Rehabilitation Nursing: Scope of Practice; Process and Outcome for Selected Diagnoses,* was published with ANA in 1988 (ANA & ARN, 1988).

Core curriculum: From the beginning, ARN leaders recognized the need to define the body of knowledge for rehabilitation nursing before ARN could begin to identify and shape the specialty. Through surveys and group work at the 1978 conference in Orlando, FL, rehabilitation nurses began to delineate what they did in their practice that made them different from nurses in other specialties.

From that early work, the components of a core curriculum began to emerge. *Rehabilitation Nursing: Concepts and Practice—A Core Curriculum* was published in 1981 (Sayles, 1981) and served the specialty until the second edition came out in 1987 (Mumma, 1987). Within 2 years, plans were being made to do a third edition in 1993, to be available at the conference that year.

Certification: An early ARN goal was to provide a program of voluntary certification for rehabilitation nurses. Certification in any nursing specialty validates the nurse's expertise in the eyes of colleagues, supervisors, and clients alike; further, it can help ensure reasonable reimbursement for nursing services. Finally, it adds immeasurably to the nurse's confidence and competence in practice. For these reasons, ARN's leaders felt a program of certification in rehabilitation nursing was important.

In 1980, a credentialing task force recommended that the organization pursue its goal. A contract was signed with The Psychological Corporation, a testing company that would administer the examination, and the certification board set the process in motion. On December 7, 1984, 965 rehabilitation nurses took the first certification examination to become certified rehabilitation registered nurses (CRRNs). The program grew rapidly, as almost 2,000 nurses took the test in 1990. CRRNs renew their certification every 5 years by taking the test again or accumulating points of credit earned for participation in continuing education or other activities.

A job analysis completed in 1990 (Dungan & McCourt, 1991) supplied further information to validate the examination. The results of the analysis were used in several other projects, such as development of the 1993 edition of the core curriculum.

Accreditation: In 1978, ARN was accredited as a provider and approver of continuing education in nursing by ANA. It was one of the youngest specialty organizations to achieve such recognition. Since then, accreditation has been achieved three times, after a rigorous review of educational programs and a site visit by ANA's accrediting body, the American Nurses Credentialing Center's Commission on Accreditation.

Provider accreditation validates that ARN designs programs according to professional standards for continuing education in nursing and ensures that the continuing education credit earned can be used in most situations required for relicensure and recertification. ARN's approval accreditation has provided chapters and other entities the ability to give approved contact hours by applying to ARN and having programs reviewed by rehabilitation nurses.

The Rehabilitation Nursing Foundation

In 1976, the ARN board established the Rehabilitation Nursing Institute, a tax-exempt foundation focusing on education and research in rehabilitation nursing. Ten years later, the institute's name was changed to the Rehabilitation Nursing Foundation (RNF) to better reflect its focus, particularly its increased concentration on research.

Through the first few years, foundation leaders devoted most resources to developing and implementing educational programs. The foundation directed conference programming through 1988; in 1984, it began providing an intermediate-level seminar preparing nurses for certification. An independent study program developed from this seminar was made available in 1985 (Rehabilitation Nursing Institute, 1985).

A basic rehabilitation nursing course was developed and cosponsored by the University of Illinois for the first time in 1988 (RNF, 1988). The course has been offered several times each year since then and was completely revised in 1992.

RNF developed its first independent study modules in 1987. The modules consisted of audiotapes and study guides and were developed from workshops held prior to ARN conferences. One or more modules have been developed each year since then.

In 1989, the foundation embarked on video production with a video for independent study on nursing care of the patient exhibiting aggressive behavior after head injury. The video was well received, and in 1991, RNF produced a comprehensive educational program on incontinence, which included two video programs and two audio modules for independent study based on preconference workshops. The incontinence program focused on the new guidelines for patient care developed by the federal Agency for Health Care Policy and Research (AHCPR).

Research became a major part of the foundation's activities with the development of the Rehabilitation Nurses Research Fund in 1987. Members, chapters, and corporations contributed the $50,000 to establish the fund, and the first annual grant was awarded in 1988. Some of the first grant topics were "Developmental Competence in Adolescents with an Acquired Disability," "Health-Promoting Knowledge, Attitudes, and Behaviors of Adults with Disabilities," "Managing the Trajectory: Determinants of Self-Care in Individuals with Parkinson's Disease," and "Quality of Life in Spinal Cord Injured Persons After Colostomy." In addition, the foundation sponsored a symposium on rehabilitation nursing research in 1992 that was a tremendous success (with an attendance of 100). The symposium was scheduled to be offered biennially.

A major rehabilitation nursing diagnosis study was conducted, beginning in 1992, that provided information for many other foundation and association projects.

External involvement with other professional organizations and agencies

ARN leaders have always recognized the need to communicate with other organizations. Informal liaison relationships were established soon after the organization's inception. In 1976, ARN was accepted as a member of the Federation for Specialty Nursing Organizations and ANA, later to become the National Federation for Specialty Nursing Organizations

(NFSNO). It was the first major step in becoming involved externally.

As ARN matured and established its credibility, it became one of the most visible specialty nursing organizations in the country. ARN officers and representatives assumed leadership roles in organizations such as NFSNO, ANA's Nursing Organization Liaison Forum (NOLF), the Commission on Accreditation of Rehabilitation Facilities (CARF), the American Hospital Association Section for Rehabilitation Hospitals and Programs (AHASRHP), the National Rehabilitation Caucus (NRC), the Certified Insurance Rehabilitation Specialist Commission (CIRSC), and the Agency for Health Care Policy and Research (AHCPR). In 1992, ARN was one of the first three specialty organizations to be accepted as ANA affiliate members.

ARN is constantly called upon to support various initiatives and to provide rehabilitation nursing thought and opinion to other agencies and groups. ARN members provide testimony for government projects, and rehabilitation nurses sit on healthcare panels and committees throughout the country.

The mission of the Association of Rehabilitation Nurses is to promote and advance professional rehabilitation nursing practice through education, advocacy, and research to enhance the quality of life for those affected by disability. Since 1974, the organization has maintained its focus on that mission.

References

American Nurses' Association (ANA) & Association of Rehabilitation Nurses (ARN). (1977). *Standards of rehabilitation nursing practice.* Kansas City, MO: Author.

American Nurses' Association & Association of Rehabilitation Nurses. (1986). *Standards of rehabilitation nursing practice* (rev. ed.). Kansas City, MO: Author.

American Nurses' Association & Association of Rehabilitation Nurses. (1988). *Rehabilitation nursing: Scope of practice; process and outcome criteria for selected diagnoses.* Kansas City, MO: Author.

Dungan, L., & McCourt, A. (1991). *Report on the Rehabilitation Nurses Job Analysis.* Skokie, IL: Association of Rehabilitation Nurses and Rehabilitation Nursing Certification Board.

Mumma, C.M. (Ed.). (1987). *Rehabilitation nursing: Concepts and practice—A core curriculum* (2nd ed.). Evanston, IL: Rehabilitation Nursing Foundation.

Rehabilitation Nursing Foundation (RNF). (1988). *Directions for practice: A basic rehabilitation nursing course.* Evanston, IL: Author.

Rehabilitation Nursing Institute. (1985). *Application of rehabilitation concepts to nursing practice.* Evanston, IL: Author.

Sayles, S.M. (Ed.). (1981). *Rehabilitation nursing: Concepts and practice—A core curriculum.* Evanston, IL: Rehabilitation Nursing Institute.

Section II
Common Disorders Among Rehabilitation Clients

Rehabilitation nurses care for people who have a variety of neurological and musculoskeletal disorders. The etiology, incidence, pathophysiology, residual deficits, and recovery patterns of these disorders vary. The purpose of this section is to provide an overview of these changes and their relationship to resulting health problems.

Specifically, this section focuses on four healthcare problems: stroke, selected musculoskeletal/orthopedic conditions, traumatic brain injury, and spinal cord injury. These problems were chosen for inclusion in this section as a result of the 1990 Rehabilitation Nurses Job Analysis Survey (Dungan & McCourt, 1991). The survey indicated that people with these four disorders represent 75% of the clients cared for by rehabilitation nurses. Persons with stroke represented the largest population (36%), followed by those with musculoskeletal/orthopedic problems (15%), then traumatic brain injury and spinal cord injury (12% each). In addition, the job analysis indicated that 59% of persons receiving rehabilitation services are elderly. Aging persons with a disability represent a new and rapidly growing segment of the rehabilitation client population. Therefore, the last chapter in this section addresses rehabilitation considerations related to caring for the aging client.

Altered physiological responses following stroke, traumatic brain injury, and spinal cord injury severely affect the ability of individuals to exercise normal motor control. Chapter 5 provides a review of normal physiology specific to motor control of movement. This chapter further discusses the relationship among the mechanisms necessary for normal voluntary movement, the basis of abnormal muscle tone and altered movement patterns, and specific treatment approaches for normalizing muscle tone and movement. The succeeding chapters are dedicated to four disorders commonly dealt with in rehabilitation and to the aging process. Chapter 6 presents information regarding stroke; Chapter 7 reviews selected musculoskeletal disorders, including osteoporosis, arthritis, and amputations; Chapter 8 reviews traumatic brain injury; and Chapter 9 provides an overview of spinal cord injury. Each of these chapters addresses the definition, epidemiology, etiology, pathophysiology, and residual deficits of the disorder it covers and lists possible nursing diagnoses associated with the disorder. Chapter 10 focuses on the impact of the aging process on disability, with a specific emphasis on meeting the unique needs of the aging population of rehabilitation clients.

Reference

Dungan, L.A., & McCourt, A.E. (1991). *Report on the Rehabilitation Nurses Job Analysis 1989-1990.* Skokie, IL: Association of Rehabilitation Nurses and Rehabilitation Nursing Certification Board.

CHAPTER 5

Normal Motor Control and Neurophysiological Approaches to Care

Normal movement is a complex and precise set of processes essential to physical activity, functional ability, and productivity. Knowledge of normal movement helps nurses comprehend the pathology of abnormal movement and muscle control, as both frequently emerge with neurological, neuromuscular, and musculoskeletal disorders. This chapter briefly summarizes nervous system processing necessary for motor activity and explains the impact upper neuron damage has on reflex activity, movement, and muscle tone. Also included is a description of four neurophysiological treatment approaches used to help normalize tone, movement, and function after neurological injury.

I. The Control of Voluntary Movement

A. Normal movement and voluntary movement
   1. Normal movement: Ability to interact with the environment in a purposeful and adaptable way
   2. Voluntary movement: Result of integrated functioning of several levels of motor control

B. Patterns of voluntary movement necessary for functional activities
   1. Developmentally acquired: Develop in a cephalocaudal (head-to-foot) sequence and proximally to distally; for example, upper extremity exhibits withdrawal reflex before lower, voluntary head movement precedes voluntary trunk movement, movements of the shoulder appear before hand function (Trombly & Scott, 1989)
   2. Learned: Develop as a result of repetition and sensory experiences

II. Levels of Motor Control

A. Spinal reflexes
   1. Occur at each level of the spinal cord
   2. Keep muscles prepared for action and for making quick adjustments during movement

B. Sensory tracts of the spinal cord (e.g., spinothalamic and spinocerebellar) transmit information to higher brain centers to guide and modify movement (see Table 5.1)

C. Motor tracts of the spinal cord (e.g., lateral and ventral corticospinal) transmit signals from the cortex, basal ganglia, brainstem, and cerebellum to the spinal cord to direct and coordinate movement (see Table 5.1)
   1. Cortex
      a. Association areas in the cortex (somesthetic and premotor areas) control movement based on sensory input regarding state of the body, state of the environment, and memories of successful past movement (see Figure 5.1)
      b. Motor cortex initiates movement, sending messages to muscles via the motor tracts (Trombly & Scott, 1989)
   2. Basal ganglia
      a. Located deep in tissues below the cortex
      b. Control postural adjustments
      c. Make anticipatory adjustments needed to initiate movement
      d. Influence the automatic execution of learned movements
   3. Brainstem
      a. Consists of midbrain, pons, and medulla
      b. Is responsible for vital motor functioning
         1) Control and reflexes of pupils, eyes, head and neck, and trunk
         2) Breathing
         3) Vasomotor control
         4) Pharyngeal reflexes
   4. Cerebellum: Modifies speed, force, and accuracy of motor movements

III. Reflex Activity

A. Definitions
   1. Reflex: A stereotypical involuntary motor response by the nervous system to a specific stimulus (Hickey, 1992)
   2. Reflex arc: Complete loop consisting of these components (Hanak, 1992, p. 44)
      a. Sensory receptors
      b. Afferent or sensory fibers
      c. Connecting neuron in the spinal cord
      d. Efferent or motor fibers
      e. Skeletal muscle or gland

B. Types of reflexes
   1. Segmental reflexes: Involve one spinal segment

2. Intersegmental reflexes: Involve several spinal cord segments
3. Suprasegmental or supraspinal reflexes: Involve brain centers that override lower-level spinal reflexes

C. Basic reflex arc (see Figure 5.2)
1. Sensory receptors receive a stimulus and send an impulse via an afferent fiber to the dorsal portion of the spinal cord
2. Afferent fibers synapse in spinal cord with efferent fibers
3. Efferent fibers send a motor message from anterior

Table 5.1. Spinal Cord Tracts

The white matter of the spinal cord is composed of tracts that carry sensory and motor impulses to/from the brain. A basic understanding of their function helps nurses to better understand dysfunction after spinal cord injury. Most tract names indicate where they start and end; for example, the spinocerebellar tract originates in the spine and terminates in the cerebellum.

Major sensory (ascending) tracts

Posterior column—a large area in the posterior cord; relays information about conscious proprioception (position and movement), localization of touch, two-point tactile discrimination, and vibration

Dorsal spinocerebellar—in the posterior and lateral cord; conveys reflex proprioceptive (balance, muscle tone, for example) information from the arms and/or legs

Ventral spinocerebellar—lies anteriorly and laterally in the cord; transmits reflex proprioceptive information from the legs

Lateral spinothalamic—in the lateral part of the cord; conducts impulses for pain, heat, and cold; probably also transmits nervous impulses for tickle, itch, muscle fatigue, bladder fullness, desire to urinate, and sexual sensations; crosses in segments of the cord near the entry level, and then ascends to the thalamus

Ventral spinothalamic—in the anterior, lateral part of the cord; conducts impulses for coarse touch/pressure

Major motor (descending) tracts

*Lateral corticospinal**—lie in the lateral cord; transmit impulses for voluntary movement, especially in the limbs; cross in the medulla—thus, motor control is from the opposite cerebral hemisphere

*Ventral corticospinal**—in the anterior and medial part of the cord; control voluntary movement in the neck and trunk; do not cross midline until about the point they end in the cord

Extrapyramidal—descending tracts that control involuntary muscle movement and modify muscle tone; integrate motor activity with vestibular and visual input; include tracts such as the rubrospinal and vestibulospinal pathways

*Corticospinal tracts also are known as *pyramidal tracts.* The terms are used interchangeably and refer to tracts that start from pyramid-shaped neurons in the motor area of the cortex and descend within the pyramid of the medulla. They control most voluntary movements.

Source Consulted

Marshall, S.B., Marshall, L.F., Vos, H.R., & Chesnut, R.M. (1990). *Neuroscience critical care: Pathophysiology and patient management.* Philadelphia: W.B. Saunders Company.

Figure 5.1. Lobes and Functional Areas of the Cerebral Hemisphere

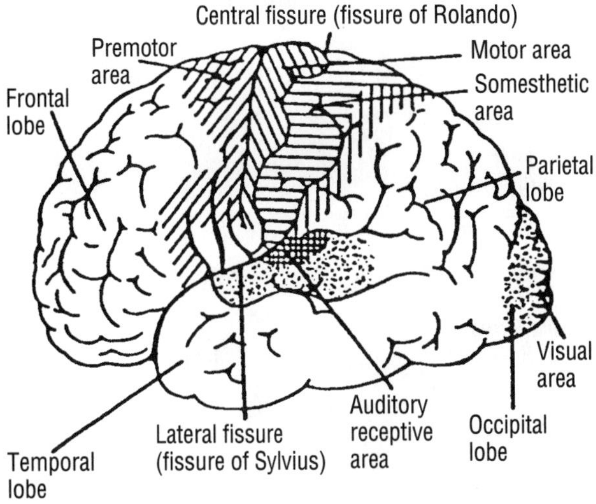

Reprinted with permission from Hickey, J. (1992). *The clinical practice of neurological and neurosurgical nursing* (3rd ed.) (p. 3). Philadelphia: J.B. Lippincott Company.

Figure 5.2. Pathway of the Lower Motor Neuron (Reflex Arc)

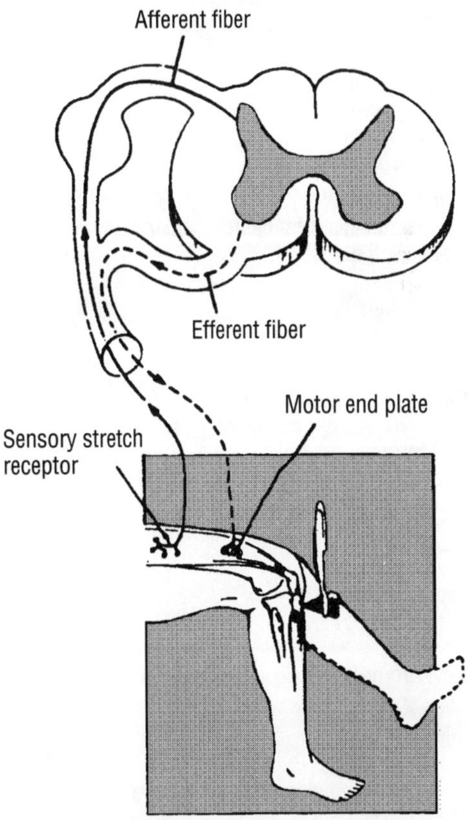

Reprinted with permission of Jones and Bartlett Publishers from Zejdlik, C.P. (1991). *Management of spinal cord injury* (2nd ed.) (p. 71). Boston: Jones and Bartlett Publishers. Copyright © 1991 Jones and Bartlett Publishers.

Table 5.2. Disorders of the Cranial Nerves and Their Clinical Manifestations

Cranial Nerves and Their Related Disorders	Clinical Manifestations
Olfactory Nerve I Head trauma Intracranial tumor Intracranial surgery	Unilateral or bilateral loss of or impairment of sense of smell Diminished taste for food
Optic Nerve II Optic neuritis Increased intracranial pressure Pituitary tumor	Homonymous hemianopia produced by lesions of optic tract
Oculomotor Nerve III ***Trochlear Nerve IV*** ***Abducens Nerve VI*** Vascular: Brainstem ischemia; hemorrhage/infarct Neoplasm Trauma Infection	Dilation of pupil with loss of light reflex on one side Impairment of ocular movement Diplopia Gaze palsies Ptosis of eyelid
Trigeminal Nerve V Trigeminal neuralgia Head trauma Cerebellopontine lesion Sinus tract tumor/metastatic disease Compression of trigeminal root by tumor	Pain in face Diminishment or absence of corneal reflex Chewing dysfunction
Facial Nerve VII Bell's palsy Facial nerve tumor Intracranial lesion Herpes zoster	Facial dysfunction; weakness and paralysis Hemifacial spasm Diminished or absent taste
Vestibulocochlear Nerve VIII Tumors/acoustic neuroma Vascular compression of nerve Ménière's syndrome	Tinnitus Vertigo Hearing difficulties
Glossopharyngeal Nerve IX Glossopharyngeal neuralgia from neurovascular compression of IXth and Xth nerves Trauma Inflammatory conditions Tumor Vertebral artery aneurysms	Pain at the base of the tongue Difficulty in swallowing Loss of the gag reflex Palatal, pharyngeal, and laryngeal paralysis
Vagus Nerve X Spastic palsy of larynx; bulbar paralysis; high vagal paralysis Guillain-Barré syndrome Carotid endarterectomy Vagal body tumors Nerve paralysis from malignancy, surgical trauma	Voice changes (temporary or permanent hoarseness) Vocal paralysis
Spinal Accessory Nerve XI Spinal cord disorder Amyotrophic lateral sclerosis Trauma Guillain-Barré syndrome	Dropping of affected shoulder with limited shoulder movement Weakness and/or paralysis of head rotation, flexion, extension; shoulder elevation
Hypoglossal Nerve XII Medullary lesions Amyotrophic lateral sclerosis Possible destruction of hypoglossal nuclei in polio and motor system disease Multiple sclerosis Trauma	Abnormal movements of the tongue Weakness and/or paralysis of the tongue muscles

Reprinted with permission of J.B. Lippincott Company from Brunner, L., & Suddarth, D. (1988). *Textbook of medical-surgical nursing* (6th ed.) (pp.1519-1520). Philadelphia: J.B. Lippincott Company.

horn cell of spinal cord out to muscle
4. Efferent fibers stimulate motor end plate of muscle, causing it to contract

D. Development of reflexes
1. Reflex responses to stimuli begin to develop in fetal stage of life and are evident in motor activity in infants
2. Primitive movement patterns are modified during the first several years of life as the nervous system matures

E. Impact of neurological damage on reflex activity
1. Limb synergies (gross patterns of flexion and extension around a joint) occur as a result of central nervous system (CNS) damage
2. Previously integrated reflexes and reactions may dominate the motor performance of people with brain injury
3. Release of primitive reflexes occurs in response to body or head position or as a result of cutaneous stimulation, which alters postural muscle tone
4. Muscle tone abnormalities include flaccidity, spasticity, and rigidity (Pedretti & Zoltan, 1990)
   a. Flaccidity, or muscle hypotonia, occurs as a result of loss of muscle innervation or disruption of the reflex arc, and as a temporary shock phenomenon following cerebral or spinal damage
   b. Spasticity, or muscle hypertonia, occurs as a result of abnormal spinal and brainstem reflexes
   c. Rigidity, or increased muscle tone, of both agonist and antagonist muscles occurs as a result of extrapyramidal system damage (see Table 5.1)
5. Brain damage can affect muscle tone
   a. Brain damage occurring early in life
      1) Can produce cerebral palsy (Tromby & Scott, 1989)
      2) Development of control of voluntary movement is delayed and motor behavior is dominated by spinal cord or brainstem reflexes
      3) Therapy focuses on establishing higher-level maturational motor patterns
   b. Brain damage occurring in focal cortical areas (e.g., stroke)
      1) Primitive reflexes reemerge due to damage in higher brain centers, especially during episodes of stress
      2) Therapeutic goal is that the client relearn control of higher-level voluntary motor patterns
   c. Brain damage occurring from generalized cortical damage (e.g., traumatic brain injury)
      1) Spinal cord and brainstem reflexes dominate
      2) Goal of therapy is to prevent or decrease the effects of primitive spinal cord and brainstem reflexes and to stimulate higher-level control and reactions
      3) Goal of therapy is to prevent primitive spinal cord and brainstem reflexes and to stimulate higher level reactions
   d. Brain damage also can impair cranial nerve functioning, as the nerves' nuclei arise in brainstem (midbrain, pons, medulla) (see Table 5.2)

Figure 5.3. Upper and Lower Motor Neuron Pathways

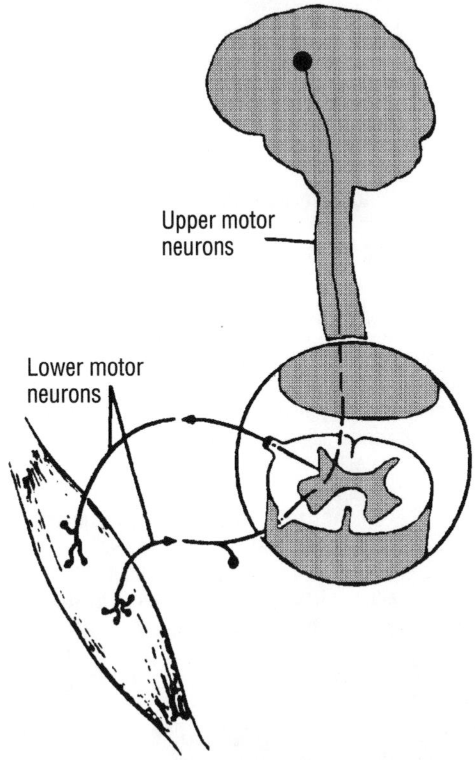

Reprinted with permission of Jones and Bartlett Publishers from Zejdlik, C.P. (1991). *Management of spinal cord injury* (2nd ed.) (p. 70). Boston: Jones and Bartlett Publishers.

IV. Upper and Lower Motor Neurons (see Figures 5.2 and 5.3)

A. Upper motor neurons (UMNs)
1. Structure and function
   a. UMNs are long tracts that travel from the brain to the spinal cord (Zejdlik, 1991); cell bodies of UMNs are located in the motor strip of the cerebral cortex
   b. UMNs synapse with lower motor neurons (LMNs) in the anterior horn cell of the spinal cord at each segmental level
   c. UMNs exert supraspinal control over LMNs by suppressing reactions to local stimuli at the spinal cord reflex level
   d. Damage to any part of the UMN system, from the brain down to and including the T12/L1 segments of the spinal cord, creates an UMN lesion (examples of UMN damage are stroke, brain injury, spinal cord injury above T12/L1, multiple sclerosis)
2. Result of UMN lesions: Reflex arc is intact but supraspinal control over spinal reflexes is damaged or destroyed, resulting in the following:
   a. Hyperactive reflexes
   b. Spastic paralysis
   c. Positive plantar (Babinski) reflex
   d. Minimal muscle atrophy

Table 5.3. Neurophysiological (Neurodevelopmental) Treatment Approaches

Bobath's Neurodevelopmental Treatment Approach (Bobath, 1978, 1990)
Used primarily for patients with hemiplegia caused by stroke, brain injury, or cerebral palsy

Major Goals and Premises
1. Normalization of tone, posture, movement, and function is a primary goal.
2. Hemiplegics are positioned in opposition to the spastic patterns of flexion and adduction in the upper extremity and extension in the lower extremity.
3. Individuals are allowed the opportunity to feel and, thus, relearn normal movement patterns and postures.
4. Reintegration of the two sides of the body is emphasized so that the hemiplegic is not allowed to function in a one-sided manner.
5. Relearning of normal bilateral segmental movements will occur.

Major Principles of Treatment
1. Bilateralness is emphasized during movement, functional activities, and bed and/or chair positioning.
2. Proximal-to-distal positioning is recommended, as tone in the limbs can be reduced from proximal points such as the head, neck, spine, shoulder, and pelvic girdles.
3. Protraction of the shoulder and pelvic girdle is emphasized; this opposes the synergistic mass pattern of retraction.
4. Weight bearing on the affected side is a major means of normalizing tone. (This can occur in sitting, lying, rising from the supine position, and bridging, for example).
5. Movement toward the affected side is emphasized (e.g., during transfers, getting into and out of bed).
6. Elongation of the trunk and neck is stressed to promote symmetry and normalize tone and posture.
7. Normal sensory information is provided to the hemiplegic side (including tactile, auditory, and visual input).
8. Tasks begin from a symmetrical midline position with equal weight bearing on both the involved and the uninvolved sides of the body.

Potential Application to Nursing
Nurses can therapeutically incorporate the above principles during repositioning, turning, transferring, dressing, grooming, and hygiene tasks.

Brunnstrom's Movement Therapy Approach (Pedretti, 1990)
Used primarily for hemiplegia

Major Goals and Premises
1. Limb synergies and abnormal reflex activity are viewed as normal; they must be experienced and can be built upon to facilitate more normal movement patterns.
2. Movement of the patient through recovery stages is facilitated.
3. Mass grasp and release of grasp will be achieved in the affected hand and/or digits.
4. A safe standing balance and an almost normal gait pattern will be accomplished.

Major Principles of Treatment
1. Evaluation and treatment are based on six specific and predictable stages of motor recovery.
2. Interventions focus on moving the patient through each succeeding stage of recovery.
3. Patients' motor performance can level off in any of the recovery stages; treatment is commensurate with the patients' stage of motor recovery.
4. Recovery occurs in six motor stages:
   a. Stage 1—Flaccidity
   b. Stage 2—Development of spasticity
   c. Stage 3—Increased spasticity (may be excessive); seen in synergy patterns
   d. Stage 4—Decreased spasticity so that gross movements apart from limb synergies can be performed
   e. Stage 5—Further decreased spasticity with ability to do more complicated combinations of movements (i.e., synergies no longer dominate movement)
   f. Stage 6—Almost normal performance of isolated joint motions that is coordinated in nature
5. Postural and attitudinal reflexes are used to enhance or reduce tone in specific muscles.

Potential Application to Nursing
Bed and chair positioning are primary activities in which this approach may be implemented.

(continued on next page)

B. Lower motor neurons (LMNs)
   1. Structure and function
      a. LMNs originate in the anterior horn cell in the ventral spinal cord at each segmental level; LMNs exit from the spinal cord to form the spinal nerves and branches of the peripheral nervous system
      b. LMNs transmit efferent (motor) messages to muscles and transmit afferent (sensory) messages back to the spinal cord
         1) Sensory/motor loop of the LMN constitutes a reflex arc
         2) All portions of the LMN must be functional for a reflex to occur
      c. LMN lesions: Occur when the reflex arc is destroyed and communication with UMNs is lost
         1) Poliomyelitis (damage to anterior horn cell)
         2) Peripheral nerve damage
         3) Spinal cord injury at the level of injury where the reflex arc is interrupted
   2. Results of LMN lesions: Reflex arc is absent and innervation of muscles is lost, possibly resulting in several conditions
      a. Flaccid paralysis
      b. Hypoactive or absent reflexes below the level of injury
      c. Severe muscle atrophy
      d. Significant problems with bladder, bowel, and sexual functioning if the LMN lesion is at the sacral segments of the cord

V. Neurophysiological Approaches to Care

A. Relationship between upper motor neuron damage, tone, and movement
   1. UMN damage disinhibits primitive brainstem reflexes, typically resulting in upper extremity flex-

Table 5.3. *(continued)*

Proprioceptive Neuromuscular Facilitation (PNF) Approach (Knott & Voss, 1968; Pope-Davis, 1990; Voss, 1967)
Particularly useful for persons with neurological and orthopedic problems—for example, amputation, low back pain, and arthritis

Major Goals and Premises

1. The response of the neuromuscular mechanism is promoted or hastened through stimulation of the proprioceptors. The principal focus of this approach is diagonal patterns of movement.
2. A primary goal is to develop balance between the agonist and antagonist muscles so the reverse of the movement pattern can be performed; for example, one learns the motor movements for dressing and then for undressing.
3. Auditory, visual, and tactile input are incorporated therapeutically to help obtain the desired motor response.
4. Trunk control is a goal so that the individual can achieve balance when sitting and standing.

Major Principles of Treatment

1. The patients' abilities, rather than their disabilities, are the focus of this approach.
2. Treatment is directed toward the head, neck, and trunk rather than toward control and function of extremities.
3. Early reflexes are important for progressive motor development and its influence on tone in the arms and legs.
4. The patient must learn to do an activity and undo, or reverse, the movements or activity.
5. An infant progressively learns movement patterns such as rolling, crawling, creeping, standing, and walking. Infants learn to use their hands with their body in various postures. When extremities move, there is a close interaction between the head, the neck and trunk, and the arms and legs.
6. When imbalance (improper flexion or extension) occurs, the opposite or antagonistic pattern should be facilitated.
7. Normal motor development sequencing and postures are taken into consideration as a patient attempts a functional activity.
8. During functional movement and activity, a balance between antagonist muscles must be established.
9. Sensory input can aid in the patient's motor learning.
10. Repetition and practice help the patient successfully learn motor skills.
11. The therapist touches the patient to correct an error or to promote a desired response.

Potential Application to Nursing
Incorporation of this approach can occur during range-of-motion activity or respiratory care, as well as when placing personal items in the patient's environment.

Rood's Sensorimotor Approach (Farber, 1982; McCormack, 1990)
Can be used to provide sensory experience to persons who have muscle tone problems or who are unresponsive or unconscious

Major Goals and Premises

1. Normalization of muscle tone, including both heavy and light muscle work groups, is a major goal. Heavy work muscles are reactivated first, except for the light muscles involved in eating and speaking.
2. Treatment starts at the developmental level of functioning. Treatment begins at the head and moves downward sequentially to the sacrum.
3. Repetition is a necessary component for training muscular responses.

Major Principles of Treatment

1. Therapeutic movement is directed toward purposeful goals—i.e., all therapy activities are designed to be meaningful so that the patient develops subcortical programs to perform motor acts.
2. Sensory input and/or stimulation is used frequently to elicit major reaction.
3. Sensory stimulation is used to activate both stabilizing and mobilizing muscles.
4. Eight sequences of motor development are used to achieve purposeful responses.
5. Cutaneous facilitation techniques, such as icing and brushing, which stimulate the exteroceptors of the skin, are used.
   a. Light moving touch is used to stimulate the light work muscles.
   b. Fast brushing (with a battery-operated device) is used carefully by experienced professionals. It stimulates the C fibers, which travel slowly because they are thin and unmyelinated.
6. Heavy joint compression, quick stretch, intrinsic stretch, and secondary ending stretch are techniques used to activate and/or facilitate the proprioceptors.
7. Stretch pressure, heavy resistance, vestibular stimulation, inversion, vibration, and osteopressure are commonly used facilitatory techniques in this approach.
8. Olfactory and gustatory stimulation is used to facilitate the cranial nerves and the autonomic nervous system.

Potential Application to Nursing
Can be used therapeutically to manipulate the environment (decor, lighting, sounds, aromas), to enhance arousal with sensory stimulation, and as preswallowing stimulation techniques.

Sources Consulted

Bobath, B. (1978). *Adult hemiplegia: Evaluation and treatment.* London: William Heinemann Medical Books, Ltd.
Bobath, B. (1990). *Adult hemiplegia: Evaluation and treatment* (3rd ed.). Oxford, England: Butterworth-Heinemann.
Farber, S. (1982). *Neurorehabilitation: A multisensory approach.* Philadelphia: W.B. Saunders Company.
Knott, M., & Voss, D.E. (1968). *Proprioceptive neuromuscular facilitation: Patterns and techniques* (2nd ed.). New York: Harper & Row Publishers, Inc.
McCormack, G.L. (1990). The Rood approach to the treatment of neuromuscular dysfunction. In L.W. Pedretti & B. Zoltan (Eds.), *Occupational therapy: Practice skills for physical dysfunction* (3rd ed.) (pp. 311-333). St. Louis: The C.V. Mosby Company.
Pedretti, L.W. (1990). Movement therapy: The Brunnstrom approach to treatment of hemiplegia. In L.W. Pedretti & B. Zoltan (Eds.), *Occupational therapy: Practice skills for physical dysfunction* (3rd ed.) (pp. 334-350). St. Louis: The C.V. Mosby Company.
Pope-Davis, S.A. (1990). The proprioceptive neuromuscular facilitation approach. In L.W. Pedretti & B. Zoltan (Eds.), *Occupational therapy: Practice skills for physical dysfunction* (3rd ed.) (pp. 363-379). St. Louis: The C.V. Mosby Company.
Voss, D.E. (1967). Proprioceptive neuromuscular facilitation. *American Journal of Physical Medicine, 46*(1), 838-898.

ion and adduction and lower extremity extension

2. UMN lesions can occur congenitally (as in cerebral palsy) or after acute neurological injury (e.g., stroke or traumatic brain injury)
3. After acute cerebral insult, hemiplegia frequently occurs in the opposite side of the body
   a. Initially, hemiplegic side is flaccid
   b. Within hours to days, tone returns and is often exaggerated; this increase in tone is known as *hypertonicity* or *spasticity*
4. Any state of discomfort or alteration in homeostasis can create an undesirable increase in muscle tone
5. Gee and Passarella (1985) and Davis (1990) emphasized that an increase in muscle tone has various causes
   a. Fear
   b. Pain
   c. Fatigue

B. Appropriate rehabilitation nursing goals
   1. Preventing increased tone from causing contractures
   2. Understanding what triggers, relaxes, counteracts, and prevents tone during patient care

C. Using appropriate treatment approaches to abnormal tone (e.g., hemiplegia)
   1. Compensatory approach
      a. Traditional method of treatment
      b. Emphasize treatment of unaffected side exclusively
      c. Focuses on preventing further medical complications
   2. Neurophysiological (neurodevelopmental) approach
      a. Current physiologically based approaches include treatment of both affected and unaffected sides of body
      b. Many rehabilitation teams use a specific neurophysiological approach to treating movement problems resulting from cortical and subcortical damage
      c. Four most commonly used approaches (see Table 5.3)
         1) Bobath's Neurodevelopmental Treatment (NDT) Approach
         2) Brunnstrom's Movement Therapy Approach
         3) Proprioceptive Neuromuscular Facilitation (PNF) Approach
         4) Rood's Sensorimotor Approach

References

Bobath, B. (1978). *Adult hemiplegia: Evaluation and treatment.* London: William Heinemann Medical Books, Ltd.

Bobath, B. (1990). *Adult hemiplegia: Evaluation and treatment* (3rd ed.). Oxford, England: Butterworth-Heinemann.

Brunner, L., & Suddarth, D. (1988). *Textbook of medical-surgical nursing* (6th ed.). Philadelphia: J.B. Lippincott Company.

Davis, J.Z. (1990). Neurodevelopmental treatment: The Bobath approach to the treatment of adult hemiplegia. In L.W. Pedretti & B. Zoltan (Eds.), *Occupational therapy: Practice skills for physical dysfunction* (3rd ed.) (pp. 351-362). St. Louis: The C.V. Mosby Company.

Farber, S. (1982). *Neurorehabilitation: A multisensory approach.* Philadelphia: W.B. Saunders Company.

Gee, Z.L., & Passarella, P.M. (1985). *Nursing care of the stroke patient: A therapeutic approach.* Pittsburgh: American Rehabilitation Educational Network Publications

Hanak, M. (1992). *Rehabilitation for the neurological patient.* New York: Springer Publishing Company.

Hickey, J. (1986). *The clinical practice of neurological and neurosurgical nursing* (2nd ed.). Philadelphia: J.B. Lippincott Company.

Hickey, J. (1992). *The clinical practice of neurological and neurosurgical nursing* (3rd ed.). Philadelphia: J.B. Lippincott Company.

Knott, M., & Voss, D.E. (1968). *Proprioceptive neuromuscular facilitation: Patterns and techniques* (2nd ed.). New York: Harper & Row Publishers, Inc.

Marshall, S.B., Marshall, L.F., Vos, H.R., & Chesnut, R.M. (1990). *Neuroscience critical care: Pathophysiology and patient management.* Philadelphia: W.B. Saunders Company.

McCormack, G.L. (1990). The Rood approach to the treatment of neuromuscular dysfunction. In L.W. Pedretti & B. Zoltan (Eds.), *Occupational therapy: Practice skills for physical dysfunction* (3rd ed.) (pp. 311-333). St. Louis: The C.V. Mosby Company.

Pedretti, L.W. (1990). Movement therapy: The Brunnstrom approach to treatment of hemiplegia. In L.W. Pedretti & B. Zoltan (Eds.), *Occupational therapy: Practice skills for physical dysfunction* (3rd ed.) (pp. 334-350). St. Louis: The C.V. Mosby Company.

Pedretti, L.W., & Zoltan, B. (Eds.). (1990). *Occupational therapy: Practice skills for physical dysfunction* (3rd ed.). St. Louis: The C.V. Mosby Company.

Pope-Davis, S.A. (1990). The proprioceptive neuromuscular facilitation approach. In L.W. Pedretti & B. Zoltan (Eds.), *Occupational therapy: Practice skills for physical dysfunction* (3rd ed.) (pp. 363-379). St. Louis: The C.V. Mosby Company.

Trombly, C.A., & Scott, A.D. (1989). Evaluation of motor control. In C.A. Trombly (Ed.), *Occupational therapy for physical dysfunction* (3rd ed.) (p. 64-65). Baltimore: Williams & Wilkins.

Voss, D.E. (1967). Proprioceptive neuromuscular facilitation. *American Journal of Physical Medicine, 46*(1), 838-898.

Zejdlik, C.P. (1991). *Management of spinal cord injury* (2nd ed.). Boston: Jones and Bartlett Publishers.

Suggested Readings

Borgman, M.F., & Passarella, P.M. (1991). Nursing care of the stroke patient using Bobath principles: An approach to altered movement. *Nursing Clinics of North America, 26,* 1019-1035.

Bouman, H.D. (1967). Exploratory and analytical survey of therapeutic exercise: Delineating the dilemma. *American Journal of Physical Medicine, 46*(1), 26-31.

Brunnstrom, S. (1970). *Movement therapy in hemiplegia.* New York: Harper & Row Publishers, Inc.

Carr, J.H., & Shepard, R.B. (1987). *A motor relearning programme for stroke* (2nd ed.). Rockville, MD: Aspen Publishers, Inc.

Hirt, S. (1967). Exploratory and analytical survey of therapeutic exercise. Historical bases for therapeutic exercise. *American Journal of Physical Medicine, 46*(1), 32-38.

Heininger, M., & Randolph, S. (1981). *Neurophysiological concepts in human behavior.* St. Louis: The C.V. Mosby Company.

Sullivan, P., Markos, P., & Minor, M.A. (1982). *An integrated approach to therapeutic exercise: Theory and clinical application.* Norwalk: Appleton & Lange.

Trombly, C.A., & Scott, A.D. (1975). *Occupational therapy for physical dysfunction.* Baltimore: Williams & Wilkins.

Voss, D.E., Ionta, M.K., & Myers, B.J. (1985). *Proprioceptive neuromuscular facilitation* (3rd ed.). Philadelphia: Harper & Row Publishers, Inc.

CHAPTER 6

Stroke

Many individuals survive strokes. They and their significant others must cope with numerous sensorimotor, visual, perceptual, and language deficits. Rehabilitation cannot eliminate the deficits; however, it can drastically influence the person's return to independence, especially in the management of self-care, activities of daily living, safety, and socialization. Rehabilitation also plays a major role in helping to prevent secondary complications. To intervene effectively as a member of the rehabilitation team, the nurse should understand the physiological, perceptual, and psychological changes that occur after stroke.

I. Stroke

A. Definition: A general term for acute brain damage caused by disease of blood vessels (Caplan, 1988); onset is rapid and produces focal injury (Gundersen, 1990)

1. When a stroke occurs, blood flow to that part of the brain is disrupted, resulting in tissue anoxia and death of brain cells (infarction)
2. The stroke process is dynamic and can have a variety of results
   a. Persistent biochemical changes in and around the damaged cell
   b. Autolysis with accumulation of lactic acid and phosphokinase
   c. Edema: Anoxia increases blood flow to the damaged area, which can increase intracranial pressure and injure fragile cells surrounding the lesion; if edema is severe, it can cause herniation and death (Bronstein, Popovich, & Stewart-Amidei, 1991; Dolan, 1991; Gundersen, 1990; Hickey, 1992; Mumma, 1987)

B. Epidemiology (Bronstein et al., 1991; Kelly-Hayes, 1991; Millikan, McDowell, & Easton, 1987)

1. Third most common cause of death in Western countries
2. Rise in mortality rate and incidence as age increases, but incidence has declined in recent years in the United States; mortality rate is higher for hemorrhagic stroke
3. More common occurrence in elderly people, males, and blacks
4. Prevalence in the United States ranges from 150 to 200 per 100,000 population

C. Etiology

1. Ischemic or hemorrhagic disruption of cerebral arteries is the major cause of stroke
   a. Normal arterial blood supply to brain involves the internal carotid artery (which ultimately becomes the middle cerebral artery) and the vertebral artery
   b. These major arteries (internal carotid, middle cerebral, and vertebral) form anterior and posterior circulatory systems that compose the circle of Willis
2. Systemic hypoperfusion (see p. 36) or a cerebral compression (for example, a tumor) less frequently produce stroke syndromes
3. Potential risk factors (many preventable)
   a. Hypertension
   b. Obesity
   c. Smoking
   d. Elevated cholesterol
   e. Heavy ingestion of alcohol
   f. Diabetes
   g. Blood disorders (e.g., sickle-cell anemia, polycythemia)
   h. Cardiac disorders
   i. Family history of stroke
   j. Older age
   k. Gender (most prevalent in males; however, females on oral contraceptives who smoke and have migraines are at higher risk [Gundersen, 1990])
   l. Race (more common in blacks)
   m. Substance abuse (heroin, cocaine, talwin, and amphetamines) (Bronstein et al., 1991; Hickey, 1992; Licata-Gehr, 1991)

D. Pathophysiology

1. Ischemic stroke (about 80% of all strokes)
   a. Process
      1) Focal area of the brain receives little or no blood flow due to occlusion of a blood vessel
      2) Focal area of the brain and adjoining brain tissue are deprived of oxygen and glucose
      3) When the deprivation is severe enough to impair gray matter function and lasts long enough, permanent damage occurs
   b. Classification of ischemic stroke
      1) Transient ischemic attack (TIA)
         a) Characteristics
            (1) Short, reversible ischemic event
            (2) Signs and symptoms that occur rapidly and last less than 24 hours
         b) Possible precursor to major stroke, myocardial infarction, or death
      2) Reversible ischemic neurological deficit (RIND): A TIA process that takes a few

days to resolve and is reversible
3) Systemic hypoperfusion: Condition in which the small distal cerebral arteries do not receive enough blood flow due to cardiac pump failure or hypovolemia related to blood loss (Caplan, 1988); also referred to as *ischemic-anoxic encephalopathy*
4) Cerebral thrombus (Bronstein et al., 1991; Caplan, 1988; Dolan, 1991; Gundersen, 1990; Licata-Gehr, 1991)
   a) Most common cause of stroke
   b) Is a stationary clot in a large blood vessel, usually caused by atherosclerotic plaque
      (1) Plaque
         (a) Plaque forms when calcium and lipids collect and attach to the vessel wall, especially in bifurcations of a large artery (see Figure 6.1)
         (b) Plaque formations produce narrowing and, thus, impede or obstruct blood flow
      (2) Atherosclerosis
         (a) Can produce degeneration of blood vessel walls
         (b) A weakened wall or plaque itself can tear, thus triggering the normal clotting process; such congestion further reduces circulation
5) Cerebral embolism
   a) Traveling clot that typically originates from thrombi in the heart, from plaque in the aortic arch or carotid or vertebral arteries; clot becomes lodged and obstructs cerebral blood flow
   b) Commonly associated with history of cardiac disease, especially atrial fibrillation in the elderly
6) Lacunar infarct (Caplan, 1988; Hickey, 1992)
   a) Thrombotic occlusion in penetrating (small) cerebral arteries
   b) Lesions are small, oval-shaped, pitting, and deep within brain
   c) Frequently develop in the pons or thalamic pathways
   d) Often result in pure motor or sensory deficits
   e) Commonly associated with history of diabetes and hypertension

Figure 6.1 Common Sites of Atherosclerotic Involvement of the Extra- and Intracranial Cerebral Arteries

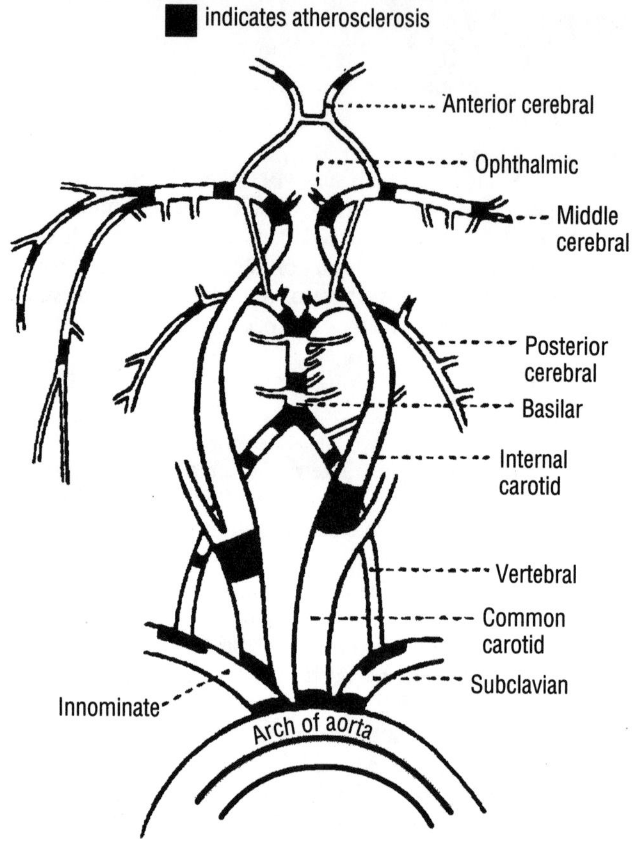

Reprinted with permission of Charles C. Thomas, Publisher, from Meyer, J.S. (1961). Changes in cerebral blood flow resulting from vascular occlusion. In W.S. Fields (Ed.), *Pathogenesis and treatment of cerebrovascular disease* (p. 96). Springfield, IL: Charles C. Thomas, Publisher.

2. Hemorrhagic stroke (about 20% of strokes) (Caplan, 1988; Dolan, 1991; Gundersen, 1990; Hickey, 1992; Loen, 1991)
   a. Process
      1) Spontaneous rupture of a cerebral vessel occurs; blood enters brain tissue or subarachnoid space
      2) "Because arteriosclerotic arteries lose most of their elasticity, they rupture easily. The hemorrhage occurs in areas where degenerative changes in the vessel walls permit rupture of small vessels" (Loen, 1991, p. 240)
      3) Wall degeneration, especially in small cerebral vessels, is thought to stem from chronic hypertension
   b. Classifications (subarachnoid hemorrhage and intracerebral hemorrhage are the most common types)
      1) Subarachnoid hemorrhage
         a) Blood from a ruptured vessel enters the subarachnoid space
         b) Usually related to saccular or congenital aneurysm rupture, most of which are in the carotid artery circulation; has several potential results
            (1) Increased intracranial pressure
            (2) Vasospasms
            (3) Ischemia, which further reduces cerebral blood flow
         c) Less commonly related to arteriovenous

Table 6.1. Clinical Features of Aphasia

Type	Involved Anatomy	Expression	Auditory Comprehension	Written Comprehension	Naming	Word/Phrase Repetition	Ability to Write
Broca's (motor, expressive)	Precentral gyrus, Broca's area	Nonfluent, telegraphic, may be mute	Subtle deficits	Subtle deficits	Impaired	Impaired	Impaired
Wernicke's (receptive, sensory)	Superior temporal gyrus	Fluent but content inappropriate	Impaired	Impaired	Severely impaired	Impaired	Impaired
Global (mixed)	Frontal-temporal area	Nonfluent	Severely impaired	Impaired	Severely impaired	Impaired	Severely impaired
Conductive (central)	Arcuate fasciculus	Fluent	Intact	Intact	Impaired	Severely impaired	Impaired
Anomic (amnesic)	Angular gyrus	Fluent	Intact	Intact	Severely impaired	Intact	Subtle deficits
Transcortical sensory (TCSA)	Periphery of Broca's and Wernicke's areas (watershed zone)	Fluent	Impaired	Impaired	Impaired	Intact	Severely impaired
Transcortical motor (TCMA)	Anterior, superior, or lateral to Broca's area	Nonfluent, speech initiation difficult	Intact	Subtle deficits	Impaired	Intact	Impaired

Reprinted with permission of Mosby-Year Book, Inc., from Bronstein, K.S., Popovich, J., & Stewart-Amidei, C. (1991). *Promoting stroke recovery: A research-based approach for nurses* (p. 202). St. Louis: Mosby-Year Book, Inc.

malformation, anticoagulants, drugs, and trauma

2) Intracerebral (intraparenchymal) hemorrhage
   a) Involves small deep-penetrating blood vessels that rupture, releasing blood directly into the brain tissue
   b) Usually invades deep white matter first
   c) The released blood puts pressure on tissue and surrounding small arterioles and capillaries, which, too, can tear
   d) Resulting hematoma acts as a space-occupying lesion and, if large enough, can cause brain shifting and/or herniation

E. Residual deficits of stroke

1. Significant alterations in many psychosocial areas
   a. Diminished affect
   b. Increased dependence in activities of daily living
   c. Decreased self-esteem
   d. Altered role performance
   e. Sexual dysfunction
   f. Change in leisure and/or social activity
   g. Decreased financial earning or vocational capability
2. General sequelae (all of which can influence safety)
   a. Weakness or paralysis contralateral to the lesion (hemiplegia)
   b. Abnormal tone, including flaccidity at first and then hypertonicity in the affected side
   c. Sensorimotor problems, ataxia, imbalance
   d. Language deficits if lesion is in the dominant hemisphere
   e. Visuospatial perception impairments
   f. Cognitive deficits
   g. Memory changes
   h. Inability to control emotions, especially crying and laughter (emotional lability)
   i. Fatigue
   j. Depression: There is controversy about whether this has an organic or an emotional basis
   k. Seizure activity
3. *Left-hemispheric stroke*: Common impairments and deficits
   a. Right hemiparesis or hemiplegia
   b. Impaired ability to think analytically
   c. Inability to do mathematical computations or interpret symbols
   d. Right homonymous hemianopsia

Figure 6.2. Lesions in Various Types of Aphasia

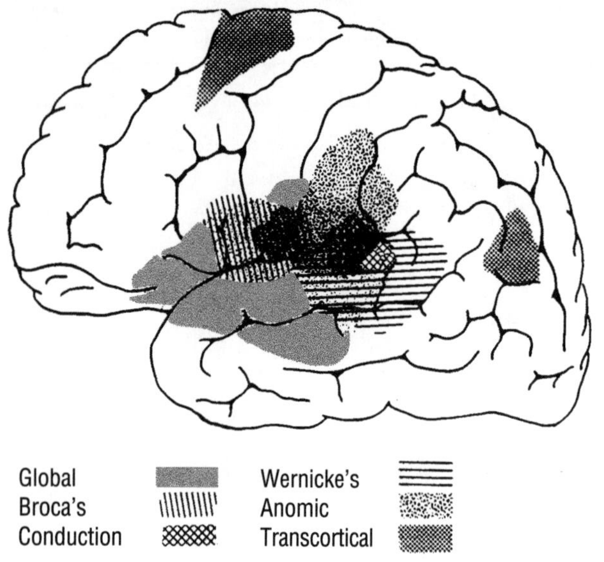

Reprinted with permission of J.V. Basmajian and Williams & Wilkins from Brandstater, M.E., & Basmajian, J.V. (Eds.). (1987). *Stroke rehabilitation.* Baltimore: Williams & Wilkins.

e. Behavioral changes, including cautiousness and hesitancy

f. *Language problems*: Language is not only speech, but also involves conveying and comprehending thoughts and ideas as well as understanding and using symbols sequentially and grammatically (Boss, 1991) (see Table 6.1)

1) Nonfluent aphasia (Broca's, or expressive, aphasia)
   a) Location of damage: Occurs with lesions in the posterior part of the dominant frontal lobe (precentral gyrus) (see Figure 6.2)
   b) Characteristic symptoms
      (1) Speech is slow, effortful to produce, and punctuated by long pauses between words; there also may be other problems with language skills
         (a) Finding words and naming objects (anomia)
         (b) Repeating words or phrases upon command (conductive aphasia)
         (c) Sentence construction
         (d) Improper use of small words (e.g., *or, and, but, if, to, from*) and/or verb endings
         (e) Unintentional repetition of a word or phrase due to impaired motor processing (perseveration)
      (2) The ability to read letters, numbers, or written material may be impaired
      (3) Writing skills—that is, translating one's thoughts into symbols—may be impaired (this is not to be confused with the physical act of writing, or penmanship)
      (4) Language comprehension may be altered (Bronstein et al., 1991; Damasio, 1992)
      (5) Automatic speech may be intact—that is, the person may be able to express a word, phrase, profanity, or song unexpectedly and clearly
2) Fluent aphasia (Wernicke's or receptive aphasia)
   a) Location of damage: Occurs with damage in the posterior, superior temporal dominant lobe (superior temporal gyrus) (see Figure 6.2)
   b) Characteristic symptoms
      (1) Involves problems with comprehension of words and sounds
      (2) The person is able to speak fluently, but speech may not be correct or appropriate in terms of the context of the conversation; mispronunciation of words and anomia also can evolve because the person cannot comprehend what he or she has said and cannot detect his or her own errors
      (3) Reading problems are also common
3) Global aphasia
   a) Location of damage: Frontal-temporal dominant lobes (see Figure 6.2)
   b) Characteristic symptoms
      (1) Both comprehension and speaking problems occur
      (2) Comprehension of written language also impaired
      (3) One or a few words may be said repeatedly in an effort to communicate a thought
      (4) Automatic speech for routines (e.g., counting, stating days of the week, or singing the lyric of a song) may be intact
4) Apraxia of speech
   a) Location of damage: Motor centers in the cortex that control speech
   b) Characteristic symptoms
      (1) Purposeful speech is hard to produce because the muscles in the mouth and throat, although they are not paralyzed, do not respond the way the person intends them to
      (2) Speech may be clear one moment and undecipherable the next
      (3) Perseveration and inconsistency are common
5) Dysarthria
   a) Location of damage: Brainstem and/or cranial nerves
   b) Characteristic symptoms

(1) Articulation problem
(2) Abnormal muscle control of the palate, tongue, labia, and/or pharynx
(3) Speech is slow, commonly slurred, hard to understand, and may be too soft or loud
(4) Voice quality also may be abnormal

6) Anarthria: Total loss of articulation capability due to absent muscle control; location of damage is brainstem

4. *Right hemispheric stroke*: Common impairments and deficits
   a. Left hemiplegia or hemiparesis
   b. Problems with depth perception and spatial relationships
   c. Visual disturbances (including left homonymous hemianopsia)
   d. Inability to distinguish directional concepts such as up/down, front/back, in/out
   e. Difficulty distinguishing foreground from background information (figure-ground spatial-temporal perception)
   f. Decreased ability to distinguish between similar shapes and forms (form-constancy spatial-temporal perception)
   g. Denial of the extent of paralysis and physical disability (anosognosia) and reduced insight into ramifications of impairments
   h. Inability to localize and/or recognize one's own body parts and how they relate to other parts (somatognosia)
   i. Lack of awareness of others' nonverbal communications—for example, facial expressions, tone of voice, territorial space, and gestures (pragmatic skills); display of a flat affect
   j. Inability to integrate sensory and perceptual stimuli from one side of the body or environment (unilateral neglect)
   k. Behavioral changes, including impulsiveness, egocentricity, quickness to try things
   l. Social inappropriateness: Sexual disinhibition and inappropriate self-disclosure
   m. Difficulty in finding locations, such as one's room, and understanding maps and objects (geographic-topographic memory)

5. *Brainstem strokes*
   a. Result from ischemic or hemorrhagic process in the midbrain, pons, or medulla
   b. There are many vital centers and nuclei of cranial nerves; thus, deficits can vary greatly
   c. Potential deficits
      1) Dysarthria
      2) Chewing and/or swallowing problems (dysphagia)
      3) Ataxia, difficulty walking, staggered gait; quadriparesis or quadriplegia
      4) Poor balance and/or coordination
      5) Double and/or blurred vision; pinpoint pupils; horizontal gaze palsy (eye moves to side away from cerebral lesion)
      6) Vertigo (with nausea)
      7) Abnormal respiratory patterns
      8) Hyperthermia
      9) Coma or persistent vegetative state (see Chapter 8)
      10) Locked-in syndrome
         a) Characteristics
            (1) Quadriplegia and facial paralysis except for eye and/or eyelid movement
            (2) Intact cognition
         b) Occurs when stroke is in the pons

F. Nursing diagnoses frequently associated with stroke (see Section III for detailed information about nursing diagnoses)

1. Impaired physical mobility
2. Self-care deficits (specify level)
3. Sensory-perceptual alteration
4. Impaired verbal communication
5. Altered urinary elimination
6. High risk for aspiration and/or impaired swallowing
7. Potential for injury (trauma)
8. Impaired home maintenance management
9. Unilateral neglect
10. Impaired thought processes
11. Disturbance in body image
12. Altered sexuality pattern
13. Caretaker stress syndrome
14. Spiritual distress

References

Boss, B.J. (1991). Managing communication disorders in stroke. *Nursing Clinics of North America, 26*, 985-996.

Brandstater, M.E., & Basmajian, J.V. (Eds.). (1987). *Stroke rehabilitation.* Baltimore: Williams & Wilkins.

Bronstein, K.S., Popovich, J., & Stewart-Amidei, C. (1991). *Promoting stroke recovery: A research-based approach for nurses.* St. Louis: Mosby-Year Book, Inc.

Caplan, L.R. (1988). Stroke. *Clinical Symposia, 40*(4), 1-32.

Damasio, R. (1992). Medical progress: Aphasia. *The New England Journal of Medicine, 326*(8), 531-539.

Dolan, J.T. (1991). *Critical care nursing: Clinical management through the nursing process.* Philadelphia: F.A. Davis Company.

Gundersen, C.H. (1990). *Essentials of clinical neurology.* New York: Raven Press.

Hickey, J.V. (1992). *The clinical practice of neurological and neurosurgical nursing* (3rd ed.). Philadelphia: J.B. Lippincott Company.

Kelly-Hayes, M. (1991). A preventive approach to stroke. *Nursing Clinics of North America, 26*, 931-942.

Licata-Gehr, E.E. (1991). Etiology of stroke subtypes. *Nursing Clinics of North America, 26*, 943-956.

Loen, M. (1991). Impairment in verbal communication. In M. Snyder (Ed.), *A guide to neurological and neurosurgical nursing* (2nd ed.) (pp. 235-256). Albany, NY: Delmar Publishers, Inc.

Meyer, J.S. (1961). Changes in cerebral blood flow resulting from vascular occlusion. In W.S. Fields (Ed.), *Pathogenesis and treatment of cerebrovascular disease* (pp. 80-105). Springfield, IL: Charles C. Thomas, Publisher.

Millikan, C.H., McDowell, F., & Easton, J.D. (1987). *Stroke.* Philadelphia: Lea & Febiger.

Mumma, C.M. (Ed.). (1987). *Rehabilitation nursing: Concepts and practice—A core curriculum* (2nd ed.). Evanston, IL: Rehabilitation Nursing Foundation.

Suggested Readings

Baggerly, J. (1991). Sensory perceptual problems following stroke: The "invisible" deficits. *Nursing Clinics of North America, 26*, 997-1005.

Doolittle, N.D. (1988). Stroke recovery: Review of the literature and suggestions for future research. *Journal of Neuroscience Nursing, 20*(3), 169-173.

◆Doolittle, N.D. (1992). The experience of recovery following lacunar stroke. *Rehabilitation Nursing, 17*, 116-120.

Goldberg, G. (Ed.). (1991). Physical medicine and rehabilitation. *Clinics of North America, 2*(3).

Gorelick, P.B. (1986). Cerebrovascular disease: Pathophysiology and diagnosis. *Nursing Clinics of North America, 21*, 275-287.

◆Greshem, G.E. (Ed.). (1990). Methodologic issues in stroke outcome research. *Stroke: A Journal of Cerebral Circulation, 21*, Supp. II(9), 1-73.

Hanak, M. (1992). *Rehabilitation nursing for the neurological patient.* New York: Springer Publishing Company.

Kane-Carlsen, P.A. (1990). Transient ischemic attacks: Clinical features, pathophysiology and management. *Nurse Practitioner, 15*(7), 9-14.

Wertz, R.T. (1990). Communication deficits in stroke survivors: An overview of classification and treatment. *Stroke: A Journal of Cerebral Circulation, 21*, Supp. II(9), 16-18.

◆ indicates a research-based work

CHAPTER 7

Musculoskeletal/Orthopedic Disorders

As reflected in the results of the Rehabilitation Nurses Job Analysis conducted in 1991 by Dungan and McCourt, almost 20% of the disorders noted in rehabilitation populations are musculoskeletal. These data are supported by U.S. governmental statistics, which identify musculoskeletal diseases as the number one cause of disability (Hicks, 1988). The incidence of musculoskeletal disorders is expected to increase as changing demographics in North America reflect a growing number of people living until an advanced age. This chapter addresses three specific disorders: osteoporosis, arthritis, and amputations. An obvious overlap exists between orthopedics and rehabilitation. But, as Dunn (1980) wrote, "Although all rehabilitation is not necessarily concerned with orthopedics, it may be said that all orthopedics is concerned with rehabilitation" (p. 444).

I. Osteoporosis

"Osteoporosis is a condition that is more effectively prevented than treated....It is often sad that osteoporosis is a condition presenting to the geriatrician, but with its roots in pediatrics" (Lindsay, 1990, p. 174). It is expected that the incidence of this debilitating disease will climb as the life expectancy increases and the baby boom generation reaches old age during the next 20 years.

Individuals with disability are at greater risk for developing osteoporosis. This is due to a lack of local stresses on bone resulting from disuse and impaired mobility.

A. Definition

1. Osteoporosis ("porous bone"): Disease process in which there is a reduction of bone density (thus making bone more susceptible to fracture)
2. First clinical indicator of osteoporosis usually is a fracture (Evans, 1990)

B. Epidemiology

1. Incidence
    a. More than 20 million Americans have osteoporosis, resulting in direct and indirect costs estimated at $7 to $10 billion annually (National Association of Orthopedic Nurses, 1990)
    b. Incidence is greater for women than men by a 5:1 ratio; men do not begin to reach the same incidence until after age 70
2. Types of osteoporosis (Melton, 1988)
    a. Type I (postmenopausal) osteoporosis
        1) Occurs in women between the ages of 55 and 70; is related to decreased estrogen
        2) Common fractures: Colles' fracture of the wrist and vertebral fractures
    b. Type II (senile) osteoporosis
        1) Related to the aging process and a chronic lack of calcium; occurs in men and women older than 70
        2) Common fractures: Hip and vertebral fractures
    c. Disuse osteoporosis (Chestnut, 1988): Individuals with disability are at greater risk because immobility or disuse increases bone loss due to decreased muscle action and weight-bearing stress
        1) Paraplegics experience a 33% bone loss 6 months following onset of their condition (Minaire et al., 1982)
        2) Polio patients experience bone loss primarily in weight-bearing bones (Shambaugh & Marciniak, 1990)
        3) Hemiplegic patients experience reduced bone density on the involved side

C. Etiology

1. Exact cause is unknown (Evans, 1990)
2. Identified contributing risk factors
    a. Genetic risk factors
        1) Female gender
        2) Asian or Caucasian (especially Northern European) ancestry
        3) Family history of hip fracture or kyphosis
        4) Mother who had osteoporosis
        5) Red or blond hair
        6) Fair skin
        7) Scoliosis
        8) Rheumatoid arthritis
    b. Nutritional risk factors
        1) Lifelong low calcium diet
        2) High sodium and protein diet
        3) Strict vegetarian diet (Heaney, 1987)
        4) Poor gastrointestinal absorption
    c. Lifestyle risk factors
        1) Low level of activity
        2) Use of tobacco
        3) Regular alcohol intake
        4) High caffeine intake
    d. Endocrine risk factors (Hickox, 1991)
        1) Nulliparity

2) Early menopause
3) Exercise-induced amenorrhea
4) Abnormally low weight or leanness
5) Hyperthyroidism

e. Pharmacological risk factors
1) Antacids containing aluminum: Cause calcium loss in stool
2) Seizure medications, such as phenytoin, phenobarbital, and primidone: Interfere with metabolism of vitamin D and decrease calcium absorption
3) Tetracycline and isoniazid: Cause increased calcium loss in urine
4) Furosemide (Lasix®): Increases calcium loss in urine
5) Vitamin A: In excess of 5,000 international units/day, increases calcium loss in urine
6) Corticosteroids such as Decadron® and prednisone: Long-term use results in severe osteoporosis

D. Pathophysiology: Exact pathophysiology is not fully understood; bone remodeling, decreasing bone density, and bone loss are involved

1. Bone remodeling
a. A normal process in which old bone breaks down (resorption) and is replaced with new bone (formation)
b. Normally occurs so that there is no change in bone density; in osteoporosis, bone resorption is increased without a corresponding increase in bone formation
c. Helps the body maintain an adequate calcium level for biologic functions such as heartbeat and muscle contraction
d. Prevents body from using calcium stored in bones

2. Bone density
a. Bone acts as a storehouse for calcium, which makes bone hard; when calcium blood levels drop, calcium is taken out of bones
b. Bone density, or mass, is determined by genetic, mechanical, nutritional, and hormonal factors
c. In both men and women, peak bone density is reached between the ages of 30 and 35; peak bone density is important in predicting occurrence of osteoporosis (Sardana, 1992)

3. Bone loss
a. Rapid bone loss and menopause
1) In women, there is a postmenopausal bone loss over a 2-year period, reducing total skeletal mass by 20% to 30% (Heaney, 1987)
2) Bone density decreases rapidly as estrogen levels decrease
3) In obese women, bone loss is lessened, perhaps due to increased weight and stress on the skeleton and the presence of adipose tissue as a source of estrogen (Stevenson et al., 1990)

b. Slow bone loss and aging: By age 65, both men and women develop impairment of calcium absorption potential (Heaney, 1987); loss of bone mass then proceeds at a similar rate for both sexes

Figure 7.1. Progression of Complications from Osteoporosis

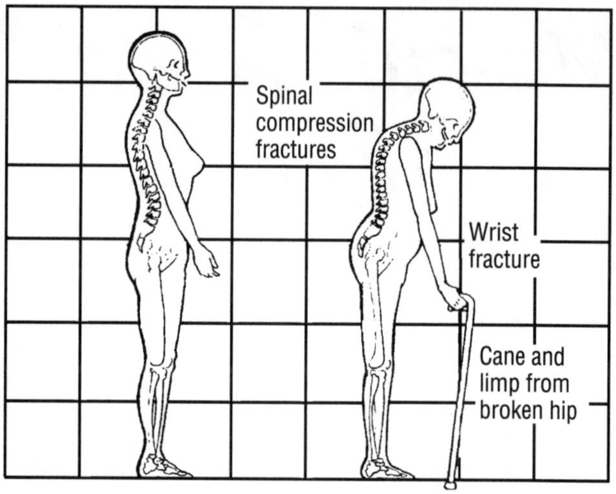

Reprinted with permission of Macmillan Publishing Company from Fardon, D.F. (1985). *Osteoporosis: Your head start on the prevention and treatment of brittle bones* (p. 13). New York: Macmillan Publishing Company. Illustrations copyright © 1985 Mitzi Dishman.

E. Residual deficit

1. Progression of complications from osteoporosis (see Figure 7.1)
2. Hip fractures
a. Osteoporotic hip fractures are associated with more deaths from complications than any other osteoporotic fracture (Liscum, 1992)
b. Due to the increasing prevalence of osteoporosis, the incidence of hip fracture may be increasing by 40% each decade (Lindsay, 1987)
c. An estimated 30% to 50% of patients with hip fractures never regain their prefracture functional level
d. Surgical repair (open reduction and internal fixation) provides hip stabilization and promotes early ambulation
e. Effective pain management is essential to ensure optimum participation in the rehabilitation process (Nelson, Taylor, Adams, & Parker, 1990)
3. Osteoporosis of the spine
a. Twenty-five percent of women over age 60 have spinal compression fractures from osteoporosis; up to 40% have some fractures after age 65
b. Spinal fracture occurs when one of the vertebrae, often cervical or lumbar, loses height and is compressed (see Figure 7.2)
c. Collapsed vertebrae may lead to deformity of the back, loss of height, and chronic back pain
d. Nonsurgical treatment (Salmond, Mooney, & Verdisco, 1991): Includes rigid cervical collar,

Figure 7.2. Normal Spine and Spine with Compression Fracture

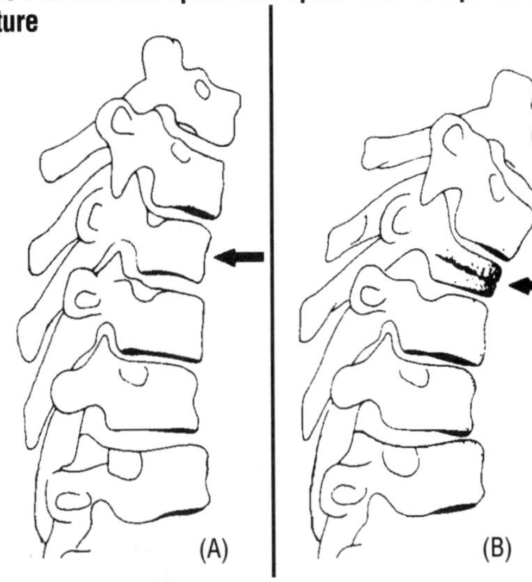

(A) = normal spine
(B) = spine with compression fracture (note shortening of vertebra and abnormal curve of spine)

Reprinted with permission of John Wiley & Sons, Inc., from McIlwain, H.H., Bruce, D.F., Silverfield, J.C., & Burnette, M.C. (1988). *Osteoporosis: Prevention, management, treatment* (p. 2). New York: John Wiley & Sons, Inc. Copyright © 1988 John Wiley & Sons, Inc.

thoracolumbarsacral orthosis (TLSO), or halo apparatus

e. Surgical treatment: Spinal fusion

F. Management measures: Prevention is more effective than current treatment; the following management measures are recommended

1. Administration of calcium
   a. Recommended intake: Recommended dietary allowance (RDA) published by the National Research Council (1989)
      1) 800 mg/day for children 1 to 10 years of age
      2) 1,200 mg/day for those 11 to 24 years of age
      3) 800 mg/day for those 25 years of age and older
      4) 1,200 mg/day for pregnant or lactating women
   b. Recommendation of the National Institutes of Health Consensus Conference on Osteoporosis in 1984 (U.S. Department of Health and Human Services, 1991)
      1) 1,000 mg/day for premenopausal women and older women taking estrogen
      2) 1,500 mg/day for postmenopausal women not taking estrogen
   c. Sources of calcium
      1) Dietary sources such as milk, yogurt, fish, and leafy dark green vegetables
      2) Calcium supplement tablets
   d. Consideration: Calcium should be used with caution in those at risk for immobilization hypercalcemia, renal function impairment, and kidney stones (Shambaugh & Marciniak, 1990)
2. Ingestion of vitamin D
   a. Can be done simply by exposing body to sunlight (vitamin D production is body's natural response to sunlight)
   b. Needed for optimal absorption of calcium in the intestines
3. Weight-bearing exercises
   a. Promote remodeling and increase bone density
   b. Include walking, swimming, and aerobics
4. Estrogen replacement therapy
   a. Estrogen decreases calcium loss from the bone but does not restore bone loss to the premenopausal level (Weinerman & Bockman, 1990)
   b. "Epidemiologic evidence indicates that estrogen can reduce the incidence of hip fractures, while adequate calcium and regular exercise appear to reduce the minimum effective dose of oral estrogen" (U.S. Department of Health and Human Services, 1991, p. 467)
5. Newer experimental treatments (Hay, 1991): Research studies are investigating medications that could rebuild bone mass once osteoporosis occurs
   a. Calcitonin to decrease bone resorption
   b. Sodium fluoride to increase bone formation
   c. Thiazide diuretics to decrease urinary excretion of calcium
   d. Anabolic steroids to increase bone formation

II. Arthritis

Although there are more than 100 separate identified diseases classified under the heading of arthritis, the outline that follows focuses on two major forms: osteoarthritis and rheumatoid arthritis. The Arthritis Health Professionals Association (1988) provided several significant statistics: After heart disease, arthritis is the second leading cause of limitation of movement. It is the leading cause of absenteeism in the workplace and the second leading reason for disability payments (after mental illness). Its annual cost in lost wages and medical bills exceeds $8.6 billion. As Conn (1990) wrote, "Arthritis and rheumatic disorders constitute an important health problem...one that rehabilitative efforts can positively affect" (p. 182). Not surprisingly, patients with arthritis are a growing population both in rehabilitation facilities and in the community. Treatment plans need to be individualized, practical, economical, and valued by the patient to promote compliance.

A. Definitions and major forms of arthritis

1. Definitions
   a. Articular: Pertaining to a joint
   b. Cartilage: Nonvascular, supporting connective tissue found in joints
   c. Joint: Connection between two bones that normally move freely, allowing for gliding and rotation
   d. Synovium: Transparent, viscous fluid secreted by synovial membrane, which lubricates joints
2. Major forms of arthritis
   a. Juvenile rheumatoid arthritis (JRA) (Cassidy &

Petty, 1990): A systemic disease affecting children under 16 years of age; manifested by three disease types
   1) Systemic, or Still's disease: Joint and systemic involvement similar to rheumatoid arthritis
   2) Polyarthritic: Arthritis in five or more joints
   3) Pauciarticular: Arthritis in four or fewer joints
   b. Osteoarthritis (OA): A noninflammatory, slowly progressive degenerative disease primarily affecting weight-bearing joints—for example, hips, knees, and spine; joint involvement is asymmetrical; also called *degenerative joint disease* (DJD)
   c. Rheumatoid arthritis (RA): A chronic inflammatory systemic condition that affects small joints (e.g., wrists); joint involvement is symmetrical and is accompanied by symptoms such as fatigue, weight loss, and other systemic manifestations

B. Epidemiology (Arthritis Health Professionals Association, 1988)
1. Arthritis in general
   a. Affects 37 million Americans, or 1 out of 7 individuals
   b. Affects 1 out of 3 families
   c. Affects 50% of all persons over age 65
   d. Women are twice as likely to experience the condition as men
2. Specific types of arthritis
   a. Osteoarthritis
      1) Most common form of arthritis
      2) Males below the age of 45 are affected more than women; women over the age of 45 are affected more often and tend to have more severe disease than males
      3) Incidence is higher in Caucasians
      4) Increased prevalence with older age, at which time it affects women and men equally
   b. Rheumatoid arthritis (Lisse, 1988)
      1) Affects 1.5% of Americans
      2) Affects more women than men by a ratio of 3:1
      3) Incidence higher in Caucasians
   c. Juvenile rheumatoid arthritis
      1) Most common arthritis found in children
      2) Prevalence rate of 0.16 to 1.1 per 1,000 persons
         a) Systemic type affects boys and girls equally
         b) Polyarthritis and pauciarticular arthritis predominantly affect girls

C. Etiology (Mankin & Brandt, 1985)
1. Osteoarthritis
   a. Unclear etiology
   b. Contributing risk factors
      1) Age
         a) Strongest risk factor, but not alone responsible for causing osteoarthritis
         b) Changes related to aging in cells and tissues may induce development of the disease
      2) Trauma
         a) Responsible for fragments in the joint secondary to fractures that were poorly reduced
         b) Recurrent dislocation of patella
         c) Congenital dislocation of hip
      3) Obesity: Increases load on joints with changes in posture and gait
      4) Preexisting joint abnormalities
         a) Rheumatoid arthritis
         b) Legg-Calvé-Perthes disease
         c) Congenital hip dislocation
         d) Avascular necrosis
2. Rheumatoid arthritis (RA)
   a. Unclear etiology
   b. Possible causes under investigation
      1) Infectious agents: Can initiate an inflammatory response; in a susceptible person, inflammation leads to continual disease activity
      2) Autoimmunity: Abnormal condition in which the body produces antibodies that attack its own joints and tissues
      3) Genetics: Familial trend; women with family history are two to three times more likely to have RA

D. Pathophysiology (Salmond et al., 1991)
1. Osteoarthritis: Hallmark is cartilage destruction (see Figure 7.3)
   a. Cartilage surface becomes disrupted and detaches from the joint
   b. Fragments of cartilage set up a low-grade, chronic inflammation within the joint or synovial lining
   c. As cartilage continues to degenerate, underlying bone produces osteophytes, or bone spurs, which cause pain and affect joint mobility as they increase in size
   d. With advanced disease, all cartilage may be destroyed
2. Rheumatoid arthritis: Synovium is the primary site of inflammation (synovitis)
   a. Synovitis causes increased synovial exudate, which leads to increased thickening of synovial fluid
   b. The inflammatory process causes increased blood flow or vascular permeability to the joint, resulting in classic symptoms of RA—joint swelling and warmth
   c. Congestion of synovial fluid accumulates with rest, resulting in the classic symptom of stiffness, which is relieved by activity
   d. As the inflammatory condition of the joints persists, the synovium thickens and proliferates inside and outside the joint; also called *pannus formation*
   e. Ligaments and tendons become inflamed, causing shortening, stiffening, and scarring

Figure 7.3. Cartilage Destruction in Osteoarthritis

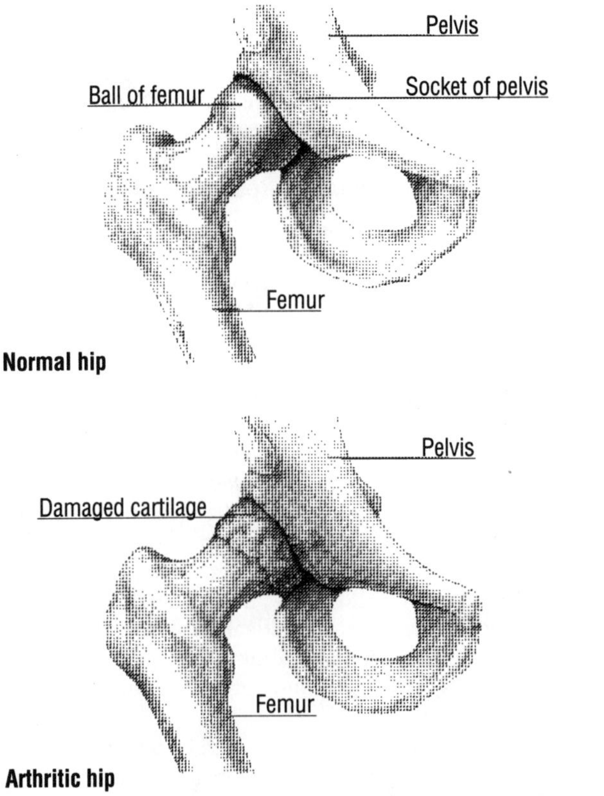

Reprinted with permission of the American Academy of Orthopaedic Surgeons from American Academy of Orthopaedic Surgeons. (1988). *Arthritis* [Public information brochure] (p.3). Park Ridge, IL: Author. (Available from American Academy of Orthopaedic Surgeons, 6300 N. River Road, Rosemont, IL 60018)

E. Residual deficits

1. Osteoarthritis: Articular deficits
   a. Joint contracture
   b. Loss of joint function
   c. Decreased range of motion
   d. Pain following activity and improving with rest
2. Rheumatoid arthritis
   a. Articular deficits
      1) Joint destruction
      2) Joint inflammation and effusion
      3) Decreased range of motion
      4) Pain and stiffness at rest
      5) Joint contractures, subluxation, and ankylosis
   b. Systemic deficits
      1) General: Fatigue, anorexia, weight loss
      2) Neurologic: Spinal cord compression, footdrop
      3) Ocular: Uveitis
      4) Cardiovascular: Cardiomyopathy, vasculitis, pericarditis
      5) Hematologic: Lymph gland enlargement
      6) Integumentary: Rheumatic nodules
      7) Pulmonary: Pleural effusion, pleuritis
      8) Mental: Depression, anxiety

F. Management measures

1. Osteoarthritis (Hicks & Gerber, 1988)
   a. Rest and supportive care
      1) Rest for affected joints to relieve pain and provide stability
      2) Application of heat or cold modalities (e.g., hot packs, heating pads, and paraffin baths) to relieve discomfort
      3) Use of girdle or corset to relieve back strain or soreness
      4) Wearing of sturdy, well-fitting shoes to help maintain posture and ambulation
      5) Use of a cane or a walker to lessen pressure and strain on joints
   b. Nutritional management: Weight reduction and management of optimal weight to decrease strain on joint
   c. Drug therapy
      1) Aspirin
      2) Nonsteroidal antiinflammatory drugs (NSAIDs)
      3) Steroids: Local intra-articular injections for severely involved joints
   d. Surgery: Total joint replacement performed to relieve pain, restore motion, and increase joint stability
      1) Total knee replacement (TKR)
         a) Involves replacement of either the medial or lateral compartment of the femorotibial joint
         b) Continuous passive motion (CPM) machine is used during rehabilitation to promote optimal joint extension and passive muscle motion to lessen stiffness and aid venous return
      2) Total hip replacement (THR)
         a) Involves replacement of both the femoral head and acetabulum
         b) Prevent dislocation through proper positioning: Hip abduction, neutral rotation, and slight external rotation
         c) Patient should not flex hip more than 60°, cross legs, or sit in a low chair
         d) Symptoms for dislocation include acute groin pain, shortened extremity in external rotation, "popping" sensation heard or felt by physician
      3) Laminectomy and spinal fusion (Chore, 1991)
         a) Laminectomy: The removal of bony arches or laminae and osteophytes of vertebrae; relieves compression of the spinal cord secondary to spinal stenosis and arthritic-related changes
         b) Spinal fusion, preferably using bone from the patient's iliac crest, increases spinal stability
2. Rheumatoid arthritis
   a. Self-care activities
      1) "Self-care is the mainstay for treatment for

preventing disability and dysfunction" (Kane & Kane, 1986, p. 251)
2) Assistive devices and adaptive aids—for example, gait aids, transfer aids, kitchen devices, clothing, and optimal environmental design—are required

b. Rest and supportive care
1) Local rest: Use of splints for inflamed joints
2) Systemic rest: 1-hour naps one to two times per day plus 8 to 10 hours of sleep at night
3) Moist heat alternating with cold applications
4) Resting splints and orthotics: Used to relieve weight on joints, stabilize joints, decrease joint motion, and preserve joint in a position of maximal function

c. Energy conservation
1) Conserving energy reduces fatigue and maximizes function
2) Techniques include the use of assistive and adaptive aids, rest, and supportive care

d. Joint protection: Includes modifying tasks to decrease stress on the joint

e. Exercise
1) Important because patients with arthritis lose muscle mass and strength due to disuse
2) Benefits of an individualized exercise program
a) Increases and maintains range of motion
b) Increases endurance
c) Strengthens muscles
d) Improves function
e) Increases bone density
f) Increases sense of well-being

f. Pharmacological therapy: Often requires the combined use of a variety of drugs
1) Antiinflammatory
a) Aspirin: Foundation of management for symptoms of inflammation, pain, and fever
b) Nonsteroidal antiinflammatory drugs (NSAIDs): Decrease vascular permeability and edema
2) Remission-inducing and immunosuppressive
a) Gold salts and D-penicillamine: Suppress immune response by inhibiting release of enzymes into the joint
b) Antimalarial medications: Suppress synovitis
c) Corticosteroids: Should be used cautiously and preferably only for the short term
d) Cytoxic medications: Used only in advanced stages of rheumatoid arthritis

g. Surgery
1) Total joint replacements
2) Laminectomy and spinal fusion
3) Arthrodesis, or fusion, of the bone of the joint

h. Psychological care
1) Impact of rheumatoid arthritis on mobility, self-care, self-concept, work, and leisure is tremendous
2) Reaction can include denial, anger, and depression
3) Premorbid personality can be a determinant of the patient's reaction to the disease
4) Unpredictability of disease's course complicates the coping process
5) Psychological counseling for patient and family is often indicated

i. Sexual adjustment: Arthritis can impose limitations or alterations that influence a person's sexual life as it does other activities of daily living (see Chapter 19)

III. Amputations

In the United States, one out of every 300 individuals has had a major amputation, and the incidence of new cases is 30,000 each year (Dernham, 1986). Patients with amputations account for a significant part of the population in most rehabilitation centers. Loss of a body part is permanent, leaving the patient with alterations in mobility and body image, as well as self-care deficits. Rehabilitation nursing interventions are critical for successful adaptation and reintegration into the community.

A. **Definition:** Types of amputations (Leonard & Meier, 1988)
1. Congenital (congenital skeletal deficiency): Absence of part or all of an extremity at birth
2. Acquired: Loss of part or all of an extremity as a direct result of disease, trauma, or surgery; higher incidence than congenital

B. **Epidemiology**
1. Age
a. Rate of amputation increases with age
b. Peak incidence occurs between 41 and 70 years of age; 75% of all amputations occur in people aged 65 or older
2. Sex: Incidence of amputation is higher in males
3. Race: African Americans with diabetes have an amputation rate 2.3 times greater than Caucasians with diabetes (Fylling & Knighton, 1989)

C. **Etiology**
1. Disease-related: Lower extremity
a. 75% of lower extremity amputations are disease-related
b. 80% of patients with amputations have peripheral vascular disease (PVD) and 75% of this group also has diabetes (Burgess, 1983); commonly the diabetic with one amputation eventually requires a contralateral amputation (Fylling & Knighton, 1989)
c. Other related diseases
1) Osteomyelitis
2) Acute embolic disease
3) Venous thrombosis
2. Trauma-related: Upper extremity
a. Seventy-five percent of upper extremity amputations are trauma-related
b. Result from motor vehicle accidents, gunshot wounds, falls, frostbite, explosions, war in-

Figure 7.4. Levels of Amputation of Extremities

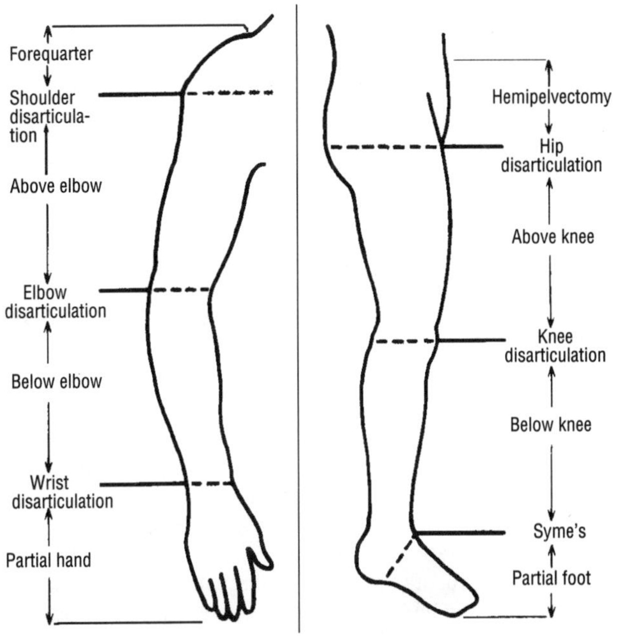

Reprinted with permission of Columbia University Press from Garrett, J.F., & Levin, E. (Eds.). (1973). *Rehabilitation practices for the physically disabled* (p. 401). New York: Columbia University Press. Copyright © 1973 Columbia University Press, New York.

Figure 7.5. Correct and Incorrect Positioning for the Below- and Above-Knee Amputee

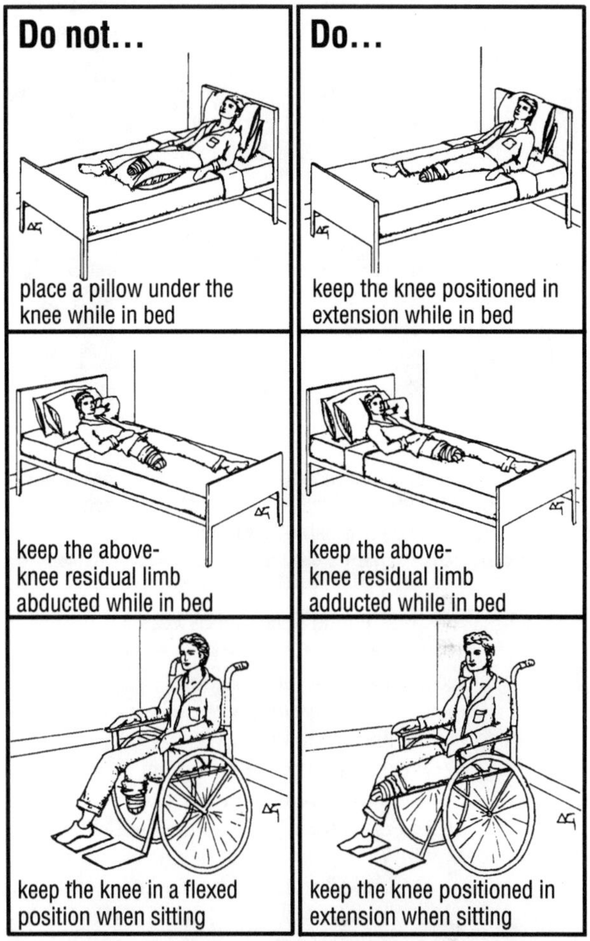

Reprinted with permission of F.A. Davis Company from Sanders, G.T. (1986). *Lower limb amputation: A guide to rehabilitation* (p. 370). Philadelphia: F.A. Davis Company.

juries, and burns (electrical, thermal, and chemical)
- c. Occur most commonly in males 17 to 55 years of age
- d. Account for 30% of amputations

3. Tumor-related: 5% of amputations due to sarcomas, most commonly in children ages 10 to 20

D. Amputation surgery

1. Disease- and trauma-related
   - a. Surgery is performed to reduce tissue damage due to trauma or progression of disease, often only after extensive efforts made to preserve limb; surgical procedure is either open (guillotine) or closed (flap)
     - 1) Open procedure
       - a) Performed when infection is present or likely to develop
       - b) End of stump is open with no skin covering it; flaps can be sutured later when healing is more likely
     - 2) Closed procedure: Distal end of bone is covered with a full thickness of skin
   - b. With trauma, body parts can be severed unexpectedly and accidentally (as in farm accidents); severe tissue injury from flame or electrical burns can necessitate amputation
   - c. Replantation referral is considered in the following cases (O'Hara & Lineaweaver, 1990)
     - 1) Amputations of thumbs or multiple digits
     - 2) Amputations in children
     - 3) Clean amputations at the palm, wrist, or forearm
     - 4) Complex injuries that might benefit from acute microsurgical reconstruction, such as revascularization and free-flap coverage
     - 5) Highest success rates are with upper extremity and digit replantation
   - d. Tumor-related (Piasecki, 1991)
     - 1) Amputation surgery is an alternative treatment done less frequently due to advances in limb-salvage surgical procedures
     - 2) Indicated when tumor margins are not microscopically clean
2. Levels of amputation (see Figure 7.4)
   - a. Amputation should be performed at the lowest level possible; poor healing may require revision to a higher level
   - b. Upper extremity amputation: Hands and arms are highly specialized in function; their loss cre-

Figure 7.6. Bandaging a Residual Limb

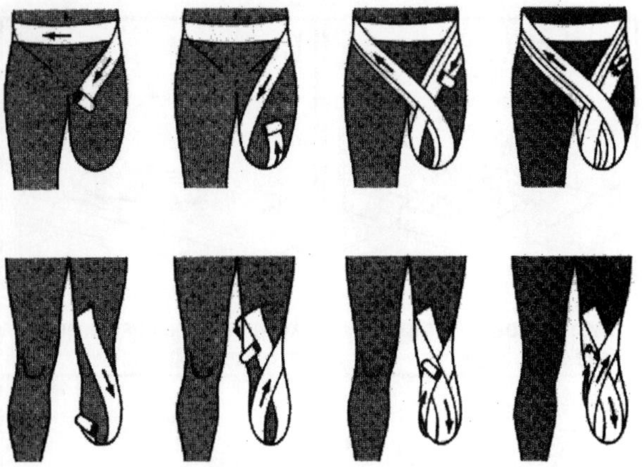

Reprinted with permission of Mosby-Year Book, Inc., from Beare, P.G., & Myers, J.L. (1990). *Principles and practice of adult health nursing* (p. 1398). St Louis: Mosby-Year Book, Inc.

ates immediate dependency coupled with a deforming change in body image

c. Lower extremity amputations
    1) Lower extremities are used for weight bearing and locomotion
    2) Preservation of the knee joint is preferred for optimal mobility and function
    3) Energy expenditure is an issue (Meier, 1985)
        a) Use of unilateral below-knee prosthesis requires about 25% to 45% more energy than normal
        b) Use of an above-knee prosthesis requires 65% to 100% more energy than normal
        c) Energy requirements are compounded for the bilateral amputee

E. Residual deficits
1. Pain
    a. Phantom sensation and pain are explained to patient as normal phenomenon related to severing of nerves at amputation site
    b. Types (Bowser, 1991)
        1) Phantom sensation
            a) Awareness of nonpainful sensation in amputated limb
            b) Feeling that limb is still present
            c) Duration is approximately 6 months
        2) Phantom pain
            a) Awareness of pain in amputated, or phantom, limb
            b) Can be triggered by touch, concurrent illness, fatigue, or emotional stress
            c) Experienced more frequently when pain is present in an extremity prior to amputation (e.g., in peripheral vascular disease, and also following severe electrical burns with extensive neurovascular damage)
        3) Neuroma: Sensitive benign tumor composed of severed nerve fibers entangled in the healing scar
2. Contractures
    a. Devastating, yet preventable barrier to optimal rehabilitation: Goal is extension of elbow or knee and hip joint and hip adduction (see Figure 7.5)
    b. Hip and knee flexion contracture can be prevented if patient lies prone for 30 minutes, as tolerated, every 3 to 4 hours
3. Psychological discomfort related to amputation
    a. Receives inadequate attention
    b. Along with physical discomfort, is cited as major reason for nonuse of prosthesis (Medhat, Huber, & Medhat, 1990)
    c. Signs of actual disturbance
        1) Refusal to look at or touch residual limb
        2) Unwillingness to discuss predicted limitations or use of prosthesis
        3) Refusal to participate in self-care
        4) Social withdrawal
    d. True test of successful rehabilitation is manner in which amputee incorporates natural body parts, with or without prosthesis, into his or her lifestyle; support groups can be helpful in this (Yetzer, Winfree, & Scaglione, 1989)

F. Amputation management: Residual limb and prosthetic care
1. Residual limb care
    a. Wound healing at the amputation site is critical
    b. Frequent inspection for skin irritation and breakdown of residual limb and of opposite extremity, especially foot, is critical
    c. Daily hygiene routines, such as washing and drying residual limb, are preferably done in the evening to help ensure that residual limb has adequate time to dry before contact with prosthesis
    d. Stroking massage keeps skin loose and mobile and prevents scar tissue from adhering to underlying bone
    e. Desensitizing residual limb by massaging and tapping improves patient's tolerance to pressure of prosthesis; also promotes sensory feedback so that tactile stimulus is not interpreted as noxious
    f. Modalities used to reduce edema and shape residual limb for eventual prosthetic fitting
        1) Figure 8 elastic bandage wrap
            a) Wrapped with greater compression applied distally and less proximally
            b) Frequent rewrapping (every 4 hours or as needed) to prevent slipping and bunching (see Figure 7.6)
        2) Stump shrinker: Heavy elastic sock
            a) Used for the patient who has difficulty keeping an elastic bandage in place
            b) Is replaced with a smaller one as shrinking occurs to maintain adequate compression

3) Removable rigid dressing: Dressing similar to a cast used to encase and protect residual limb and permit fitting of a temporary prosthesis so that ambulation can begin soon after surgery (Wu & Krick, 1987)

2. Prostheses
   a. Initially, prosthesis is worn only for 15- to 20-minute periods and is removed to check condition of the skin
   b. Prostheses can be functional and/or cosmetic
   c. Weight loss or gain of as little as 5 lbs can affect prosthetic fit and function
   d. Numerous prostheses may be needed for the long term due to specific requirements related to work, school, home, sport, and leisure activities
   e. Lower-extremity prostheses
      1) Prosthetics are less complex and more uniform from amputee to amputee
      2) Gait training begins on parallel bars and progresses to use of a walker, crutches, cane, or to unassisted ambulation
   f. Upper-extremity prostheses
      1) Prosthesis attempts to replace very complex appendage, especially when it is replacing the dominant hand or arm
      2) Prostheses are generally body powered (operated by cable) or externally powered (e.g., electric, as in the Utah elbow)

G. Pediatric considerations (Whaley & Wong, 1991)
   1. Child's developmental level and attention span must be considered when prosthetic training sessions are provided
   2. Prosthetic training can be incorporated into play activities
   3. Children who have lost a limb may develop a problem of bony overgrowth requiring surgical revision prior to skeletal maturity

H. Geriatric considerations
   1. Many patients with amputations are over age 65, and effects of aging process can affect amputation rehabilitation
   2. Osterman and Pinzur (1987) wrote, "When limb loss is accompanied by perceptual and balance deficits, visual and auditory losses, and cognitive disorders, all common problems in the older population, the challenge to become ambulatory is much greater" (p. 248)
   3. Due to longer life spans, the phenomenon of dual disability—such as the concurrence of lower extremity amputation and hemiplegia in the same patient—is increasingly being recognized as a significant and unique rehabilitation problem (O'Connell & Gnatz, 1989).

IV. Nursing Diagnoses Associated with Musculoskeletal/Orthopedic Disorders (see Section III for detailed information on nursing diagnoses)

A. Alteration in family process
B. Altered sexual patterns
C. Anxiety
D. Body image disturbance
E. Chronic pain
F. Colonic constipation
G. Distress of the human spirit
H. Disturbance in role performance
I. Disuse syndrome
J. Diversional activity deficit
K. Health management deficit
L. High risk for falls
M. High risk for injury
N. Impaired mobility
O. Ineffective family coping
P. Ineffective individual coping
Q. Knowledge deficit
R. Nutritional deficit
S. Self-care deficit
T. Self-esteem disturbance
U. Social isolation

References

American Academy of Orthopaedic Surgeons. (1988). *Arthritis* [Public information brochure]. Park Ridge, IL: Author. (Available from American Academy of Orthopaedic Surgeons, 6300 N. River Road, Rosemont, IL 60018)

Arthritis Health Professionals Association. (1988). *Teaching slide collection manual* (2nd ed.). Atlanta: Arthritis Foundation.

Beare, P.G., & Myers, J.L. (1990). *Principles and practice of adult health nursing*. St Louis: Mosby-Year Book, Inc.

Bowser, M.S. (1991). Giving up the ghost: A review of phantom limb phenomena. *Journal of Rehabilitation, 57*(3), 55-62.

Burgess, E.M. (1983). Amputations: Symposium on orthopædic surgery. *Surgical Clinics of North America, 63*(3), 749-770.

Cassidy, J., & Petty, R. (1990). *Textbook of pediatric rheumatology*. New York: Churchill Livingston.

Chase, J.A. (1991). Spinal stenosis. *Nursing Clinics of North America, 26*, 53-63.

Chestnut, C.H. (1988). Osteoporosis. In J.A. DeLisa (Ed.), *Rehabilitation medicine: Principles and practice* (pp. 865-875). Philadelphia: J.B. Lippincott Company.

Chore, J.A. (1991). Spinal stenosis. *Nursing Clinics of North America, 26*, 53-63.

Conn, V. (1990). Joint self-care by older adults. *Rehabilitation Nursing, 15*, 182-186.

Dernham, P. (1986). Phantom limb pain. *Geriatric Nursing, 7*(1), 34-37.

Dungan, L.A., & McCourt, A.E. (1991). *Report on the Rehabilitation Nurses Job Analysis 1989-1990.* Skokie, IL: Association of Rehabilitation Nurses and Rehabilitation Nursing Certification Board.

Dunn, B.H. (1980). Rehabilitation: Philosophy, concepts, and principles. In N. Hilt (Ed.), *Manual of orthopedics* (pp. 444-448). St. Louis: The C.V. Mosby Company.

Evans, J.G. (1990). The significance of osteoporosis. In R. Smith (Ed.), *Osteoporosis* (pp. 1-8). Oxford, England: LR Printing Services Limited.

Fardon, D.F. (1985). *Osteoporosis: Your head start on the prevention and treatment of brittle bones.* New York: Macmillan Publishing Company.

Fylling, C.P., & Knighton, D.R. (1989). Amputation in the diabetic population: Incidence, causes, cost, treatment, and prevention. *Journal of Enterostomal Therapy, 16*(6), 247-255.

Garrett, J.F., & Levin, E. (Eds.). (1973). *Rehabilitation practices for the physically disabled.* New York: Columbia University Press.

Hay, E.K. (1991). That old hip. *Nursing Clinics of North America, 26*, 43-52.

Heaney, R.P. (1987). Prevention of osteoporotic fracture in women. In L.V. Avioli (Ed.), *The osteoporotic syndrome: Detection, prevention, and treatment* (pp. 67-90). Orlando, FL: Grune & Stratton.

Hickox, P.G. (1991, June). Hormone replacement therapy guidelines. *Consultant*, pp. 35-44.

Hicks, J.E. (1988). Rehabilitation of musculoskeletal disorders in the geriatric population. In J.D. Frengley, P. Murray, & M.L. Wykle (Eds.), *Practicing rehabilitation with geriatric clients* (pp. 110-134). New York: Springer Publishing Company.

Hicks, J.E., & Gerber, L.H. (1988). Rehabilitation of the patient with arthritis and connective tissue disease. In J.A. DeLisa (Ed.), *Rehabilitation medicine: Principles and practice* (pp. 765-794). Philadelphia: J.B. Lippincott Company.

Kane, R.A., & Kane, R.L. (1986). Self-care and health care: Inseparable but equal for well-being of the old. In J.K. Dean, T. Hickey, & B. Holstein (Eds.), *Self-care and health in old age* (pp. 251-283). Dover, NH: Croom Helm.

Leonard, J.A., & Meier, R.H. (1988). Prosthetics. In J.A. DeLisa (Ed.), *Rehabilitation medicine: Principles and practice* (pp. 330-345). Philadelphia: J.B. Lippincott Company.

Lindsay, R. (1987). Prevention of osteoporosis. *Clinics of Orthopedics, 222*, 44-59.

Lindsay, R. (1990). Practical aspects of osteoporosis. In R. Smith (Ed.), *Osteoporosis* (pp. 173-180). Oxford, England: LR Printing Services Limited.

Liscum, B. (1992). Osteoporosis: The silent disease. *Orthopedic Nursing, 11*(4), 21-25.

Lisse, J.R. (1988). Rheumatic disorders in adults under fifty. *Postgraduate Medicine, 84*(5), 113-121.

Mankin, H.J., & Brandt, K.B. (1985). Pathogenesis of osteoarthritis. In W.N. Kelley, E.D. Harris, S. Ruddy, & C.B. Sledge (Eds.), *Textbook of rheumatology* (pp. 1469-1479). Philadelphia: W.B. Saunders Company.

McIlwain, H.H., Bruce, D.F., Silverfield, J.C., & Burnette, M.C. (1988). *Osteoporosis: Prevention, management, treatment.* New York: John Wiley & Sons, Inc.

Medhat, A., Huber, P.M., & Medhat, M.A. (1990). Factors that influence the level of activities in persons with lower extremity amputation. *Rehabilitation Nursing, 15*, 13-18.

Meier, R.H. (1985). Rehabilitation of the patient with amputation. In L.S. Halstead & M. Grabois (Eds.), *Medical rehabilitation* (pp. 133-145). New York: Raven Press.

Melton, L.J. (1988). Epidemiology of fractures. In B.L. Riggs & L.J. Melton (Eds.), *Osteoporosis: Etiology, diagnosis, and management* (pp. 133-154). New York: Raven Press.

Minaire, P., Meunier, P., Edouard, C., Messy, P., Depassio, J., Caulin, F., Pilonchery, G., & Berard, E. (1982). Acute osteoporosis in paraplegic patients: Pathophysiology and effects of treatment with calcitonin or dichlorodimethylene diphosphonate. In J. Menczel, G.C. Robin, M. Makin, & R. Steinberg (Eds.), *Osteoporosis* (pp. 421-432). New York: John Wiley & Sons.

National Association of Orthopedic Nurses. (1990). *The impact of orthopaedic conditions on the health and economy of the United States.* Pitman, NJ: Author.

National Research Council. (1989). *Recommended dietary allowances* (10th ed.). Washington, DC: National Academy Press.

Nelson, L., Taylor, F., Adams, M., & Parker, D.E. (1990). Improving pain management for hip fractured elderly. *Orthopedic Nursing, 9*(3), 79-83.

O'Connell, P.G., & Gnatz, S. (1989). Hemiplegia and amputation. *Archives of Physical Medicine and Rehabilitation, 70*, 451-454.

O'Hara, M., & Lineaweaver, W.C. (1990). Microsurgical replantation: Development and current status. *Critical Care Nursing Quarterly, 13*(1), 1-11.

Osterman, H.M., & Pinzur, M.S. (1987). Amputation: Last resort or new beginning? *Geriatric Nursing, 8*(5), 246-248.

Piasecki, P. (1991). Limb-salvage procedures for osteosarcoma. *Nursing Clinics of North America, 26*, 33-41.

Salmond, S.W., Mooney, N.E., & Verdisco, L.A. (Eds.). (1991). *Core curriculum for orthopedic nursing* (2nd ed.). Pitman, NJ: Anthony J. Jannetti.

Sanders, G.T. (1986). *Lower limb amputation: A guide to rehabilitation.* Philadelphia: F.A. Davis Company.

Sardana, R. (1992). Nutritional management of osteoporosis. *Geriatric Nursing, 13*, 315-319.

Shambaugh, G.E., & Marciniak, C. (1990). Osteoporosis. In D. Green (Ed.), *Medical management of long term disability* (pp. 101-124). Rockville, MD: Aspen Publishers, Inc.

Stevenson, J.C., Lees, B., Fielding, C., Cust, M.P., Ganger, K.F., & Hillard, T.C. (1990). Exercise and the skeleton. In R. Smith (Ed.), *Osteoporosis* (pp. 119-124). Oxford, England: LR Printing Services Limited.

U.S. Department of Health and Human Services. (1991). *Healthy people 2000: National health promotion and disease prevention objectives.* Washington, DC: U.S. Government Printing Office.

Weinerman, S.A., & Bockman, R.S. (1990). Medical therapy of osteoporosis. *Orthopedic Clinics of North America, 21*, 109-124.

Whaley, L.F., & Wong, D.L. (1991). *Nursing care of infants & children* (4th ed.). St. Louis: Mosby-Year Book, Inc.

Wu, Y., & Krick, H. (1987). Removable rigid dressing for below-knee amputees. *Clinical Prosthetics and Orthotics, 11*(1), 33-44.

Yetzer, E.A., Winfree, M., & Scaglione, C. (1989). An amputee support group. *Rehabilitation Nursing, 14*, 141-142.

Suggested Readings

Atkins, D.J., & Meier, R.H. (1989). *Comprehensive management of the upper-limb amputee.* New York: Springer-Verlag.

Bild, D.E., Selby, J.V., Sinnock, P., Browner, W.S., Braveman, P., & Showstack, J.A. (1989). Lower-extremity amputation in people with diabetes: Epidemiology and prevention. *Diabetes Care, 12*(1), 24-31.

◆Cook, B., Noteloviz, M., Rector, C., & Krischer, J.P. (1991). An osteoporosis patient education and screening program: Results and implications. *Patient Education and Counseling, 17*, 135-145.

◆Crouse, S.F., Lessard, C.S., Rhodes, J., & Lowe, R.C. (1990). Oxygen consumption and cardiac response of short-leg and long-leg prosthetic ambulation in a patient with bilateral above-knee amputation: Comparisons with able-bodied men. *Archives of Physical Medicine and Rehabilitation, 71*, 313-317.

Dacher, J.E. (1989). Rehabilitation and the geriatric patient. *Nursing Clinics of North America, 24*(1), 225-237.

◆Doucette, M.M., Fylling, C., & Knighton, D.R. (1989). Amputation prevention in a high-risk population through comprehensive wound-healing protocol. *Archives of Physical Medicine and Rehabilitation, 70*, 780-785.

Ehrlich, G.E. (Ed.). (1986). *Rehabilitation management of the rheumatic conditions.* Baltimore: Williams & Wilkins.

Garvey, R.S. (1989). Individuals with amputations find rehabilitation in competitive sports. *Journal of Rehabilitation, 55*(1), 19-20.

◆Hallal, J.C. (1991). Life satisfaction in women with postmenopausal osteoporosis of the spine. *Health Care for Women International, 12*(1), 99-110.

Hamerman, D. (1989). The biology of osteoarthritis. *The New England Journal of Medicine, 320*, 1322-1330.

Harris, H.D. (1990). Rheumatoid arthritis, pathophysiology and implications for therapy. *The New England Journal of Medicine, 322*(18), 1277-1289.

◆Huber, M.P., Medhat, A., & Carter, M.C. (1988). Prosthetic problem inventory scale. *Rehabilitation Nursing, 13*, 326-329.

Kirkpatrick, M.K., Edwards, M.K., & Finch, N. (1991). Assessment and prevention of osteoporosis through the use of a client self-reporting tool. *Nurse Practitioner, 16*(7), 16-26.

Leek, J.C., Gershwin, M.E., & Fowler, W.M. (Eds.). (1986). *Principles of physical medicine and rehabilitation in the musculoskeletal diseases.* Orlando, FL: Grune & Stratton.

Nazaroff, K.S., Stanton, J.H., Magana, K.R., & Kaufman, R.L. (1989). Halo-body jacket immobilization in rheumatoid arthritis patients with cervical myelopathy. *Nursing Clinics of North America, 24*, 209-223.

Odderson, I.R., & Czerniecki, J.M. (1990). Reflex sympathetic dystrophy in an amputee: Case study. *Archives of Physical Medicine and Rehabilitation, 71*, 161-163.

Olson, B., & Ustanko, L. (199). Self-care needs of patients in a halo brace. *Orthopedic Nursing, 9*(1), 27-33, 52.

◆Pollock, S.E., Christian, B.J., & Sands. D. (1990). Responses to chronic illness: Analysis of psychological and physiological adaptation. *Nursing Research, 39*, 300-304.

◆Schiaffino, K.M., Revenson, T.A., & Gibofsky, A. (1991). Assessing the impact of self-efficacy beliefs on adaptation to rheumatoid arthritis. *Arthritis Care and Research, 4*(4), 150-157.

Sheon, R.P., Moskowitz, R.W., Goldberg, V.M., & Heuter, B. (1987). *Coping with arthritis.* New York: McGraw-Hill.

◆Stone, L.R., Keenan, M.A., & Shin, D.Y. (1990). Acquired limb loss in patients with traumatic brain injury. *American Journal of Physical Medicine and Rehabilitation, 69*(3), 135-139.

Swogger, G. (1987). The emotional effects of the osteoporotic syndrome. In L.V. Avioli (Ed.), *The osteoporotic syndrome: Detection, prevention, and treatment* (pp. 143-148). Orlando, FL: Grune & Stratton.

◆ indicates a research-based work

CHAPTER 8

Traumatic Brain Injury

There are more than 2 million traumatic brain injuries (TBIs) per year in the United States; 500,000 of them are serious enough to require hospital admission (Interagency Head-Injury Task Force, 1989). TBI is characterized by primary impact and secondary insult. Outcome is dependent upon numerous factors including, but not limited to, severity, location of damage, extent of secondary insults, complications, premorbid health status and personality, age, learning ability, emergency care, access to and participation in rehabilitation, and social support systems.

Patient outcomes related to neurological, functional, cognitive, behavioral, and psychosocial deficits are evaluated on an ongoing basis. Rehabilitation after TBI is a multiphasic process that can span the remainder of the individual's life and pervade all of its aspects.

I. Traumatic Brain Injury

A. Definition and related terminology

1. Definition: Cerebral cell damage to neurons and axons resulting in irreversible injury (Miller, Pentland, & Berrol, 1990)
2. Related terminology
   a. *Closed head injury* (CHI): Nonpenetrating injury
   b. *Open head injury* (OHI): Penetrating injury resulting in brain tissue exposure and disruption of normal protective barriers
   c. *Coma*: State of unconsciousness in which there is no arousal or awareness and no response to stimulation; score is equal to or less than 8 on the Glasgow Coma Scale (see Figure 8.1)
   d. *Vegetative state*
      1) Individual can be aroused but awareness level cannot be determined (term originated by Jennett & Plum, 1972)
      2) Responses that are present (Berrol, 1990)
         a) Sleep-wake cycle
         b) Spontaneous eye opening
         c) Blood pressure, respirations, digestion
         d) Corneal, pupillary, occulocephalic reflexes
         e) Reflexive, but not localized, response to stimulation
      3) Berrol (1990) listed other terms used to describe this state
         a) *Prolonged coma*
         b) *Protracted awareness*
         c) *Low level*
   e. *Persistent vegetative state* (PVS): Refers to the vegetative state in its chronic form
      1) Medical classification that indicates prognosis, *not* diagnosis
      2) Responses are the same as those of someone in a vegetative state

B. Epidemiology: Difficult to collect data due to inconsistencies in identifying severity of injury and in treatment and hospitalization of persons with TBI; statistics available from the Interagency Head-Injury Task Force (1989) (and others as indicated)

1. Jennett (1990) reported that in the United States, there are about 400 persons severely disabled by brain injury per 100,000 population
2. Approximately 70,000 to 90,000 of those who survive TBI will have lifelong debilitating loss of function; another 2,000 will exist in a persistent vegetative state
3. Males are more likely to suffer serious head injury than are females
4. Young males 15 to 24 years of age have the highest rate of injury
5. TBI is the leading killer and cause of disability in children and young adults
6. Young people with head injuries commonly have a history of social deviancy, risk-taking behavior, and substance abuse before injury (Jennett, 1990)
7. According to the 1987 National Head Injury Foundation Task Force findings, 40% of all head-injured rehabilitation patients had moderate-to-severe problems with substance abuse prior to their head trauma (Spaaradeo, Strauss, & Barth, 1990)
8. In another study, 50% of head-injured persons had returned to preinjury levels of drinking 1 year after injury (Spaaradeo et al., 1990)

C. Etiology

1. Indirect or direct force applied to the head, causing brain to move within skull
2. Related causes
   a. Motor vehicle crashes: Cause 50% of all TBIs
   b. Falls: Responsible for 21%
   c. Assaults and violence: Account for 12%
   d. Sports and recreation: Account for 10%
   e. Child abuse: Responsible for 64% of infant head injuries

D. Pathophysiology

1. Difficult to distinguish all of the structural and neurochemical components associated with mechanisms of injury to brain during trauma
   a. In the literature, the terms used to describe in-

Figure 8.1. Glasgow Coma Scale

Eye opening (E)	
Spontaneous	4
To speech	3
To pain	2
Nil	1
Best motor response (M)	
Obeys	6
Localizes	5
Withdraws	4
Abnormal flexion	3
Extensor response	2
Nil	1
Verbal response (V)	
Oriented	5
Confused conversation	4
Inappropriate words	3
Incomprehensible sounds	2
Nil	1

Coma score (E + M + V) = 3 to 15

Reprinted with permission of the F.A. Davis Company from Jennett, B., & Teasdale, G. (1981). *Management of head injuries* (p. 78). Philadelphia: F.A. Davis Company.

jury vary among authors

b. Categorizations and definitions can be overlapping and confusing
c. It is widely acknowledged that the same basic mechanisms are operant for all ranges or severities of brain injury; that is, the person who presents with more severe symptoms has merely sustained more of the same type of damage than a person with less severe symptoms

2. The pathological events in TBI were summarized by Gilroy (1990): "The head and intracranial contents may be injured by forces of acceleration—the sudden linear movement of the skull; deceleration—the sudden reduction in velocity of linear movement; rotation—sudden rotary movements of the skull and contents; and lastly, missile penetration" (p. 329)
   a. Acceleration and deceleration occur when mechanical forces applied to the head or body cause movement within the skull
      1) Once movement ceases, the soft brain collides with the bony interior of the skull
      2) Intracranial mass lesions can develop (Miller et al., 1990)
      3) Frontal and temporal lobes typically are injured first, and the damage progresses inward, reaching the brainstem area (Pang, 1985)
   b. Concomitant rotation during impact causes shearing of the axons (white matter); this is known as *diffuse axonal injury* (DAI)
   c. TBI may result from a focal injury (see description in next column)
   d. Ultimately, TBI may be caused by acceleration, deceleration, or diffuse axonal injury in isolation or any combination of the three processes
3. Primary damage involves events that occur at the time of impact; these events can be extracranial or intracranial (Charness, 1986; Marshall, Marshall, Vos, & Chesnut, 1990; Miller et al., 1990; Salazar, 1992; Smith & Winkler, 1990)
   a. Extracranial damage involves mainly the scalp, skull, and dura mater
   b. Intracranial damage to cerebral tissue may be focal or diffuse
      1) Focal damage: Localized contusion (hemorrhage into the tissue) or laceration (Miller et al., 1990); produces localized deficits
         a) Vision problems
         b) Motor dysfunctions
         c) Speech impairments
      2) Diffuse damage: Widespread and scattered throughout the brain
         a) Because there is extensive shearing of white matter axons, or diffuse axonal injury, the neurological deficits vary considerably
         b) Important points to remember about DAI
            (1) Frequently related to acceleration and/or deceleration events; rotational acceleration of the skull produces shearing and strains within the intracranial contents (Ylvisaker, 1985)
            (2) Initial shearing also triggers secondary neurological changes in the axons at the cellular level; this, over time, can affect the extent of injury
            (3) Recent clinical findings suggest that an individual does not have to lose consciousness to experience DAI; conversely, if the reticular activating system in the brainstem is disturbed, it may cause enough damage to produce coma (Salazar, 1992; Teasdale & Mendelow, 1984)
4. Secondary insult of TBI: After initial impact, secondary results occur that interrupt the supply of oxygen and glucose, thus depriving the brain of energy
   a. Miller et al. (1990) grouped such secondary factors into systemic and intracranial insults (see Figure 8.2)
      1) *Systemic insult* pertains to bodily injuries from the trauma
      2) *Intracranial insult* refers specifically to changes occurring in the brain tissue and identifies secondary damage to the injured brain
         a) Brain distortion
         b) Brain shift
         c) Herniation
         d) Hypoxia and/or ischemia
   b. Conclusions found in Salazar (1992)
      1) There is delayed secondary injury in terms

Figure 8.2. Secondary Systemic and Intracranial Insults in the Injured Brain

Systemic
- Arterial hypoxemia
- Arterial hypotension
- Hypercapnia
- Anemia
- Pyrexia
- Hyponatremia
- Hypoglycemia

Intracranial
- Hematoma—extradural, subdural, intracerebral
- Raised pressure—brain swelling, brain edema, acute hydrocephalus
- Infection—meningitis, abscess/empyema
- Epilepsy
- Vasospasm

Reprinted with permission of F.A. Davis Company from Miller, J.D., Pentland, B., & Berrol, S. (1990). Early evaluation and management. In M. Rosenthal, E.R. Griffith, M.R. Bond, & J.D. Miller (Eds.), *Rehabilitation of the adult and child with traumatic brain injury* (2nd ed.) (p. 27). Philadelphia: F.A. Davis Company.

Table 8.1. Severity of Minor Concussional Head Injury and Assessment for Related Long-Term Dysfunction

Length of Posttraumatic Amnesia (PTA)	Severity	Expected Long-Term Dysfunction
PTA < 1 hour	Mild	Early return to work with no sequelae
PTA 1-24 hours	Moderate	Problems of headache, dizziness, incoordination, persisting abnormal neurological signs
PTA 1 day-1 week	Severe	Posttraumatic sequelae with some degree of permanent disability
PTA > 7 days	Very severe	Full return of neuropsychologic function would be the exception, not the rule

Adapted with permission of F.A. Davis Company from Miller, J.D., & Jones, P.A. (1990). Minor head injury. In M. Rosenthal, E.R. Griffith, M.R. Bond, & J.D. Miller (Eds.), *Rehabilitation of the adult and child with traumatic brain injury* (2nd ed.) (pp. 238-239). Philadelphia: F.A. Davis Company.

of changes occurring at the cellular level of the brain
   a) Metabolites
   b) Electrolytes
   c) Excitatory neurotransmitters
2) Brain loss after trauma may be from a cycle (ongoing cascade) of "biochemical events set in motion by the trauma" (p. 58)

5. Classification of TBI
   a. Mild TBI (referred to by many as *minor TBI* or *postconcussional syndrome*)
      1) Commonly results from contusive injuries and can occur without associated loss of consciousness (Gennarelli, 1986)
      2) Mild TBI accounts for approximately 80% of all TBIs (Anderson & McLaurin, 1980; Miller & Jones, 1985)
      3) Usually is manifested by at least one of several responses
         a) Loss of consciousness that lasts no longer than 20 minutes (a score of 13 to 15 on Glasgow Coma Scale) (see Figure 8.1)
         b) Loss of memory: Either retrograde (prior to trauma) or anterograde (after the trauma); commonly referred to as posttraumatic amnesia (PTA)
            (1) Characteristics of PTA: Loss of acute memory, disorientation, and disturbed learning
            (2) Return of continuous memory for day-to-day happenings signals that PTA is ending (Bond, 1990)
            (3) Duration of PTA has prognostic value for long-term disability (see Table 8.1)
         c) Alteration in mental status at the time of injury (even if the person remained conscious and did not have amnesia)
         d) Physical symptoms
            (1) Nausea
            (2) Headache
            (3) Dizziness
            (4) Tinnitus
            (5) Visual disturbance
            (6) Olfactory deficit
            (7) Extended periods of fatigue
         e) Cognitive deficits, which cannot be completely accounted for by emotional factors
            (1) Poor short-term memory and concentration
            (2) Irritability
            (3) Depression
   b. Moderate TBI: Represents a more extensive pattern of injury than mild TBI
      1) Loss of consciousness and a score of 9 to 12 on the Glasgow Coma Scale (see Figure 8.1)
      2) Usually requires treatment in a formal rehabilitation setting
      3) Individuals typically are able to return to an altered preinjury lifestyle despite the fact that long-term deficits (either pronounced or subtle) may persist
      4) Postconcussive symptoms can be extensive (see the five manifestations listed under "Mild TBI")

Figure 8.3. Sequelae of TBI

Neurological	Motor impairments: ataxia, spasticity, paralysis, paresis
	Neurological impairments: altered level of consciousness, seizure disorder, hydrocephalus (often requiring shunting), hyperphagia, hypothalamic fever, altered sleep-wake cycle, headache
Sensory/Perceptual	Diplopia, strabismus, ptosis; altered or loss of auditory, olfactory, gustatory processes; chronic pain
Nutritional/Metabolic	Dysphagia (aspiration risk, feeding tube may be necessary), infection (urinary or respiratory), syndrome of inappropriate antidiuretic hormone (SIADH), diabetes insipidus (DI), fluid volume excess or deficit, endocrine (hormonal) dysfunctioning, impaired skin integrity (stoma, poor wound healing, pressure ulcer)
Elimination	Neurogenic bowel and/or bladder
Musculoskeletal	Heterotopic ossification (HO), multiple fractures
Respiratory	Risk of infection, respiratory distress and/or arrest (requiring tracheostomy); tracheal granuloma and/or stenosis
Cardiovascular	Decreased activity tolerance, at risk for pulmonary emboli, deep venous thromboses
Cognitive/Behavioral	Reduced level of awareness, attention, memory, executive functioning; personality changes, agitation
Communicative	Aphasia, dysarthria
Sexual	Disinhibition, sexual dysfunction, changes in hormonal regulation

c. Severe TBI: Effects of extensive diffuse axonal injury spread throughout cortex and upper and lower brainstem
   1) Focal damage, in the form of hemorrhage and hematoma, plus secondary complications also are frequently present
   2) Clinical hallmarks: Length of unconsciousness lasting more than 6 hours and a score of 8 or lower on the Glasgow Coma Scale
   3) May result in numerous potential deficits (see Figure 8.3 for an in-depth list)

E. Residual deficits

1. Many residual deficits occur after TBI; many may not be resolved; recovery is ongoing and may last for months or years
2. Physiological deficits are somewhat universal and predictable; cognitive, behavioral, and social disturbances are variable for each individual (see Figure 8.3 for common sequelae of TBI)

Figure 8.4. Rancho Los Amigos Levels of Cognitive Function Scale: Adapted Version, 1979

I. No response to pain, touch, sound, or sight

II. Generalized reflex response to stimulation/pain

III. Localized response—blinks to strong light, turns toward/away from sound, responds to physical discomfort, gives inconsistent response to commands

IV. Confused-agitated—alert; very active, aggressive, or bizarre behaviors; performs motor activities but behavior is nonpur-poseful; extremely short attention span

V. Confused-nonagitated—gross attention to environment, highly distractible, requires continual redirection, difficulty learning new tasks, agitated by too much stimulation

VI. Confused-appropriate—inconsistent orientation to time and place, retention span/recent memory impaired, begins to recall past, consistently follows simple directions, goal-directed behavior with assistance

VII. Automatic-appropriate—performs daily routine in highly familiar environment in a nonconfused but automatic robot-like manner, skills noticeably deteriorate in unfamiliar surroundings, lack of realistic planning for own future

VIII. Purposeful-appropriate

Reprinted with permission of Rancho Los Amigos Medical Center from Rancho Los Amigos Medical Center, Adult Brain Injury Service. (1979). *Levels of cognitive function scale* (adapted version) (pp. 78-80). Downey, CA: Author.

F. Progress and prognosis

1. There are many tools for determining progress, prognosis, and evaluation of outcomes
2. Prognosis related to numerous variables (see the introductory paragraph of this chapter on page 52)
3. Below is a list of evaluation instruments currently in use
   a. Rancho Los Amigos Levels of Cognitive Function Scale—general assessment tool (see Figure 8.4) (Rancho Los Amigos Medical Center, Adult Brain Injury Service, 1979)
   b. Glasgow Coma Scale (GCS), useful in acute care (see Figure 8.1) (Jennett & Teasdale, 1981)
   c. Glasgow Coma Outcome Scale (Jennett & Bond, 1975)
   d. Disability Rating Scale (DRS) (Rappaport, Hall, Hopkins, Belleza, & Cope, 1982)
   e. Neuropsychological Battery (e.g., Halstead-Reitan, WAIS-R/WISC-R) (Reitan & Wolfson, 1985)
   f. Coma-Near Coma (Rappaport, Dougherty, & Kelting, 1992)

   g. Coma Recovery Scale (CRS) (Giacino, Kexmarski, DeLuca, & Cicerone, 1991)
   h. SSAM (Mediplex) (Ellis & Rader, 1990)
   i. Western Neuro Sensory Stimulation Profile (WNSSP) (Ansell & Keenan, 1989)

G. Pediatric considerations

1. A child who has sustained a head injury and has residual physical, cognitive, or social deficits has a developmental disadvantage
2. In evaluating the effects of pediatric brain injury and making predictions about recovery and prognosis, the following must be assessed
   a. Premorbid developmental, functional, and psychodynamic levels
   b. Premorbid living situation
   c. Deficits due to TBI
   d. Cognitive and developmental ability after TBI
3. Ability to learn (especially new information) depends greatly on the abilities to attend and to concentrate, both of which may be impaired after TBI
4. Educational achievement after TBI—which should be assessed by special educators, psychologists, and therapists—depends on several factors
   a. Attention span and ability to concentrate
   b. Ability to tolerate classroom stimulation
   c. Ability to communicate
   d. Ability to follow commands, process basic information, and integrate learning
5. Social interactions
   a. Pediatric client, in relating to others outside the family, uses play and social activities to aid in establishing his or her identity
   b. Special environments can help child in social and academic settings
   c. To help children develop skills to monitor their own behavior, it may be necessary to institute a formalized behavioral management program with the following components
      1) Target behaviors
      2) Contingencies
      3) Positive reinforcement
6. Adolescent TBI clients
   a. May have their future academic goals altered due to cognitive, behavioral, and neurological impairments
   b. Can be helped to attain feasible goals by early vocational assessment and appropriate education and/or training

H. Nursing diagnoses for TBI (both adults and children) (see Section III for detailed information on nursing diagnoses)

1. Altered health maintenance
2. Potential for injury
3. Altered nutrition—less and/or more than body requirements
4. Potential for aspiration
5. Fluid volume deficit
6. Impaired skin integrity
7. Hyperthermia
8. Bowel incontinence/functional incontinence
9. Caregiver role strain (North American Nursing Diagnosis Association, 1992)
10. Impaired physical mobility
11. Total or limited self-care deficit
12. Impaired home maintenance management
13. Ineffective airway clearance
14. Sleep pattern disturbance
15. Chronic pain
16. Sensory–perceptual alteration
17. Knowledge deficit
18. Impaired thought processes
19. Impaired social interaction
20. Self-esteem disturbance
21. Impaired verbal communication
22. Altered family processes
23. Sexual dysfunction

References

Anderson, D.W., & McLaurin, R.L. (1980). The National Head and Spinal Cord Injury Survey. *Journal of Neurosurgery, 53,* S1-S43.

Ansell, B.J., & Keenan, J.E. (1989). The Western Neuro Sensory Stimulation Profile: A tool for assessing slow-to-recover head-injured patients. *Archives of Physical Medicine and Rehabilitation, 70*, 104-108.

Berrol, S. (1990). Persistent vegetative state. In M.E. Sandel & D.W. Ellis (Eds.), *The coma-emerging patient* (pp. 559-567). Philadelphia: Hanley & Belfus, Inc.

Bond, M.R. (1990). Standardized methods of assessing and predicting outcome. In M. Rosenthal, E.R. Griffith, M.R. Bond, & J.D. Miller (Eds.), *Rehabilitation of the adult and child with traumatic brain injury* (2nd ed.) (pp. 59-64). Philadelphia: F.A. Davis Company.

Charness, A. (1986). *Stroke/head injury: A guide to functional outcomes in physical therapy management.* Rockville, MD: Aspen Publishers, Inc.

Ellis, D.W., & Rader, M.A. (1990). Structured sensory stimulation. *Physical Medicine and Rehabilitation: State of the Art Reviews, 4*, 465-477.

Gennarelli, T.A. (1986). Mechanisms and pathophysiology of cerebral concussion. *Journal of Head Trauma Rehabilitation, 1*, 23-29.

Giacino, J.T., Kexmarski, M., DeLuca, J., & Cicerone, K.D. (1991). Monitoring rate of recovery to predict outcome in minimally responsive patients. *Archives of Physical Medicine and Rehabilitation, 72*, 897-901.

Gilroy, J. (1990). *Basic neurology* (2nd ed.). New York: Pergamon Press.

Interagency Head-Injury Task Force. (1989). *Interagency Head-Injury Task Force Report.* Bethesda, MD: National Institute of Neurological Disorders and Stroke, National Institutes of Health.

Jennett, B. (1990). Scale and scope of the problem. In M. Rosenthal, E.R. Griffith, M.R. Bond, & J.D. Miller (Eds.), *Rehabilitation of the adult and child with traumatic brain injury* (2nd ed.) (pp. 3-7). Philadelphia: F.A. Davis Company.

Jennett, B., & Bond, M. (1975). Assessment of outcome after severe brain damage. *Lancet, 1*(1905), 480-484.

Jennett, B., & Plum, F. (1972). Persistent vegetative state after brain damage: A syndrome in search of a name. *Lancet, 1*(753), 734-737.

Jennett, B., & Teasdale, G. (1981). *Management of head injuries.* Philadelphia: F.A. Davis Company.

Marshall, S.B., Marshall, L.F., Vos, H.R., & Chesnut, R.M. (1990). *Neuroscience critical care: Physiology and patient management.* Philadelphia: W.B. Saunders Company.

Miller, J.D., & Jones, P.A. (1985). The work of a regional head injury service. *Lancet, 1*, 1141.

Miller, J.D., & Jones, P.A. (1990). Minor head injury. In M. Rosenthal, E.R. Griffith, M.R. Bond, & J.D. Miller (Eds.), *Rehabilitation of the adult and child with traumatic brain injury* (2nd ed.) (pp. 238-239). Philadelphia: F.A. Davis Company.

Miller, J.D., Pentland, B., & Berrol, S. (1990). Early evaluation and management. In M. Rosenthal, E.R. Griffith, M.R. Bond, & J.D. Miller (Eds.), *Rehabilitation of the adult and child with traumatic brain injury* (2nd ed.) (pp. 21-37). Philadelphia: F.A. Davis Company.

North American Nursing Diagnosis Association. (1992). *NANDA nursing diagnoses: Definitions and classification 1992-1993.* St. Louis: Author.

Pang, D. (1985). Pathophysiological correlates of neurobehavioral syndromes following closed head injury. In M. Ylvisaker (Ed.), *Head injury rehabilitation: Children and adolescents* (pp. 3-70). Boston: College-Hill Press, Inc.

Rancho Los Amigos Medical Center, Adult Brain Injury Service. (1979). *Levels of cognitive function scale* (adapted version). Downey, CA: Author.

Rappaport, M., Dougherty, A.M., & Kelting, D.L. (1992). Evaluation of coma and vegetative states. *Archives of Physical Medicine and Rehabilitation, 73*, 628-634.

Rappaport, M., Hall, K.M., Hopkins, H.K., Belleza, T., & Cope, D. (1982). Disability rating scale for severe head trauma patients: Coma to community. *Archives of Physical Medicine and Rehabilitation, 63*, 118-123.

Reitan, R.M., & Wolfson, D. (1985). *Halsted-Reitan Neuropsychological Test Battery: Theory and clinical interpretation.* Tucson, AZ: Neuropsychological Press.

Rosenthal, M., Griffith, E.R., Bond, M.R., & Miller, J.D. (Eds.). *Rehabilitation of the adult and child with traumatic brain injury* (2nd ed.). Philadelphia: F.A. Davis Company.

Salazar, A.M. (1992). Traumatic brain injury: The continuing epidemic. In V.C. Hachinski (Ed.), *Challenges in neurology* (pp. 55-65). Philadelphia: F.A. Davis Company.

Smith, S.S., & Winkler, P.A. (1990). Traumatic head injuries. In D.A. Umphred (Ed.), *Neurological rehabilitation* (2nd ed.) (pp. 347-396). St. Louis: The C.V. Mosby Company.

Spaaradeo, F., Strauss, D., & Barth, J. (1990). The incidence, impact, and treatment of substance abuse in head trauma rehabilitation. *Journal of Head Trauma Rehabilitation, 5*, 1-8.

Teasdale, G., & Mendelow, D. (1984). Pathophysiology of head injuries. In N. Brooks (Ed.), *Closed head injury: Psychological, social, and family consequences* (pp. 4-36). Oxford, England: Oxford University Press.

Ylvisaker, M. (1985). *Head injury rehabilitation: Children and adolescents.* Boston: College-Hill Press, Inc.

Suggested Readings

Fay, G., & Tanesheski, T. (1986). Neuropsychological assessment of head-injured children. *Journal of Head Trauma Rehabilitation, 1*, 16-21.

Jaffe, K., & Hays, R. (1986). Pediatric head injury: Rehabilitation medical management. *Journal of Head Trauma Rehabilitation, 1*, 30-40.

Lehr, E. (1990). *Psychological management of traumatic brain injuries in children and adolescents.* Rockville, MD: Aspen Publishers, Inc.

CHAPTER 9

Spinal Cord Injury

Early and effective rehabilitation of the patient with spinal cord injury (SCI) is essential for optimal recovery and quality of life. Traumatic spinal cord injury often has a permanent impact on the physiological, psychological, vocational, and social aspects of a patient's life.

Technological advances have had a positive impact on the care and treatment of SCI patients from the point of trauma through extended rehabilitation. Sophisticated lifesaving, critical care, and management techniques have increased survival rates, lengthened life spans, and improved the quality of life of SCI patients.

Dual diagnoses and treatment are not uncommon. Persons with SCI may concurrently experience extensive burns, traumatic brain injury, and substance abuse. These increase both the complexity and the cost of care. Persons with SCI are living longer and aging with a major physical disability, which continuously influences their health state and medical needs. These interrelated factors of survival, technology, and economics have mandated the need for highly effective rehabilitation nursing to deal with the spinal cord injured patient.

I. Spinal Cord Injury

A. Definition: Traumatic insult to the spinal cord resulting in alterations or complete disruption of normal motor, sensory, and autonomic function

1. Quadriplegia
   a. Loss of motor and sensory function in cervical segments causing impairment in arms, trunk, legs, and pelvic organs
   b. Usually occurs as a result of injuries at T1 or above
2. Paraplegia
   a. Loss of motor and sensory function in thoracic, lumbar, or sacral segments causing impairment in trunk, legs, and pelvic organs
   b. Usually occurs as a result of injuries at T2 or below

B. Epidemiology (Hickey, 1992; National Spinal Cord Injury Statistical Center [NSCISC], 1986; Staas et al., 1988; Walleck, 1988; Zejdlik, 1992)

1. Incidence of SCI is approximately 700 to 800 cases per million in the United States (8,000 new cases per year) (Zejdlik, 1992, p. 20)
   a. Occurs primarily in young adults (16 to 30 years of age)
   b. Eighty percent of SCI patients are male
2. Prognosis
   a. Life expectancy after SCI is approximately 30.2 years
   b. Factors affecting survival rate
      1) Level of lesion
      2) Extent of paralysis
      3) Age
      4) Medical complications (e.g., infection)

C. Etiology

1. Trauma
   a. Accidents (including motor vehicle accidents)
   b. Falls
   c. Violence
   d. Sporting or recreational injuries
2. Blunt injuries causing contusion of the spinal cord
   a. Flexion injury
      1) Occurs when head is thrown forward
      2) Occurs if head is struck from behind
      3) Occurs commonly in motor vehicle accidents and falls
   b. Flexion with rotation injury occurs when this combination of forces causes severe twisting, resulting in ruptured ligaments and dislocations
   c. Extension injury occurs in forward falls in which face or chin is struck
   d. Vertical compression injury occurs when a fall or blow to top of the head shatters vertebral body affecting the cord (commonly occurs in diving injuries)
3. Penetrating injuries that directly pierce the cord
   a. Gunshot wound
   b. Knife wound

D. Pathophysiology

1. Varying degrees of damage associated with spinal cord injury
   a. Severity of bony injury does not always correspond to the extent of neurological impairment
   b. Common sites of injury are the most mobile parts of the spine, namely, the cervical and thoracolumbar junctures
   c. Spinal cord itself may sustain contusion without vertebral fractures or dislocations
   d. Progressive tissue destruction occurs in the cord within hours and may involve several responses
      1) Decrease of microperfusion at site of injury
      2) Hemorrhage in the gray matter
      3) Development of hematoma and edema
      4) Release of biochemicals at site of injury
      5) Ischemia and necrosis in the cord, causing neurological damage
   e. Bony level of injury: Injury to the vertebral col-

umn as a result of fracture, ligament rupture, or both (also called *skeletal level of injury*)
   1) Stable injury: Occurs when the bone and/or ligaments support the injured cord area, preventing progression of neurological deficit
   2) Unstable injury: Occurs when the bone and ligaments are disrupted and unable to support and protect the injured cord area, possibly causing further neurological deficit
2. Levels of spinal cord injury
   a. Upper motor neuron (UMN) injury (see Chapter 5)
      1) Is evident in lesions above T12/L1 vertebrae
      2) Causes loss of cerebral control over all reflex activity below level of lesion
      3) Causes spastic paralysis
   b. Lower motor neuron (LMN) injury (see Chapter 5)
      1) Is evident in lesions below T12/L1 level (conus medullaris/cauda equina)
      2) Causes destruction of the reflex arc
      3) Causes flaccid paralysis
3. Neurological level of injury: Determined by level of lowest neurological segment of the cord that retains normal sensory and motor function on both sides of the body
   a. Complete injury
      1) Loss of all voluntary motor and sensory function below level of injury, including the lowest sacral segment
      2) There may be a zone of partial preservation (American Spinal Injury Association, 1992)
         a) Consists of the neurologic levels below the level of complete injury where some sensory and/or motor function is found
         b) Term used only with complete injuries (for example, a person with a complete C5 injury may have patchy sensation at C6 or C7 but not have any anal reflexes, such as sacral sparing, and thus still be classified as a complete C5 injury)
   b. Incomplete injury: Results in some preservation of sensory and/or motor function below level of injury and in lowest sacral segment
4. Neuroanatomic description of incompleteness by syndromes (see Figure 9.1)
   a. Anterior cord syndrome
      1) Caused by damage to the anterior artery, affecting anterior two thirds of the cord
      2) Produces paralysis and loss of pain and temperature sensation below the lesion with preservation of position sense
   b. Central cord syndrome
      1) Caused by damage to central part of the cord
      2) Usually in the cervical region
      3) Produces loss of motor power and sensation that affects upper limbs more than lower limbs
   c. Brown-Sequard syndrome
      1) Caused by damage to one side (hemisection) of the cord
      2) Produces loss of motor function and position sense on the same side as the damage and a loss of pain and temperature sensation on the opposite side
   d. Posterior cord syndrome
      1) Caused by damage to posterior dorsal columns of the cord
      2) Produces loss of position sense and motor function with preservation of pain sensation
   e. Conus medullaris syndrome
      1) Caused by damage to the conus and lumbar nerve roots
      2) May produce areflexia (flaccidity) in bladder, bowel, and/or lower limbs

Figure 9.1. Spinal Cord Syndromes

Syndrome	Mechanism of Vertebral Injury	Mechanism of Spinal Cord Injury
Anterior cord syndrome 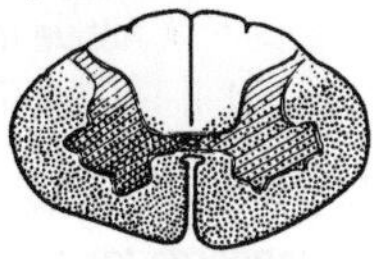	• Flexion and dislocation injuries to cervical cord	• Direct injury; compression or vessel occlusion; infarction • Compromised anterior spinal artery
Central cord syndrome 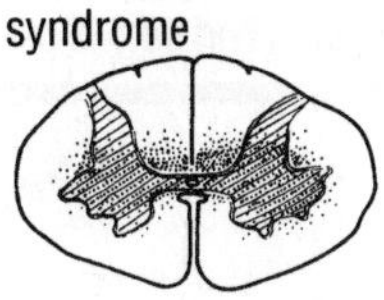	• Severe hyperextension injury to cervical cord • Spinal cord tumor	• Compression of cord between degenerated intervertebral disks • Centralized cord edema
Brown-Sequard syndrome (hemisection of spinal cord) 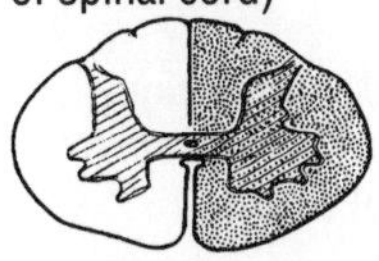	• Direct penetrating injury such as stab wound or gunshot	• Laceration and hemisection of spinal cord
Conus medullaris cauda equina injury 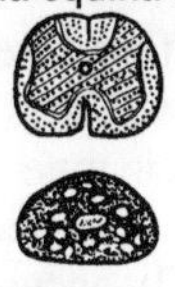	• Fracture dislocation	• Compression, contusion, or laceration of conus and sacral spinal nerve roots
Sacral sparing 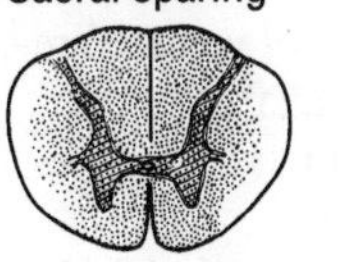		• Direct trauma to major portion of cord • Spinal cord ischemia or infarction caused by disruption of spinal cord circulation • Radicular arteries remain intact

Reprinted with permission of F.A. Davis Company from Dolan, J.T. (1991). *Critical care nursing: Clinical management through the nursing process* (p. 212). Philadelphia: F.A. Davis Company.

Figure 9.2. Motor Grading Scale

Grade	Rating of Level of Movement	Description of Motor Abilities
0	Absent	Total paralysis
1	Trace	Palpable and/or visible contraction
2	Poor	Active movement and full range of motion (ROM) when gravity is eliminated
3	Fair	Active movement and full ROM against gravity
4	Good	Active movement and full ROM against moderate resistance
5	Normal	Active movement and full ROM against full resistance

Sources Consulted

American Spinal Injury Association (ASIA). (1992). *Standards for neurological and functional classification of spinal injury patients* (rev. ed.). Chicago: Author.

Zejdlik, C.P. (1992). *Management of spinal cord injury* (2nd ed.). Boston: Jones and Bartlett Publishers.

f. Cauda equina syndrome
   1) Caused by damage below conus to lumbosacral nerve roots
   2) May produce areflexia in bladder, bowel, and/or lower limbs

g. Sacral sparing: Damage that affects a major part of the cord but preserves radicular arteries, which allow sensation in sacral area

5. Spinal shock
   a. Immediate response to traumatic or sudden spinal cord injury
   b. Temporary suppression of spinal reflexes below level of injury in combination with loss of sensation, motor function, and muscle tone
      1) May subside within 1 hour or last for weeks
      2) Recovery of reflex activity usually occurs in an ascending pattern
      3) Spinal shock ends with return of perianal reflexes (bulbocavernosus and anal reflexes)
      4) Incomplete injury may result in varying degrees of spinal shock
      5) Spinal shock resolves to spasticity in UMN lesions; flaccidity will remain permanently in LMN lesions

E. **Assessing impairment**: American Spinal Injury Association (ASIA) Impairment Scale (American Spinal Injury Association, 1992)
   1. Frequently used scale that reflects severity of impairment
   2. Modified version of the Frankel Grading System for SCI
   3. Levels of ASIA scale (see Figure 9.2)
      a. A—Complete: No sensory or motor function preserved in sacral segments 4-5
      b. B—Incomplete: Sensory function (but not motor function) preserved below the neurological level and extends through sacral segments 4-5
      c. C—Incomplete: Motor function preserved below the neurological level, and the majority of muscles below the level are Grade 3 or lower (see Figure 9.2)
      d. D—Incomplete: Motor function preserved below the neurological level, and the majority of muscles below the level are at Grade 3 or higher (see Figure 9.2)
      e. E—Normal: Normal sensory and motor function

F. **Residual deficits** and systemic dysfunctioning that may occur after spinal cord injury (Mandzak-McCarron, 1988; Mumma, 1987; Staas et al., 1988; Walleck, 1988)
   1. Neurological manifestations
      a. Loss or decrease of voluntary motor function below level of injury
      b. Loss or decrease of sensation
      c. Loss of normal reflex activity
      d. Autonomic dysfunctions due to loss of normal sympathetic nervous system functioning
         1) Autonomic dysreflexia (see Chapter 12, p. 89)
         2) Hypotension
         3) Loss of thermoregulation
         4) Loss of vasomotor tone and/or control
   2. Cardiovascular manifestations
      a. Hypotension and vasodilation, causing decreased cardiac output
         1) Orthostatic hypotension: Rapid drop in blood pressure when the erect position is assumed; patients with cervical or high thoracic injury have poor vasomotor control, so there is difficulty getting blood out of the lower extremities and back to the heart
         2) Vasodilation occurs as a result of loss of sympathetically induced vasoconstriction; triggers pooling of blood in abdomen and lower extremities
      b. Bradycardia due to unopposed vagal tone (10th cranial nerve)
      c. Impaired temperature regulation manifested by poikilothermia, a condition in which the body assumes the environmental temperature due to the inability to sweat or shiver below the injury
   3. Respiratory manifestations (see Chapter 14, p. 116)
      a. Injury above C4 results in paralysis of respiratory muscles, including the diaphragm; patient usually is dependent on a ventilator
      b. Injury between C4 and T6 results in paralysis of the intercostal and abdominal muscles; pa-

tient usually is weaned from the ventilator but requires aggressive pulmonary management
   c. Injury between T6 and T12 results in paralysis of some abdominal muscles; patient does not require a daily respiratory program unless an upper respiratory infection is present
4. Metabolic manifestations
   a. Negative nitrogen balance
   b. Decreased basal metabolic rate and expenditure of energy
   c. Hypercalcemia and/or hypercalciuria
   d. Altered secretion of pituitary-derived hormones
   e. Heterotopic ossification
5. Gastrointestinal manifestations
   a. Peristaltic slowing, causing paralytic ileus
   b. Increased acidity, causing GI bleeding
   c. Pancreatitis after injury (Sugarman, 1985)
   d. Abnormal liver function due to trauma
   e. Neurogenic bowel (see Chapter 13)
6. Genitourinary manifestations
   a. Neurogenic bladder (see Chapter 13)
   b. Urinary outlet sphincter dysfunctioning
7. Sexual manifestations (see Chapter 19)
8. Psychosocial manifestations
   a. Patients with SCI must adjust to a variety of stressors and losses
      1) Stressors
         a) Survival
         b) Quality of life
         c) Lifestyle alterations
         d) Occupational changes
         e) Participation in recreational activities
      2) Losses
         a) Sensation
         b) Mobility
         c) Bowel and bladder control
         d) Sexual function
         e) Control and independence
         f) Former roles
         g) Self-esteem
   b. Emotions and behaviors that may be exhibited after SCI
      1) Anxiety
      2) Frustration
      3) Anger
      4) Hostility
      5) Fear
      6) Sarcasm
      7) Regression
      8) Denial
      9) Guilt
      10) Depression
      11) Sensory overload

G. **Potential nursing diagnoses** (see Section III for detailed information on nursing diagnoses)
1. Health management deficit
2. Impaired physical mobility
3. Self-care deficit (total or partial)
4. Ineffective airway clearance
5. Altered urinary elimination
6. Altered bowel elimination
7. Altered nutrition
8. Autonomic dysreflexia
9. High risk for skin breakdown
10. Chronic pain
11. Sensory-perceptual alterations
12. Knowledge deficit
13. Sexual dysfunction
14. Ineffective individual and/or family coping
15. Self-esteem disturbance
16. Reactive depression

References

American Spinal Injury Association (ASIA). (1992). *Standards for neurological and functional classification of spinal injury patients* (rev. ed.). Chicago: Author.

Dolan, J.T. (1991). *Critical care nursing: Clinical management through the nursing process.* Philadelphia: F.A Davis Company.

Hickey, J.V. (1992). *The clinical practice of neurological and neurosurgical nursing* (3rd ed.). Philadelphia: J.B. Lippincott Company.

Mandzak-McCarron, K. (1988). Rehabilitation of the patient with spinal cord injury. *Trauma Quarterly, 4*(3), 45-57.

Mumma, C.M. (Ed.). (1987). *Rehabilitation nursing: Concepts and practice—A core curriculum* (2nd ed.). Evanston, IL: Rehabilitation Nursing Foundation.

National Spinal Cord Injury Statistical Center (NSCISC). (1986). *Spinal cord injury: The facts and figures.* Birmingham, AL: The University of Alabama at Birmingham.

Staas, W.J., Formal, C.S., Gershkoff, A.M., Freda, M., Hirschwald, J.F., Miller, G.T., Forrest, L., & Burkhard, B.A. (1988). Rehabilitation of the spinal cord injured patient. In J. DeLisa (Ed.), *Rehabilitation medicine: Principles and practice* (pp. 635-667). Philadelphia: J.B. Lippincott Company.

Sugarman, B. (1985). Medical complications of spinal cord injury. *Quarterly Journal of Medicine, 54*(213), 3-18.

Walleck, C.A. (1988). Central nervous system II: Spinal cord injury. In V.D. Cadona, P.D. Hurn, P.J. Mason, A.M. Scanlon-Schilpp, & S.W. Veise-Berry (Eds.), *Trauma nursing from resuscitation through rehabilitation* (pp. 419-448). Philadelphia: W.B. Saunders Company.

Zejdlik, C.P. (1992). *Management of spinal cord injury* (2nd ed.). Boston: Jones and Bartlett Publishers.

Suggested Readings

Berly, M.H., & Wilmot, C.B. (1984). Acute abdominal emergencies during the first four weeks after spinal cord injury. *Archives of Physical Medicine and Rehabilitation, 65*, 687-690.

◆Bracken, M.B., Shepard, M.J., Collins, W.F., Holford, T.R., Young, W., Baskin, D.S., Eisenberg, H.M., Flamm, E., Leo-Summers, L., Maroon, J., Marshall, L.F., Perot, P.L., Jr., Piepmeier, J., Sonntag, V.K.H., Wagner, F.C., Wilberger, J.E., & Winn, H.R. (1990). A randomized, controlled trial of methylprednisolone or naloxone in the treatment of acute spinal cord injury: Results of the second national acute spinal cord injury study. *The New England Journal of Medicine, 322*, 1405-1422.

Buchanan, L.E., & Nawoczenski, D.H. (1987). *Spinal cord injury concepts and management approaches.* Baltimore: Williams and Wilkins.

◆Geisler, F.H., Dorsey, F.C., & Coleman, W.P. (1991). Recovery of motor function after spinal cord injury: A randomized, placebo-controlled trial with CM1-ganglioside. *The New England Journal of Medicine, 324*, 1829-1838.

Gines, D.J. (1988). Long-term nutrition care for the client with spinal cord injury. *Topics in Clinical Nutrition, 3*(3), 61-69.

◆ indicates a research-based work

CHAPTER 10

Rehabilitation Across the Life Span: Gerontological Rehabilitation

As the population of older individuals increases, the unique healthcare concerns of those over 65 years of age merit special consideration. Physical limitations increase with advancing age. Of the more than five million older people hospitalized annually, many require rehabilitation services (Katov, 1990). Reports of the prevalence and severity of disability in the elderly vary considerably. One of the reasons for the variations is the failure to differentiate between functional limitations and disability (Kelly-Hayes, Jette, Wolf, D'Agostino, & Odell, 1992).

Most of the clients for whom rehabilitation nurses care are over the age of 65. In a study conducted by the Association of Rehabilitation Nurses, the respondents (rehabilitation nurses) indicated that 59% of their patients were elderly (Dungan & McCourt, 1991). Unfortunately, one of the most significant barriers to rehabilitation faced by the older adult is not the functional limitation imposed by chronic illness and disability, but rather that imposed by attitudes. Families and friends often accept the limitations of disability as an inevitable consequence of aging, rather than something that can be ameliorated through rehabilitation. Nurses and the other members of the rehabilitation team are susceptible to prejudices against the aged. Although rehabilitation of an individual who is 100 years old may not extend the client's life, it likely will make a difference in the quality of the remaining months or years of life. It is important that rehabilitation nurses advocate for consistent access to rehabilitation for older adults.

Nursing therapy with older clients in rehabilitation is holistic in nature and includes the family and other support systems. Family support is a consistent need for rehabilitation clients of all ages. Insufficient family support is likely to result in placement of the older adult in a long-term care facility or nursing home. The rehabilitation nurse focuses on increasing the older individual's functional ability, promoting motivation, maximizing community involvement, and facilitating means of support for the client.

I. The Aging Process: Related Theory

A. Theories of aging (none is universally accepted)
   1. Molecular factors: Aging changes are believed to be related to the oxidation-reduction reactions that progressively deactivate essential molecules such as DNA and proteins
   2. Cellular factors
      a. Environmental damage results in cumulative, progressive injury to cells
      b. Error theory holds that, with age, there is a loss of genetic information within the cells that results in errors in protein synthesis
   3. Organ system factors: Aging changes are believed to be the result of immune system incompetence that occurs with time

B. Characteristics of the aging process
   1. Universal: Occurs in all individuals
   2. Progressive: Changes tend to increase over time
   3. Deleterious: Many aspects viewed as negative
   4. Intrinsic: Occurs irrespective of environmental factors

II. Physiological Aspects of Aging That Can Lead to Functional Limitation

A. Hematological system (Myers-Robfogel & Bosmann, 1984)
   1. Anemia: Common problem that should always be considered in older clients
   2. Hypoalbuminemia: Can result in decreased binding for protein-binding drugs (e.g., meperidine, tolbutamide, warfarin)
   3. Decreased body water (increased fat): Can result in changes in drug absorption and distribution
      a. Water-soluble drugs (e.g., digoxin): Higher plasma concentration produces a stronger drug effect
      b. Fat-soluble drugs (e.g., diazepam, phenobarbital): Lower plasma concentration, with greater absorption and longer effect

B. Hepatic system: Decreased enzyme activity and metabolism (drugs might be metabolized more slowly)

C. Renal system
   1. Decreased renal mass
   2. Decreased renal blood flow with decreased glomerular filtration rate (results in lower creatinine clearance)

D. Pulmonary system: Primary change is a reduced reserve capacity

E. Cardiovascular system (Wenger, 1984)
   1. Reduced work capacity due to decreased maximal exercise heart rate and oxygen consumption
   2. Reduced reflex tachycardia related to decreased sensitivity of the baroreceptors, resulting in orthostatic hypotension

F. Immunological system: Primary change is a decreased resistance to infection and a decrease in hypersensitivity reactions
G. Sensory system
   1. Vision: Presbyopia, or impaired ability of the lens to focus on close objects
   2. Hearing: Presbycusis, or reduced hearing acuteness
   3. Olfactory: Anosomia, or loss of smell
   4. Taste: Reduced ability to taste (can result in diminished appetite)
   5. Other sensory modalities: Impairment of perception of deep pain, tactile sensitivity, and vibratory perception
H. Endocrine system: In general, there is a decrease in organ function or system responsiveness to hormones
   1. Primary decrease in glucose tolerance
   2. Thyroid dysfunction (more often, hyperthyroidism)
I. Neurological system
   1. Cognition: Short-term memory loss can occur with aging and can affect the older client's ability to complete the rehabilitation program successfully
   2. Proprioception (position of the body in space): Balance and coordination can decline with age
J. Musculoskeletal system
   1. Muscle fiber size and mass decrease with age
   2. Osteoarthritis and osteoporosis increase with age (see Chapter 7)

III. Special Considerations for Older Adults Participating in Rehabilitation

A. Falls (see Chapter 11)
   1. Reasons for older adults' increased risk for falls
      a. Possible delay in compensatory responses to changes in posture (Woollacott, 1990)
      b. Cardiovascular problems, such as hypotension, to which older adults are susceptible (Jonsson & Lipsitz, 1990)
      c. Medication use (Ray & Griffin, 1990)
         1) Approximately 70% to 80% of individuals over age 65 are taking one or more prescription medications; some of these can act to increase risk of falling
         2) Medications linked with falls
            a) Diuretics
            b) Antihypertensives
            c) Psychotropics
            d) Antiparkinsonian agents
            e) Antihistamines
   2. Importance of preventing falls: Falls are not a normal consequence of aging, and rehabilitation nurses must be concerned with averting them by taking preventive measures (Daleiden, 1990)
      a. Careful assessment of risk factors and identification of those at high risk for falls
      b. Analysis of any history of falls and the conditions surrounding a fall
B. Physical constraints
   1. Foot problems (Helfand, 1990)
      a. In older adults, feet are a common source of pain related to the effects of disease and the constant stress of years of use
      b. Often an area to which older adults pay little daily preventive attention (Clark, 1984)
      c. Diabetic and peripheral neuropathy may lead to maceration and infection of foot areas, particularly between the toes
      d. Rehabilitation concerns
         1) Underlying problems in nails and skin need to be corrected
         2) Modifications of shoes might correct gait problems and foot deformities that are common in aging
            a) Heel wedging
            b) Metatarsal bars for weight transfer
   2. Nutrition
      a. Older individuals requiring rehabilitation might present with nutritional deficiencies (Duchene & LeSage, 1990; Matthews, 1989; Weg, 1990)
      b. Hospitalization, which often coincides with an acute episode of illness or disability, might precipitate nutritional imbalance
         1) Individual's ability to receive adequate nutrition and hydration can be impeded by medical treatments, medications, and the unfamiliar environment of the hospital
         2) Lack of proper dental care and missing teeth add to this problem
      c. Problems resulting from malnutrition
         1) Prolonged time for wound healing
         2) Loss of energy and endurance
         3) Susceptibility to infections
         4) Muscle wasting
         5) Development of pressure ulcers
C. Motivational factors (Duchene et al., 1990): Many factors influence the older adult's motivation to participate in self-care
   1. Responses to aging, chronicity, and disability
      a. Positive responses focus on satisfaction with life, retirement, family, and hope for the future
      b. Negative responses are associated with depression and failure to adjust to multiple losses
   2. Cognitive deficits
      a. Impairment of memory
      b. Impairment of problem-solving ability
   3. Beliefs and expectations about care, prognosis, and the role and support of family members; client and family should be given reality-based information
   4. Attitudes of healthcare providers
      a. Overly helpful caregiver can decrease motivation to participate in self-care
      b. Caregiver who reinforces independent behaviors is of critical importance in increasing the individual's motivation to participate in self-care activities
D. Learning capabilities (Gardner, Greenwell, & Costich, 1991) (see Chapter 16)
   1. Older adults continue to learn
   2. Older adults must be partners in learning if teaching plans are to work
   3. Visual and auditory limitations must be considered when teaching plan is designed

IV. Possible Nursing Diagnoses: Older adults can have any number of nursing diagnoses, depending on their individual situations, physical conditions, and potential for rehabilitation (see Section III for detailed information on nursing diagnoses)

References

Clark, G. (1984). Functional assessment. In T. Williams (Ed.), *Rehabilitation in the aging* (pp. 111-124). New York: Raven Press.

Daleiden, S. (1990). Prevention of falling: Rehabilitative or compensatory interventions? *Topics in Geriatric Rehabilitation, 5*(2), 34-43.

Duchene, P., Dean-Baar, S., Cronin-Stubbs, D., DiFilippo, J., Kopanke, D., Stehlin, M., & LeSage, J. (1990). Geriatric rehabilitation: Strategies for independence. *Focus on Geriatric Care and Rehabilitation, 3*(8), 1-8.

Duchene, P., & LeSage, J. (1990). Hydration and nutrition. In D. Corr & C. Corr (Eds.), *Nursing care in an aging society* (pp. 92-113). New York: Springer Publishing Company.

Dungan, L.A., & McCourt, A.E. (1991). *Report on the Rehabilitation Nurses Job Analysis 1989-1990.* Skokie, IL: Association of Rehabilitation Nurses and Rehabilitation Nursing Certification Board.

Gardner, D., Greenwell, S., & Costich, J. (1991). Effective teaching of the older adult. *Topics in Geriatric Rehabilitation, 6*(3), 1-14.

Helfand, A. (1990). Limiting mobility loss from foot problems. In S. Brody & L. Pawlson (Eds.), *Aging and rehabilitation II: The state of the practice* (pp. 95-109). New York: Springer Publishing Company.

Jonsson, P., & Lipsitz, L. (1990). Cardiovascular factors contributing to falls in the older adult. *Topics in Geriatric Rehabilitation, 5*(2), 21-33.

Katov, C. (1990). *Access to geriatric rehabilitation services: A background paper.* Washington, DC: American Association of Retired Persons.

Kelly-Hayes, M., Jette, A., Wolf, P., D'Agostino, R., & Odell, P. (1992). Functional limitations and disability among elders in the Framingham study. *American Journal of Public Health, 82*, 841-845.

Matthews, L. (1989). Malnutrition in hospitalization: A barrier to rehabilitation. *Topics in Geriatric Rehabilitation, 5*(1), 61-68.

Myers-Robfogel, M., & Bosmann, H. (1984). Clinical pharmacology in the aged: Aspects of pharmacokinetics and drug sensitivity. In T. Williams (Ed.), *Rehabilitation in the aging* (pp. 23-41). New York: Raven Press.

Ray, W., & Griffin, M. (1990). Prescribed medications and the risk of falling. *Topics in Geriatric Rehabilitation, 5*(2), 12-20.

Weg, R. (1990). Preventive and therapeutic nutrition. In S. Brody & L. Pawlson (Eds.), *Aging and rehabilitation II: The state of the practice* (pp. 165-185). New York: Springer Publishing Company.

Wenger, N. (1984). Cardiovascular status: Changes with aging. In T. Williams (Ed.), *Rehabilitation in the aging* (pp. 1-12). New York: Raven Press.

Woollacott, M. (1990). Changes in posture and voluntary control in the elderly: Research findings and rehabilitation. *Topics in Geriatric Rehabilitation, 5*(2), 1-11.

Suggested Readings

Brotman, H. (1982). *Every ninth American: An analysis for the chairman of the Select Committee on Aging, House of Representatives* (Committee Publication No. 97-332). Washington, DC: U.S. Government Printing Office.

Clark, G., & Murray, P. (1988). Rehabilitation of the geriatric patient. In J. DeLisa (Ed.), *Rehabilitation medicine: Principles and practice* (pp. 410-429). Philadelphia: J.B. Lippincott Company.

◆Fuller, J., & Winters, J. (1991). Joint loading during stretching exercises recommended for osteoarthritis: A biomechanical analysis. *Topics in Geriatric Rehabilitation, 6*(4), 25-33.

◆Fulper, K. (1989). Easy street: Efficacy of a simulated environment in geriatric rehabilitation. *Topics in Geriatric Rehabilitation, 4*(4), 82-85.

Hiatt, L. (1990). Environmental factors in rehabilitation of disabled elderly people. In S. Brody & L. Pawlson (Eds.), *Aging and rehabilitation II: The state of the practice* (pp. 150-164). New York: Springer Publishing Company.

Kane, R. (1990). Targeting geriatric assessment. In S. Brody & L. Pawlson (Eds.), *Aging and rehabilitation II: The state of the practice* (pp. 301-314). New York: Springer Publishing Company.

Nickel, V., & McGurk-Burleson, E. (1985). Concepts of rehabilitation. In T. Sculco (Ed.), *Orthopedic care of the geriatric patient* (pp. 357-369). St. Louis: The C.V. Mosby Company.

Torres-Gil, F., & Rosenquist, L. (1990). Public policy and geriatric rehabilitation. In B. Kemp, K. Brummel-Smith, & J. Ramsdell (Eds.), *Geriatric rehabilitation* (pp. 417-428). Boston: College-Hill Press, Inc.

Trieschmann, R. (1987). *Aging with a disability.* New York: Demos Publications.

◆Woollacott, M. (1990). Changes in posture and voluntary control in the elderly: Research findings and rehabilitation. *Topics in Geriatric Rehabilitation, 5*(2), 1-11.

◆indicates a research-based work

Section III
Functional Health Patterns and Nursing Diagnoses

Section III addresses the broad spectrum of clinical activities that compose the specialty of rehabilitation nursing. Rehabilitation nursing involves caring for clients of all ages in institutional and community-based settings. Nurses practicing in the specialty need both general and in-depth knowledge. Section III is designed to facilitate the nursing process; assist with organizing nursing care plans; provide material for educational programs; and enhance communication with clients, families, and other healthcare professionals.

Section III has 11 chapters, each of which represents a functional health pattern (labeled according to *Manual of Nursing Diagnosis: 1993-1994*, Gordon, 1993). Three areas are addressed within each functional pattern: (a) related theory and concepts, (b) nursing assessment, and (c) related nursing diagnoses with major interventions and expected outcomes. Most of the nursing diagnoses in this section have been approved by the North American Nursing Diagnosis Association (NANDA). The diagnoses range from those dealing with functional activities (such as self-care deficits), to those that are physiologic (e.g., autonomic dysreflexia), cognitive (e.g., impaired thought processes), and psychosocial (such as self-esteem disturbance). The definitions used in this section are primarily from Gordon (1993) and *Nursing Diagnoses: Definitions and Classification 1992-1993* (NANDA, 1992). Interventions and outcomes for the diagnoses are presented solely as guidelines for practice. Appropriate use of the guidelines requires accurate diagnoses, relevant nursing knowledge, consideration of clients' goals, and familiarity with institutional protocols.

Editor's note: References are found at the end of each chapter and, where necessary, are listed by major topics within the chapter. Throughout the section, the ➤ symbol indicates a nursing diagnosis, and the key parts of the diagnosis (e.g., interventions) are set apart by rules. The 11 functional health patterns are used with permission of Mosby-Year Book, Inc. The nursing diagnoses are used with permission of the North American Nursing Diagnosis Association.

References

Gordon, M. (1993). *Manual of nursing diagnosis: 1993-1994.* St. Louis: Mosby-Year Book, Inc.

North American Nursing Diagnosis Association (NANDA). (1992). *NANDA nursing diagnoses: Definitions and classification 1992-1993.* St. Louis: Author.

CHAPTER 11

Health Perception–Health Management Pattern

"The goal of rehabilitation nursing is to assist the individual with disability and chronic illness in the restoration and maintenance of maximal health" (American Nurses' Association & Association of Rehabilitation Nurses, 1988, p. 4). For the rehabilitation client, effective health management is critical to achieving and maintaining an optimal quality of life. The prevention of further loss of function through avoidance of injury is essential to wellness. When disabled individuals are unable to meet their self-care needs as a result of functional impairment, they assume management of their health by supervising and/or training others. As a result of the relationship between the rehabilitation nurse and the client, the client becomes the expert in his or her own health management needs.

Providing a safe environment is essential in both institutional and home settings. The impact of falls and injuries on the client and the family cannot be underestimated. In addition to causing physical and emotional harm, injuries prolong the rehabilitation process, increase the cost of health care, and can result in questions of liability and negligence. Issues of patients' rights, advocacy, and restraint-free environments have forced professional nurses to evaluate the assessment and implementation of safety interventions for clients. Education of the client and the client's family is essential to the client's achievement of self-care management and maintenance of safety within a facility or a home setting.

The test of successful rehabilitation nursing is the transfer of knowledge and accountability for healthcare needs from nurses to clients, families, and significant others in a manner that promotes health and wellness for the individual with a disability. Included in this chapter are the concepts of health and wellness and the prevention of injuries, related assessment factors, and the nursing diagnoses of health management deficit and high risk for injury. The case study that is also included analyzes the client's level of health-seeking behaviors, participation in preventive practices, and adherence to prescribed therapy and follow-up care.

I. Related Theory and Concepts

A. Definitions of wellness

1. "Wellness, from a holistic perspective, implies integration of optimal mental, physical, emotional, and psychological functioning" (Frye, 1986, p. 6)
2. Wellness is a dynamic state that necessitates continuous balancing; Dunn (1961) stated that it is "an integrated method of functioning which is oriented toward maximizing the potential of which the individual is capable, within the environment where he is functioning" (p. 4)

B. Wellness-related theories

1. Self-responsibility (Ardell & Tager, 1982)
   a. This theory envisioned a five-dimensional framework in which the core dimension of self-responsibility is the hub of a circle, surrounded by four dimensions
      1) Physical fitness
      2) Stress awareness and management
      3) Environmental sensitivity
      4) Nutritional awareness
   b. Five beliefs denote a high level of responsibility for oneself and are summarized in the statements that follow (Ardell & Tager, 1982)
      1) I am in control of my health
      2) Whether sick or well, I am responsible for my state of health
      3) The main factors affecting my health are my attitude, my beliefs, and my behaviors
      4) If I take care of myself, I can drastically reduce my prospects for illness and dramatically improve my chances of optimal functioning
      5) If I lead a wellness lifestyle, I can come close to my best potential and derive great satisfaction
   c. Wellness is a uniquely defined personal concept (Ardell & Tager, 1982)
   d. Wellness requires active participation and is based on personal experience and observation—that is, learning through experiencing the positive or negative consequences of behavioral choices made by oneself or others (Ardell & Tager, 1982)
2. Theory of hardiness (Kobasa, Hilker, & Maddi, 1979; Kobasa, Maddi, & Zola, 1983)
   a. "Persons high in hardiness involve themselves in whatever they are doing (commitment), believe and act as if they can influence the events forming their lives (control) and consider change to be not only normal but also a stimulus to development (challenge)" (Kobasa et al.,

1983, p. 596)

b. Characteristics of persons with a low level of hardiness
    1) Alienation
    2) Sense of powerlessness
    3) Sense of threat in the dynamic, changing process of life

c. Persons with a high level of hardiness maintain and strive for wellness even in highly stressful situations

3. Locus of control
    a. Locus of control is the "individual's beliefs about whether or not a contingency relationship exists between behavior (action) and reinforcements (outcomes)" (Shillinger, 1983, p. 59)
    b. Types of control: Internal versus external (Lefcourt, 1981)
        1) Internal control: Individual's belief that his or her own actions influence outcome
        2) External control: Individual's belief that external forces determine outcome
            a) Chance as an external locus of control: Client's belief that events occur randomly and are totally divorced from individual action
            b) Powerful others as an external locus of control: Client's belief that outcomes are dominated by powerful authority figures

4. Self-efficacy (Bandura, 1977, 1982)
    a. Definition: Belief that one is capable of a behavior
    b. Characteristics of high self-efficacy include the ability to organize and mobilize cognitive, social, and behavioral skills in changing circumstances (i.e., flexibility and transfer of learning)
    c. Individuals high in self-efficacy strive to achieve their maximum potential

5. Health belief model (Becker, 1974; Clark, 1986)
    a. Attempts to explain differences among individuals in several areas
        1) Participation in health programs
        2) Response to symptoms
        3) Compliance with medical regimens
    b. Six dimensions of beliefs affect decision making and motivation
        1) Perceived susceptibility
        2) Perceived severity (consequences)
        3) Perceived benefits
        4) Perceived barriers
        5) Perceived cues to action
        6) Motivation related to general health

C. Concepts related to prevention of injury: Prevention of falls and related injuries is an essential aspect of health management for people with disabilities

1. Patients at risk for falling
    a. Number of factors that have potential impact on the risk of falling is infinite
    b. There have been numerous studies on risk factors associated with falls in the elderly population, very often associated with risk management programs or nursing diagnoses (Hendrich, 1988a, 1988b; Robbins et al., 1989; Ross, Watson, Gyldenvand, & Reinboth, 1991)
    c. Research specifically addressing risk factors related to falling in a rehabilitation setting has been minimal (Vlahov, Myers, & Al-Ibrahim, 1990)
    d. Studies that have been conducted in rehabilitation settings report various findings
        1) In a study by Mion et al. (1989) on medical rehabilitation patients, altered proprioception was the only major predictor of falling
        2) Grant and Hamilton (1987) reported on those who were most at risk for falling
            a) Patients 60 years of age and older
            b) Patients diagnosed with cerebrovascular accident (CVA)
            c) Patients diagnosed with closed head injury
            d) Patients with a previous history of falling
        3) DeVincenzo and Watkins (1987) performed a risk management study on accidental falls
            a) Patients most often fell during the 1st and 4th week of hospitalization
            b) Most falls occurred in the patients' bedrooms
            c) Patients were likely to be in wheelchairs
            d) CVA patients accounted for most of the falls
        4) A study on medical, surgical, and nursing home units (Brians, Alexander, Grota, Chen, & Dumas, 1991) at a large veterans hospital indicated that only four variables were statistically related to patient falls; patients with one or more of these four variables was at even greater risk if they were in wheelchairs
            a) Dizziness, unsteady gait, impaired balance
            b) Impaired memory or judgment
            c) Weakness
            d) A history of falling

2. Education of patient, patient's family, and all staff
    a. Is the single most important consideration in maintaining a safe environment and minimizing risk of injury
    b. Includes thorough assessment of patient's strengths and needs; always should include safety issues

3. Use of restraints
    a. Physical restraint: Defined as "any manual method or physical or mechanical device, material, or equipment attached or adjacent to the individual's body that the individual cannot remove easily which restricts freedom of movement or normal access to one's body" (Health Care Financing Administration (HCFA), 1991, p. 51)
    b. Chemical restraint
        1) Defined as "drugs prescribed to control mood, mental status or behavior" (HCFA, 1991, p. 51)
        2) Can have potential side effects in the elderly

(Hendrich, 1988a)
a) oversedation
b) increased confusion
c) orthostatic hypotension
d) Parkinsonian syndrome-type reactions

c. Neither physical nor chemical restraints necessarily lessen agitated and confused behavior
   1) Restraints can increase injury
   2) Patients continue to fall, trying to go over bed rails or getting tangled in restraints
d. An alternative is a restraint-free environment altered to maintain the patient's safety

II. Nursing Assessment

A. Client's coping status regarding responsibility for and access to health care
   1. Health and lifestyle prior to injury or illness
   2. Interest in a health management program
   3. Ability and motivation to take responsibility for health, including knowledge of nutritional needs
   4. Access to and availability of healthcare providers and facilities
   5. Knowledge of prescribed medications and their effects
   6. Knowledge of medical status and related treatment program

B. Client's emotional status
   1. Resolution of grieving process related to injury and/or disease
   2. Chemical dependency
   3. Methods of coping

C. Client's functional status
   1. Strength and endurance
   2. Self-care needs (e.g., feeding, bathing, dressing, toileting)
   3. Mobility status: Use of adaptive equipment or devices
   4. Continence and elimination needs
   5. Communication abilities
   6. Ability to monitor environment

D. Client's general health and medical status
   1. History of falls, seizures, or orthostatic hypotension
   2. Perception and sensation (including vision and proprioception
   3. Sleep and rest needs

E. Client's cognitive status
   1. Memory
   2. Judgment
   3. Reasoning
   4. Problem solving

F. Availability of family and social support systems

G. Availability of financial resources adequate to meet healthcare needs

H. Availability of community resources to help with promotion of wellness

III. Nursing Diagnoses

➤ **A. Health management deficit**

1. **Definition:** Inability to identify and manage necessary aspects of care and health promotion activities

2. Major defining characteristics

a. Verbalized or demonstrated lack of knowledge, comprehension, and/or motor skills required for meeting basic health needs and health promotion
b. Evidence of preventable complications and occurrence of undesirable outcomes
c. Evidence of noncompliance or ineffective management of therapeutic regimen
d. Verbalization of difficulty in caring for self or environment

3. Related factors/etiologies

a. Physical
   1) Loss of body part
   2) Sensory deficits
   3) Motor skills deficit
   4) Chemical dependency
   5) Debilitating disease or injury
   6) Pain
b. Emotional/maturational
   1) Depression; prolonged or dysfunctional grieving
   2) Decreased self-esteem
   3) Lack of experience in managing wellness
   4) Lack of motivation
c. Cognitive
   1) Perceptual deficits
   2) Communication deficits
   3) Inexperience with, or inability to comprehend or follow, a new or complex treatment regimen
   4) Lack of education or intellectual development
d. Social/economic
   1) Inability to gain access to the healthcare system
   2) Nontherapeutic relationships with healthcare providers (e.g., healthcare professionals, personal care attendants)
   3) Decreased social support
   4) Spiritual and cultural influences on personal health beliefs
   5) Language differences that interfere with ability to gain access to or use healthcare or self-care resources
   6) Funding resources inadequate to obtain and maintain needed equipment, supplies, and services

4. Interventions

a. Identify and designate person(s) responsible for health management—for example, client, parent, spouse
   1) Interventions are directed toward all responsible persons
   2) Other responsible persons are directed to act on behalf of the client to promote client's wellness and health management
b. Educate client at his or her learning level to fa-

cilitate health maintenance
1) Use teaching tools (written materials, audio- or videotapes, lectures, models)
2) Use demonstrations and return demonstrations
3) Use memory aids—for example, written reminders, medication dispensers, consistent location of supplies, software for life skills
4) Provide progressive sequential learning experiences that build on skills without overwhelming the learner (e.g., having the client take on progressive responsibility for bladder management)

c. For institutionalized clients, design a physical environment that minimizes dependency and the sick role
1) Have clients and healthcare providers wear street clothes
2) Make environment and activities as realistic (home-like) as possible; suggestions follow below
   a) Client should eat meals in a dining room with other people
   b) Client should have access to food and beverages between meals
3) Help clients identify and begin to resume family role responsibilities within the family structure
4) Provide privacy for client when he or she is performing physical care and interacting with others and allow time for client to be alone
5) Introduce client to role models—for example, other clients who demonstrate competence in managing their health and wellness

d. Establish a milieu that fosters self-reliance and wellness
1) Encourage client to set goals with the assistance of the healthcare provider
2) Encourage client to become involved in all phases of care planning; promote client's control of the process
3) Negotiate to simplify or alter client behaviors and outcomes; adapt program methods or schedules to client's preferred routine
4) Avoid assuming a "powerful other" role that reinforces external control
5) Create a contract with client to define agreed-upon responsibilities and conditions for program participation
6) If indicated, institute a behavioral modification program and provide rewards for positive learning and behaviors

e. Refer client to community resources and support groups

f. Involve case manager (e.g., home health agency nurse, insurance nurse case manager) in long-term follow-up and assessment of transition from inpatient to outpatient settings (see Figure 11.1)

5. Expected outcomes

a. Client demonstrates ability to manage healthcare activities necessary for optimal wellness
b. Client is able to teach caregiver skills and knowledge necessary for maintaining optimal health and wellness

➤ **B. High risk for falls and injury**

1. Definition: State in which an individual is predisposed to risk of bodily injury

2. Risk factors

a. Knowledge deficit regarding safety techniques and proper use of equipment
b. Impaired mobility
c. Neuromuscular deficit
d. Cognitive deficit
e. Impaired sensation or perception
   1) Temperature
   2) Touch
   3) Position sense (proprioception)
   4) Vision
   5) Hearing
f. Environmental hazards
g. Adverse effects of medication
h. Unmet elimination needs
i. Seizures, vertigo
j. Fatigue
k. Use of chemical or physical restraints
l. History of falling

3. Interventions

a. Teach client and family to monitor for environmental hazards; recommend changes to allow for highest level of safety
   1) Grab bars and/or handrails
   2) Mobility devices
   3) Uncluttered floors (no scatter rugs)
   4) Frequently used items kept in easily accessible places
   5) Adequate lighting, especially at night
   6) Bed in low position
b. Help client meet self-care needs until independence can be achieved or attendant or caretaker has received appropriate education
c. Teach client and family the potential side effects of medications and alcohol
d. Ensure safety for patient who has cognitive or thought process deficits by changing environment to meet safety needs
   1) Provide method to communicate with caregiver
   2) Establish a toileting program
   3) Install door locks or an escape alarm
   4) Provide an organized, consistent, uncluttered environment
e. Teach mechanisms to compensate for sensory-perceptual deficits
   1) Testing water before bathing
   2) Using compensatory strategies for visual field deficits

Figure 11.1. Client Case Study: Health Management Deficit

This case study is condensed to highlight aspects relating to the client's management of his health care.

Client's History

The client was a 28-year-old male with a C5 spinal cord injury that occurred when he was 25, after a diving accident he had while intoxicated; the case involved workers' compensation liability.

Setting

The client lived in the community.

Presenting information

The client was referred to a home health agency for around-the-clock personal care, community reintegration, and long-term case management. The client had switched agencies seven times and had a community-wide reputation for verbal abusiveness, lack of cooperation, and unrealistic goals and expectations.

Nursing Summary

The client had permanent quadriplegia. His physical rehabilitation was comprehensive and completed at a major rehabilitation center. His emotional and social rehabilitation required continued support to promote adjustment. The client was angry, denied responsibility, and rejected or sabotaged interventions that would lead to independence.

The client had no personal life goals. His focus was on controlling daily care, characterized by frequent rigidity and whimsical changes of mind. His pattern of control lacked predictability or logical reason, and he jeopardized his health by placing himself at risk of injury and complications. He placed blame on others (such as his caregivers, the payer, and the rehabilitation center) for his social isolation and physical complications.

Related Factors

- Depression and dysfunctional grieving
- Decreased self-esteem
- Motor skill deficits
- Nontherapeutic relationships with healthcare providers
- Decreased social support
- Maturational (age-related) factors

Goals and Plan of Care

The client expressed a desire to achieve several goals:

- consistent group of team members—that is, dealing with the same people consistently,
- reliable scheduling, and
- knowledgeable and competent caregivers.

The rehabilitation nurse case manager agreed to the goals and added the following:

- multidisciplinary evaluations to ensure safety and adequacy of all activities and environments,
- establishment of criteria for client's acceptance or rejection of caregivers, and
- clear communication and defined authority for both the client and the agency.

The client agreed to these goals and was accepted by the agency for care.

Implementation

Bladder management: The rehabilitation nurse case manager provided education on bladder management techniques and the minimum requirements for safety and infection control. In collaboration with the physician, the client was asked to select a method of bladder management. The client selected the times of day and specific techniques for his bladder program.

Establishing the team of caregivers: The client was asked to interview and select agency caregivers, determine their shifts, and negotiate a schedule for each caregiver. The agency screened caregivers for knowledge and skills and maintained a master scheduling calendar. The case manager maintained routine contact with the client to make sure that all shifts were covered. He also was permitted to request the removal of a caregiver from his team for defined causes; all removals had to be arranged with advance notice to allow for rescheduling of the team. If the client failed to provide advance notice, then replacement was not guaranteed.

(continued on next page)

3) Preventing burns and frostbite

f. Teach client and family the signs and symptoms of seizure activity and ways to maintain safety during and after a seizure
g. Teach safety factors associated with transfer techniques, gait training, and mobility devices
h. Provide proper, well-maintained footwear
i. Ensure that the toileting program is adequate to meet nighttime needs
j. Teach patient and family how to decrease effects of orthostatic hypotension—for example, sitting on edge of bed for several seconds before transferring
k. Provide information on community resources, as appropriate; this can include information on emergency call devices for outside assistance when client is alone
l. Use distractions, redirection, humor, and quiet areas to decrease agitated behavior without use of restraints

4. Expected outcomes

a. Client will be free of physical injury
b. Patient and family verbalize or demonstrate an awareness of risk factors related to patient's specific deficits
c. Patient and family are aware of how to seek assistance if an injury does occur

References

American Nurses' Association & Association of Rehabilitation Nurses. (1988). *Rehabilitation nursing: Scope of practice; process and outcome criteria for selected diagnoses.* Kansas City, MO: American Nurses' Association.

Ardell, D.B., & Tager, M.J. (1982). *Planning for wellness: A guidebook for achieving optimal health* (2nd ed.). Dubuque, IA: Kendall/Hunt Publishing Company.

Bandura, A. (1977). *Social learning theory.* Englewood Cliffs, NJ: Prentice-Hall, Inc.

Bandura, A. (1982). Self-efficacy: Mechanism in human agency. *American Psychologist, 32*(2), 122-147.

Figure 11.1. *(continued)*

Transportation: The rehabilitation nurse, the physical therapist, and the client discussed his transportation needs. Caregivers were permitted to drive the client and to perform car transfers into vehicles approved by the therapist as being safe for transfers. The client was asked to select an appropriate vehicle. He also was asked to accompany his caregivers on errands, such as to the grocery store, and to plan social outings.

Collaboration

In promoting the client's role in making choices, the rehabilitation professionals had to allow the client to select risky options and to learn to accept the consequences. The team members needed to exercise consistency in their behaviors with the client so that the client could not manipulate them or blame them for outcomes. The whole team's collaboration was essential for success.

Case conferences: The home health agency rehabilitation nurse case manager conducted regular case conferences at the agency office for the caregivers. This allowed the team to plan a strategy to deal with the client's behavior and developed a strong team support network. Case conferences also were held at the client's home to ensure his participation and to promote control of his care.

Contact with other involved parties: There was regular contact with the insurance case manager, the client's attorney, and the physician. These team members attended the conferences in person or by phone, when appropriate.

Evaluation

At the outset of service, the client challenged the scope of all agreements and established goals. The team developed a contract with the client that established the parameters of service. The client was given a range of options for his care, but limits were established to minimize the severity of the consequences of any poor decisions he might make. As the client demonstrated his willingness to make healthy choices, restrictions were gradually lifted.

Bladder management: The client selected intermittent catheterization for bladder management despite recommendations for an external catheter. The client had to agree to allow the caregiver to perform the catheterization at the necessary times, to arrange his outings to fit the schedule, and to structure his fluid intake. To date, there has been no incidence of urinary tract infection or episodes of incontinence (reflex emptying).

Establishing the team of caregivers: It took several weeks to establish a stable team of caregivers. The client wanted only young, attractive females. He was educated about antidiscrimination laws and the agency's policy on fair hiring and was offered the alternative of choosing another agency. The case manager assisted him in interviewing caregivers and screening them for knowledge and competence. In the first weeks, he made last-minute cancellations of visits from caregivers whom he did not like and procrastinated on outings so that shift changes occurred late. This created gaps in his schedule and caused caregivers to disrupt their own plans. He was allowed to experience being without a caregiver for several hours. Caregivers were given authority to refuse to take him on an outing if a late return would interfere with their after-hours activities. The client now communicates desired schedule changes to the agency and has learned constructive ways to have caregivers removed from his team. He is learning that treating his caregivers with respect will win their cooperation in doing tasks his way.

Transportation: The client wanted to continue using his two-seat sports car. The physical therapist instructed the client on body mechanics and the risks of using this car. Several caregivers had sustained back injuries from previous employment. Alternatives for transportation were discussed. Initially, the client asked his family and friends to transfer him. When these people began to refuse, he decided to purchase a van.

Conclusion

Developing this client's self-management skills involved an initial setting of limits and giving the client a selection of options. As the client learned to make constructive decisions, he demonstrated appropriate health management skills and was rewarded with expanded options. Note the parallels of this process to the wellness-related theories, particularly those of Ardell and Tager (self-responsibility) (1982), Kobasa, Maddi, and Zola (hardiness) (1983), and Lefcourt (locus of control) (1981).

Becker, M.H. (1974, Winter). The health belief model and sick role behavior. *Health Education Monographs,* pp. 409-419.

Brians, L. Alexander, K., Grota, P., Chen, R., & Dumas, V. (1991). The development of the risk tool for fall prevention. *Rehabilitation Nursing, 16,* 67-69.

Clark, C. (1986). *Wellness nursing: Concepts, theory, research, and practice.* New York: Springer Publishing Company.

DeVincenzo, D., & Watkins, S. (1987). Accidental falls in a rehabilitation setting. *Rehabilitation Nursing, 12,* 248-252.

Dunn, H. (1961). *High level wellness.* Arlington, VA: R.W. Beatty Company.

Frye, B. (1986). A model of wellness-seeking behavior in traumatic spinal cord injury victims. *Rehabilitation Nursing, 11*(5), 6-7, 14.

◆Grant, J., & Hamilton, S. (1987). Falls in a rehabilitation center: A retrospective and comparative analysis. *Rehabilitation Nursing, 12,* 74-76.

Health Care Financing Administration (HCFA). (1991). *Interpretive guidelines: Skilled nursing facilities and intermediate care facilities* [Standard: 483, 13(a)]. Austin, TX: Texas Department of Human Services.

Hendrich, A. (1988a). *Patient fall prevention.* Greencastle, IN: Ann Hendrich & Associates, Inc.

Hendrich, A. (1988b). An effective unit-based fall prevention program. *Journal of Nursing Quality Assurance, 3*(1), 28-36.

Kobasa, S.C., Hilker, R.R., & Maddi, S.R. (1979). Who stays healthy under stress. *Journal of Occupational Medicine, 21,* 595-598.

Kobasa, S.C., Maddi, S.R., & Zola, M.A. (1983). Type A and hardiness. *Journal of Behavioral Medicine, 6*(1), 41-49.

Lefcourt, H. (Ed.). (1981). *Research with locus of control construct.* New York: Academic Press, Inc.

◆Mion, L., Gregor, S., Buettner, M., Chwirchak, D., Lee, O., & Paras, W. (1989). Falls in the rehabilitation setting: Incidence and characteristics. *Rehabilitation Nursing, 14,* 17-22.

Robbins, A., Rubenstein, L., Josephson, K., Schulman, B., Osterweil, D., & Fine, G. (1989). Predictors of falls among elderly people. *Archives of Internal Medicine, 149,* 1628-1633.

Ross, J., Watson, C., Gyldenvand, T., & Reinboth, J. (1991). Potential for trauma: Falls. In M. Maas, K. Buckwalter, & M. Hardy (Eds.). *Nursing diagnoses and interventions in the elderly* (pp. 18-31). Redwood City, CA: Addison-Wesley Nursing.

Shillinger, F. (1983). Locus of control: Implications for clinical nursing practice. *Image: The Journal of Nursing Scholarship, 15*(2), 58-63.

◆Vlahov, D., Myers, A., & Al-Ibrahim, M. (1990). Epidemiology of falls among patients in a rehabilitation hospital. *Archives of Physical Medicine and Rehabilitation, 71*, 8-12.

Suggested Readings

Association of Rehabilitation Nurses. (1991). *The rehabilitation nurse case manager: Role description.* Skokie, IL: Author.

Becker, M.H. (Ed.). (1974). *The health belief model and personal health behavior.* Thorofare, NJ: Charles B. Slack.

Campbell, C. (1984). *Nursing diagnosis and intervention in nursing practice* (2nd ed.) (pp. 1396-1399). New York: John Wiley & Sons.

Carpenito, L. (1991). *Nursing care plans and documentation: Nursing diagnoses and collaborative problems.* Philadelphia: J.B. Lippincott Company.

Derstine, J. (1987). Wellness: A theme for an elective course in rehabilitation nursing. *Rehabilitation Nursing, 12*, 16, 33-34.

Gordon, M. (1991). *Manual of nursing diagnosis: 1991-1992.* St. Louis: Mosby-Year Book, Inc.

Hearne, J., & Klockens, A.J. (1988). Applicability of the Parcel-Meyer Children's Health Locus of Control Scale. *Journal of School Health, 58*(1), 16-19.

Kelly, M.P. (1992). Health promotion in primary care: Taking account of the patient's point of view. *Journal of Advanced Nursing, 17*(1), 93-100.

Kelly, R.B., Zyzanski, S.J., & Alemagno, S.A. (1991). Prediction of motivation and behavior changes following health promotion: Role of health beliefs, social support and self-efficacy. *Social Science Medicine, 32*, 311-320.

◆Mayo, N., Korner-Bitensky, N., Becker, R., & Georges, P. (1989). Predicting falls among patients in a rehabilitation hospital. *American Journal of Physical Medicine and Rehabilitation, 68*(3), 139-146.

Mitchell II, M. (1989). *Neuroscience nursing: A nursing diagnosis approach.* Baltimore: Williams & Wilkins.

Mumma, C.M. (Ed.). (1987). *Rehabilitation nursing: Concepts and practice—A core curriculum* (2nd ed.) (pp. 28-35, 152-155). Evanston, IL: Rehabilitation Nursing Foundation.

Myles, S. (1988). Monitoring patient safety at the bedside. *Journal of Nursing Quality Assurance, 3*(1), 57-62.

O'Brien, B., O'Such, D., & Palette, S. (1987). Setting realistic goals for quality assurance monitoring: Patient falls versus patient days. *Quality Review Bulletin, 13*, 339-342.

Palanck, C.L. (1991). Determinants of health promotive behaviors: A review of current research. *Nursing Clinics of North America, 26*, 815-832.

◆Raz, T., & Baretich, M. (1987). Factors affecting the incidence of patient falls in hospitals. *Medical Care, 25*(3), 185-194.

Reames, K. (1988). Ensuring patient safety. *Journal of Nursing Quality Assurance, 3*(1), 72-75.

Speake, D.L., Cowart, M.E., & Pettet, K. (1989). Health perceptions and health behaviors of the elderly. *Research in Nursing and Health, 12*(2), 93-100.

Weinberg, L., Babicki, C., & McIntyre, K. (1988). *Rehabilitation nursing care plan stimulators* (p. 52). Washington, DC: National Rehabilitation Hospital.

Young, H.M., Lierman, L., Powell-Cope, G., Kasprzyk, D., & Benoliel, J.Q. (1991). Operationalizing the theory of planned behavior. *Research in Nursing and Health, 14*(2), 137-144.

◆ indicates a research-based work

CHAPTER 12

Nutritional–Metabolic Pattern

Adequate nutrition is a significant goal for people with physical disabilities and chronic diseases. Clients' participation in a rehabilitation program demands strength and energy. Underweight clients risk complications such as skin breakdown and often lack the energy needed for activities of daily living. Overweight clients can experience problems with endurance that add to the difficulties of those providing their physical care. In the unresponsive patient with central nervous system (CNS) damage, nutrition is important to sustain life and potentiate recovery.

Disabled persons—whether in the community or in an institutional setting—need optimal nutrition to prevent complications and to maximize the physical quality of their lives. Rehabilitation nurses can help individuals maintain a desired level of nutrition through specific nursing interventions and consultation with other rehabilitation team members.

The nursing diagnoses of altered nutrition (less than body requirements), fluid volume deficit/fluid volume excess, and impaired swallowing are included in this chapter because they directly pertain to nourishment. The nursing diagnoses of high risk for skin breakdown and pressure ulcers relate to inadequate nutrition and metabolic changes, which predispose the human organism to skin breakdown. Autonomic dysreflexia, also the result of an alteration in metabolism, is included as a nursing diagnosis as well.

Nutrition and Metabolism

I. Related Theory and Concepts

A. Physiological principles related to nourishment

1. Normal growth and development as well as physical and mental functioning throughout the life span depend on adequate amounts of several nutrients
   a. Protein
   b. Carbohydrates
   c. Fat
   d. Calories
   e. Vitamins
   f. Minerals
   g. Fluids
   h. Electrolytes
2. Adequate nutritional intake of the above elements depends on numerous factors as specified by Drinka and Goodwin (1991)
   a. Appetite
   b. Smell
   c. Taste
   d. Access to food
   e. Attentiveness
   f. Dexterity
   g. Mastication
   h. Swallowing
   i. Digestion
   j. Absorption
   k. Transport
   l. Storage
   m. Metabolic demand
   n. Excretion

B. Nutritional considerations in neurological injury and illness

1. Especially if traumatic in nature, neurological injury or illness interferes with metabolism and places clients at risk for protein and caloric deficits (Bivins & Fath, 1990)
2. After trauma, disequilibrium typically results from decreased oral intake with simultaneous increased nutritional requirements
   a. Inadequate protein can be devastating to the recovery process because it is necessary for several activities (Williams, 1989)
      1) Building and sustaining tissue
      2) Maintaining energy
      3) Maintaining various physiological processes, including hormone, enzyme, and antibody activity
   b. According to Blissitt (1990), "carbohydrates and fat are used for energy, and protein is reserved for tissue repair synthesis" (p. 375)
3. Traumatic spinal cord injury and brain injury seem to produce acute hypermetabolic states (Bivins & Fath, 1990; Kaufman et al., 1987; Moore, Najarian, & Konvolinka, 1989)
   a. Such injuries trigger a catabolic response in which endogenous (internal) proteins are broken down
   b. Potential complications arising from catabolism
      1) Protein and/or caloric malnutrition
      2) Increased susceptibility to infection
      3) Respiratory distress
      4) Poor wound healing
      5) Slowed recovery
4. During stress (trauma), glycogen stores in the liver and muscle cells are temporarily converted to glucose for energy (glycogenolysis); because of the high energy demands, proteins—rather than stored fats—are used as energy sources; thus, further pro-

tein depletion occurs

5. Trauma and/or sepsis can also cause high nitrogen excretion from breakdown of muscle and lean body mass; the muscle flaccidity associated with acute SCI enhances nitrogen and calcium losses even more than does immobilization (Kearns, Thompson, Werner, Pipp, & Wilmot, 1992)
6. Nitrogen is normally necessary in order for tissue synthesis (growth, tissue repair, muscle development) to occur; it comes from dietary protein (Bodinski, 1987)
   a. Exogenous (food) protein is essential because once it is eaten, it is digested and turned into amino acids in the alimentary tract
   b. These amino acids are absorbed and transported to cells where they are converted to substances such as collagen and myosin
7. Effects of *traumatic brain injury* on nutrition (Yankelson, 1990)
   a. Damage to the hypothalamus, which can produce hyperphagia; this is displayed in several behaviors
      1) Loss of satiety
      2) Desire to eat and/or drink constantly—especially palatable foods such as sweets
      3) Hoarding of food
      4) Eating nonedible items
   b. Frontal lobe damage, which can create problems with initiation: for example, even though clients might be hungry, they cannot initiate the motor act of eating without being cued
8. Effects of *stroke* on nutrition
   a. Elderly stroke patients might have malnourishment and vitamin deficiencies on admission to rehabilitation (Axelsson, Asplund, Norberg, & Eriksson, 1989; Morely, 1991)
   b. Axelsson et al. (1989) found that nutritional status of those with right-arm paresis was worse than that of those with left-arm paresis
9. Effects of *respiratory disease* on nutrition
   a. Depression, anorexia, side effects of medication, fatigue, and difficulty eating during dyspneic episodes are often associated with a less-than-adequate intake of nutrients
   b. Caloric needs are increased in persons with respiratory disease due to several factors (Kersten, 1989)
      1) Increased work of breathing
      2) Increased dead space ventilation
      3) Inefficient gas exchange
      4) Increased oxygen consumption
   c. Excessive carbohydrate intake (> 500 gm/day) results in increased oxygen consumption and CO_2 production and retention, compounding already existing respiratory insufficiency (Miller, 1986)

C. Pediatric considerations

1. Nutritional management of the disabled child presents unique challenges due to alterations in growth, body composition, energy requirements, and feeding difficulties (Dudek, 1987)
2. Dietary assessment of the disabled child should include both what and how much the child eats
3. The family's perception of the child's nutritional status is a critical factor in selecting a therapeutic approach
4. Therapeutic approaches to nutritional therapy for children with disabilities include food supplements, nighttime nasogastric feedings, nasojejunal feedings if esophageal reflux is a problem, and feeding via gastrostomy
5. Oral food intake and activities involved in chewing, sucking, and swallowing help to develop the oropharyngeal musculature needed for speech; if oral intake is bypassed early in life, other interventions must substitute for the role of food intake in speech development (Dietz & Bandini, 1989)
6. Children receiving long-term anticonvulsant therapy are at high risk for vitamin D and folate deficiencies, altered calcium metabolism, and pathologic fractures

II. Nursing Assessment

A. Nutritional intake
   1. Amount and type
   2. Food preferences and/or cultural patterns
   3. Food intolerances
   4. Appetite

B. Height, premorbid and current weight

C. Activity level (voluntary and involuntary)

D. Condition of hair and skin

E. Ability to taste and smell

F. Ability to swallow

G. Dentition

H. Medications

I. Temperature

J. Affect

III. Nursing Diagnosis

➤ **A. Altered nutrition—less than body requirements**

1. **Definition:** Intake of nutrients insufficient to meet metabolic needs

2. **Major defining characteristics**
   a. Body weight 20% or more below ideal
   b. Reported or observed inadequate caloric and nutritional intake relative to minimum daily requirements
   c. Weight loss (with or without adequate intake)
   d. Pale conjunctiva and mucous membranes
   e. Fatigue
   f. Excessive hair loss, poor muscle tone

3. **Related factors/etiologies**
   a. Altered taste and olfactory sensation
   b. Inability to procure or prepare food
   c. Inability to chew, masticate, or swallow
   d. Knowledge deficit about daily requirements
   e. Anorexia
   f. Inability to digest food or absorb nutrients
   g. Impairment of cognition or consciousness
   h. Depression

i. Chemical dependency
j. Hypermetabolism after trauma, injury, stress

4. Nursing interventions

a. General
 1) Weigh client routinely or have client monitor his or her own weight
 2) Teach client and/or family importance of nutrition related to client's disease or disability; have client keep nutritional record
 3) Teach client purpose of having a high-fiber diet and adequate fluid intake to help promote optimal bowel and bladder functioning; encourage him or her to follow such a diet
 4) Intervene appropriately and supportively for depression, because it may create over- or undereating
 5) Administer vitamins and minerals as ordered
 6) Assist client with feeding as necessary
 7) Refer client to community resources, when indicated, for assistance with food procurement and preparation

b. Interventions specific to *stroke*
 1) Follow interventions listed in the "Impaired Swallowing" section of this chapter (see page 81)
 2) Insert client's dentures prior to meals; obtain referral to a dentist if dentures no longer fit
 3) Place food, drink, and pills on unaffected side of client's tongue
 4) Offer several small meals per day if client fatigues easily at mealtime; this might help with endurance levels during therapy and with attention deficits
 5) Help client to sit upright for oral intake
 6) Cue client verbally regarding feeding principles if he or she is dysphagic or if neglect or hemianopsia is present

c. Interventions specific to *orthopedic and/or musculoskeletal disorders*
 1) Amputation: Explain importance of dietary intake of protein, zinc, and vitamin C in wound healing
 2) Rheumatoid arthritis: Impact of food on rheumatoid arthritis is being researched
  a) Be supportive and communicative rather than judgmental or critical when patients inquire about topics such as nonmedical remedies involving food
  b) Recommend a balanced diet
  c) Teach overweight clients importance of weight reduction to reduce strain on joints
  d) Consult with an occupational therapist to teach client joint-saving strategies for kitchen organization and methods of joint protection and energy conservation during meal preparation and cleanup (Dudek, 1987)

d. Interventions specific to *traumatic brain injury*: Vary greatly depending on the patient's level of consciousness, behaviors, short-term memory, and learning capabilities
 1) Monitor client for dysphagia (see "Impaired Swallowing" section of this chapter on pages 79-83)
 2) Administer intermittent (or continuous) tube feedings to patients with head of bed elevated at least 30 degrees
 3) Change tube-feeding regimens in comatose patients (per order and/or protocol) based on daily assessments
  a) Posturing or spasms
  b) Constipation
  c) Infection and/or fever
  d) Medication changes
  e) Weight
  f) Skin condition
  g) Estimated nutrient needs (as calculated by a dietitian)
  h) Serum and urine laboratory values (Godbole, Berbiglia, & Goddard, 1991; Yankelson, 1990)
 4) If short-term memory is impaired, potential strategies suggested by Yankelson (1990) can be tried
  a) Use repetition; give the same information in several ways (for example, verbally, in writing, via demonstration)
  b) Develop and follow through with consistent team feeding program
  c) Use visual aids, especially in game format for those with minimal short-term memory loss
  d) Verbally cue or set a timer to remind patient to continue eating if attention is poor or there is short-term memory loss
  e) When feasible, engage patient in typical activities of daily living
   (1) Menu and meal planning
   (2) Grocery shopping
   (3) Cooking
   (4) Social skills associated with eating (for example, table manners)
 5) Give one item of food or drink at a time if patient displays impulsivity; otherwise, patient might consume too much too quickly
 6) Offer finger foods, one-to-one feeding, or verbal cuing for clients disinterested in eating or those who forget they are eating
 7) Help patient advance from eating alone in his or her room with controlled distractions, to dining with one other person, to eating in a full dining room atmosphere (Wood, 1991)
 8) Ready patient for each meal by asking preparatory questions (examples are listed below) to reinforce cognitive retraining and supply answers if patient cannot (Wood, 1991)
  a) "How long do most meals take?"
  b) "What tastes good in cereal?"

c) "Why do people use napkins?"

9) Prevent client from eating nonedible or spoiled food that might have been hoarded

e. Interventions specific to *spinal cord injury*

1) Once bowel sounds are present, ensure ingestion of foods high in nutrients soon after injury

2) Educate patient about preventive role of protein in relation to the following problems

a) Pressure ulcers

b) Infection

3) Monitor respiratory status closely

4) Teach patient regarding activities and conditions that can cause respiratory compromise

a) Parenteral or oral feedings

b) Swallowing air during meals

c) Paralytic ileus

5) Recognize possible necessity of providing iron-rich food and/or medication and avoiding overhydration (normochromic and normocytic anemia can emerge in the acute phase of SCI [Huang, DeVivo, & Stover, 1990])

6) Explain potential for signs and symptoms of hyponatremia and explain treatment

f. For patients with *respiratory disease*, provide high-protein, high-calorie foods with frequent small feedings

5. Expected outcomes

a. Client's weight is stable and appropriate

b. Client's nutritional intake is adequate to meet metabolic needs; adheres to dietary modifications

c. Client and family identify factors that might contribute to inadequate nutritional intake

d. Client and family identify factors that contribute to adequate nutritional status

Fluid Volume Deficit and Excess

Sixty percent of a child's total body weight is composed of water (Bindler & Howry, 1991). Fifty to sixty percent of adult body weight is water (Horne, Heitz, & Swearingen, 1991); in the elderly, this drops to 45% to 50% due to loss of muscle mass (Kositzke, 1990). Maintenance of an internal homeostatic balance is essential and involves the regulation of body fluids. Monitoring and regulating fluids in rehabilitation patients is vital because so many signs and/or symptoms associated with fluid disturbances are vague and nonspecific. The importance of early recognition of fluid volume changes by nurses cannot be stressed enough. Late detection can create severe—even life-threatening—physical complications and increase length of hospital stay.

The brain, the autonomic nervous system (especially the sympathetic system), and the renal and endocrine systems work synergistically to maintain fluid homeostasis. Persons with cerebral insult are at risk for changes in fluid volume because many alterations occur in the normal feedback mechanisms among these systems. Rehabilitation nurses will encounter a variety of fluid (and electrolyte) problems in patients of all ages. The elderly are particularly at risk for fluid volume deficits.

I. Related Theory and Concepts: Physiology of Fluid Balance

A. Body fluids are separated into two general categories

1. Intracellular fluid (ICF): Fluid within cells

2. Extracellular fluid (ECF): Fluid outside cells

a. ECF contains all the electrolytes; sodium is present in large quantities

b. ECF interacts with outside environment and is more likely to be lost by the body than ICF

c. All food and fluid (except undigestible wastes) are absorbed from gut into ECF

d. ECF is a combination of intravascular, interstitial, and transcellular fluids

1) Intravascular fluid: Liquid portion of blood; is contained inside blood vessels

2) Interstitial fluid: Encircles the cells; lymph is a type of interstitial fluid

3) Transcellular fluid: Smallest portion of ECF

a) Cerebrospinal (CSF)

b) Pericardial fluid

c) Pleural fluid

d) Peritoneal fluid

e) Synovial fluid

f) Intraocular fluid

g) Sweat

h) Digestive secretions

B. Water balance: Maintenance of proper proportion of salt to water in the blood

1. Salt (Na+) is a primary solute (particle) in ECF; the ratio of water to solutes is measurable and is referred to as *osmolality*

2. Serum (and urine) osmolality measurements are useful in determining fluid disturbances; for example, if serum sodium decreases (the normal range is between 135-145 mEq/liter in adults), the osmolality of the blood decreases—in other words, blood is more dilute and has excess water relative to the amount of salt

3. Fluid shifting between compartments (e.g., between blood and interstitial space or between interstitial space and cells) occurs as a result of differences in osmolality; some compartments have selectively permeable membranes that permit movement of water and some solutes, meaning that fluid moves to those compartments with higher osmolality

4. Blood-brain barrier is permeable to fluid shifts but is essentially impermeable to large particles and toxic substances

C. Fluid regulators

1. ICF is regulated by antidiuretic hormone (ADH)

a. ADH is produced in hypothalamus and stored in posterior pituitary gland; when ADH is released from pituitary gland, it ultimately causes collecting duct and distal tubule of kidney to reabsorb fluid rather than excrete it

b. When blood osmolality is concentrated (i.e., when blood has low levels of fluid compared to a high number of particles), ADH secretion increases to raise body's fluid level

c. When blood osmolality is dilute (i.e., when

blood has high level of fluid compared to a low number of particles), ADH secretion is suppressed so that fluid is not reabsorbed but is excreted

d. Many factors can stimulate ADH secretion (Dolan, 1991; Goldberger, 1986; Groer, 1981)
   1) Hypotension
   2) Pain
   3) Stress
   4) Positive pressure ventilators
   5) Some medications might influence ADH
      a) Nicotine
      b) Carbamazepine
      c) Chlorothiazide diuretics
      d) Morphine
      e) Some anesthetics
      f) Hypoglycemics
      g) Chemotherapeutic agents (e.g., vincristine and cyclophosphamide)
   6) Cerebral injury or disease
e. Alcohol ingestion blocks ADH secretion and causes diuresis
   1) Important that caregivers of SCI clients understand this concept; when SCI clients drink alcohol, they produce fluid and need to catheterize or be catheterized more frequently
   2) These clients also are at risk of developing hypokalemia, because they excrete potassium as they frequently urinate

2. ECF is regulated by several hormones and enzymes that work via simple feedback loops; a major one is aldosterone
   a. Aldosterone acts on the distal tubule of the kidney to promote reabsorption of sodium
   b. In turn, this allows for reabsorption of water, which maintains blood volume and, thus, blood pressure

D. Two types of volume disturbances: Fluid volume deficit and fluid volume excess

1. **Fluid volume deficits (1) and (2)**: Specific physiological concepts that relate to rehabilitation patients
   a. Deficits in ECF (extracellular fluid) occur when fluid is lost from body
   b. Rehabilitation patients can lose fluids in one or more ways
      1) Insensible water loss (e.g., from lungs and skin)
      2) Diarrhea
      3) Use of diuretics
      4) Diabetes insipidus
      5) Wound exudate
   c. ECF loss also can occur when fluid collects in a "third space" and cannot be used by the body; it is trapped and gradually resolves over time; in rehabilitation patients, "third spacing" accompanies the following conditions
      1) Thrombophlebitis (DVT) (Stroot, Lee, & Barrett, 1984)
      2) Intestinal obstruction
         a) Absent or diminished peristalsis produces fluid accumulation in gastrointestinal (GI) tract
         b) Traumatic spinal cord injury can result in paralytic ileus, placing clients with this condition at risk for intestinal obstruction and third spacing
   d. Intracellular fluid (ICF) loss causes cells to shrink
      1) Shrinkage of brain cells affects the central nervous system
      2) Signs and symptoms
         a) Weakness
         b) Restlessness
         c) Delirium
         d) Tetany
         e) Hyperpnea
         f) Thirst
         g) Fatigue
         h) Fever
      3) Unless ICF loss is treated, oliguria (reduced excretion of urine) may present

2. **Fluid volume excess**
   a. Exists when there is more water in comparison to particles, thus diluting the blood
      1) Serum sodium level is 134 mEq/L or less (Dolan, 1991)
      2) Serum sodium level less than 130 mEq/L is indicative of ICF volume excess, whereas a drop in hematocrit is present with ECF volume excess (Dolan, 1991)
   b. Types of fluid volume excess: Systemic and localized
      1) Systemic hypervolemia
         a) Increased circulating blood volume in intravascular and/or interstitial spaces
         b) Some common causes
            (1) Chronic or abnormal stimulation of kidney to save sodium or water; for example, in endocrine dysfunctioning after cerebral damage or hemorrhage, increased ADH stimulates kidney to reabsorb water, thus resulting in water retention; process is known as *syndrome of inappropriate antidiuretic hormone* (SIADH)
            (2) Abnormal renal function
            (3) Cardiovascular dysfunctioning (congestive heart failure or pulmonary edema)
            (4) Excessive sodium or fluid intake (oral or IV)
            (5) Hyperaldosteronism: With increased aldosterone, there is both water and sodium retention
      2) Localized fluid volume excess (edema)
         a) Accumulation of fluid in selected tissues or spaces
         b) Causes
            (1) Disruption of capillary membranes: Such edema represents extra fluid in

interstitial spaces (can occur locally or systemically)
(2) Impaired lymphatic drainage
(a) Enlarged, shiny, firm hand that commonly develops in acute hemiplegia (hand/shoulder syndrome)
(b) Pulmonary edema that develops in elderly patients who have heart failure because the lymphatic system cannot remove fluid rapidly enough
c) Also can occur in transcellular spaces—cavities and spaces of body
(1) Cerebrospinal (CSF) spaces
(2) Pericardial spaces
(3) Pleural spaces
(4) Synovial spaces
(5) Intraocular spaces
3) Cerebral edema is a unique and complex example of localized hypervolemia and/or edema; it can have several effects
a) Rise in intracranial pressure
b) Disturbance of brain cell metabolism
c) Disruption of the blood-brain barrier, causing fluid shifting
d) Hypoxia or infarction

II. Nursing Assessment

A. Energy level
B. Elimination pattern
C. Fluid consumption
D. Respiratory status (rate, patterns, secretions)
E. Vital signs
F. Condition of skin and oral mucosa
G. Neurological evaluation
H. Cognitive status
I. Weight pattern
J. Presence of seizure activity

III. Nursing Diagnoses

➤ A. Fluid volume deficit (1)

1. **Definition:** Decreased circulating volume due to failure of regulatory mechanisms (Gordon, 1993)

2. **Major defining characteristics**

a. Dilute urine, increased output
b. Sudden weight loss
c. Dry skin and mucous membranes
d. Weakness
e. Thirst
f. Increased body temperature
g. Altered serum sodium
h. Decreased skin turgor
i. Change in mental status

3. **Related factors/etiologies**

a. Hypothalamic dysfunctioning that interferes with thirst, temperature regulation, or ADH production and/or release
b. Posterior pituitary tumor
c. Neurogenic dysphagia
d. Severe chronic obstructive pulmonary disease with expulsion of extreme amounts of sputum
e. Mechanical ventilation (rare but can interfere with ADH release)

4. **Interventions**

a. Weigh patient on a scheduled basis
b. Monitor intake and output; report large output that is consistently greater than intake
c. Monitor urine specific gravity and osmolality
d. Monitor serum electrolytes (e.g., sodium sedimentation rate, blood urea nitrogen)
e. Offer patients, especially the elderly, about 2,000-3,000 ml of fluids per 24 hours unless contraindicated; offer fluids every hour while patients are awake and with their evening snack
f. Teach patients that caffeine acts as a diuretic and, thus, caffeinated beverages should not be sole source of liquid intake
g. Actively assist elderly, cognitively impaired, infant, and dysphagic patients with fluids they like, liquid dense foods, and thick liquids
h. Administer replacement fluids as ordered
i. Teach SCI patients about implications of ingesting alcohol (i.e., diuretic effect requiring frequent catheterization; potential hypokalemia)
j. Provide safety during episodes of impaired level of consciousness

5. **Expected outcomes**

a. Client's fluid imbalances are restored
b. Client and/or family verbalize(s) signs and symptoms of possible fluid volume deficit

➤ B. Fluid volume deficit (2)

1. **Definition:** Decreased circulating volume due to active loss of body fluid (Gordon, 1993)

2. **Major defining characteristics**

a. Decreased urine output
b. Concentrated urine
c. Sudden weight loss
d. Dry skin and mucous membranes
e. Weakness
f. Thirst
g. Increased body temperature
h. Increased serum sodium
i. Hypotension
j. Change in mental status

3. **Related factors/etiologies**

a. Vomiting (can result from increased intracranial pressure)
b. Diarrhea (a complication of enteral feedings, antibiotics, bowel impactions)
c. Excessive use of diuretics
d. Hemorrhage
e. Paralytic ileus
f. Deep vein thrombosis (DVT)
g. Wound drainage

4. **Interventions**
   a. Administer intravenous or oral fluids as ordered
   b. Closely monitor intake and output
   c. Monitor weight regularly
   d. Monitor for hypoactive or absent bowel sounds, tarry stools, coffee-ground or bright red emesis; report significant findings to physician
   e. Assess for signs and symptoms of DVT (calf pain, swelling, warmth, redness, positive Homan's sign)
   f. Monitor extremities for potential fluid accumulation
   g. Provide graded compression stockings (antiembolic)
   h. Observe for changes in vital signs (elevated pulse and respiratory rate, decreased pressure) (Reedy, 1988)
   i. Instruct patient in proper hydration for his or her specific disability or impairment

5. **Expected outcomes**
   a. Client's fluid imbalances are restored
   b. Client and/or family verbalize(s) signs and symptoms of possible fluid volume deficit

➤ C. **Fluid volume excess**

1. **Definition:** Increased local or total body fluid volume (Gordon, 1993)

2. **Major defining characteristics**
   a. Edema, effusion, anasarca (accumulation of great amounts of fluid in all body tissues)
   b. Sudden weight gain
   c. Change in mental status
   d. Intake greater than output, oliguria, specific gravity changes
   e. Shortness of breath, dyspnea, orthopnea
   f. Abnormal breath sounds (crackles, rales), change in respiratory pattern
   g. Jugular vein distension; S_3 heart sound
   h. Decreased hematocrit and hemoglobin
   i. Alteration in electrolytes; azotemia

3. **Related factors/etiologies**
   a. Excess fluid or sodium intake
   b. Compromised regulatory mechanisms
   c. Water replacement without simultaneous salt replacement

4. **Interventions**
   a. Weigh patient on a scheduled basis
   b. As a prevention, replace fluids lost from body with a variety of liquids, but avoid tap water
   c. Strictly enforce fluid restrictions but allow patient to choose desired liquids, offer cold fluids between meals rather than with meals, involve patient in calculating intake and output
   d. Allow patient to "sham drink" (i.e., to rinse, not swallow, a mouthful of water and then spit it out) (Hornc ct al., 1991)
   e. Elevate head of bed 15 to 30 degrees if cerebral edema is present or suspected
   f. Perform or have patient perform range-of-motion exercises
   g. Elevate extremities if edematous

5. **Expected outcomes**
   a. Client's body weight will be within normal range with no evidence of sudden increase
   b. Client's electrolytes will be within normal limits
   c. Client verbalizes knowledge of fluid restrictions and participates in achieving desired intake

Impaired Swallowing

In most facilities, nurses supervise patients as they eat meals and snacks. This is especially true in the field of rehabilitation, where nurses are involved with the treatment team to provide safety and adequate nourishment for patients with impaired swallowing.

Rehabilitation nurses set up meals for patients who can feed themselves; assist or actually feed those unable to feed themselves; assess patients as they chew, drink, and swallow; and monitor and record patients' caloric and fluid intake and weight patterns.

Because rehabilitation nurses intervene with populations at high risk of developing neurogenic-related chewing and swallowing disorders, they must be confident about recognizing the associated symptomatology and signs. Normally, deglutition is controlled by the brainstem and many cranial and cervical nerves (see Figure 12.1 and Figure 12.2). In general, swallowing is a complex process that involves both voluntary and involuntary activity. If cerebral lesions are present, dysphagia, or difficulty with chewing and swallowing, can occur.

Dysphagia can be life-threatening and frightening; it can cause a number of physical complications such as aspiration (before, during, or after the swallow), dehydration, nutritional deficits, electrolyte disturbances, mucosal ulcerations, and inability to ingest oral medications. At the very least, it can be socially embarrassing and contribute to depression and/or isolation.

Chewing and swallowing impairments must be detected as early as possible. This will help to prevent choking or inadvertent aspiration leading to pneumonia. It also will ensure that therapeutic programs and remediation are initiated by the team early on in the person's rehabilitation.

I. Related Theory and Concepts

A. Three phases in a normal swallow: Oral, pharyngeal, and esophageal
   1. **Oral phase** of swallowing process (see Figure 12.3 and Figure 12.4)
      a. Is under voluntary control
      b. Salivary secretions help break down food substances (under control of cranial nerve VII)
      c. Mastication muscles and mandibular muscles (controlled by cranial nerves V and VII) act to chew and grind food into pieces
      d. Tongue movement anteriorly, posteriorly, and

Figure 12.1. Anatomy of the Pharynx

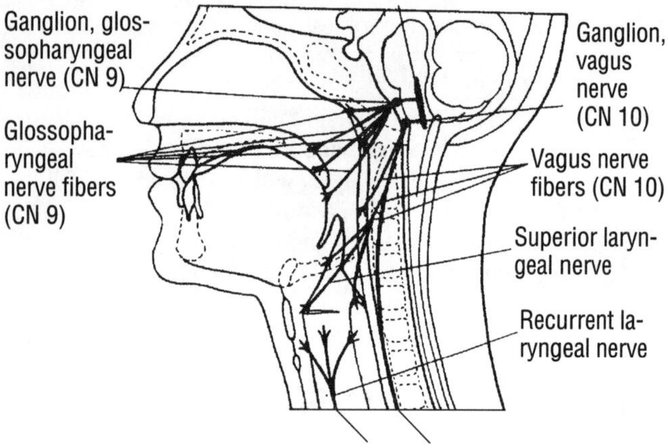

Reprinted with permission of Springer-Verlag New York, Inc., and James F. Bosma, MD, from Bosma, J.F., Donner, M.W., Tanaka, E., & Robertson, D. (1986). Anatomy of the pharynx pertinent to swallowing. *Dysphagia, 1*(1), 29.

laterally (via cranial nerve XII) moves food to the back of the mouth and retrieves food particles that have migrated elsewhere in oral cavity

e. Soft palate elevation closes off nasal passageway and prevents nasal regurgitation
f. Lower lip adduction contains food particles and saliva and ensures adequate pressure exchange for strong and efficient swallow
g. Posterior tongue movement causes pressure against posterior pharyngeal wall combined with pharyngeal elevation, so that bolus is squeezed into pharynx (throat)

2. **Pharyngeal phase** of swallowing process (see Figure 12.5 and Figure 12.6)
    a. Involuntary or reflexive actions occur as bolus moves down pharynx via motor components of cranial nerves V, VII, IX, and X
    b. Laryngeal elevation and vocal cord closure help to protect airway during the swallow
    c. Epiglottic closure inhibits food penetration into airway (trachea)
    d. Food bolus is transmitted through relaxed cricopharyngeal sphincter into esophagus
3. **Esophageal phase** of swallowing process
    a. Bolus is propelled toward stomach via peristalsis and gravity
    b. Cricopharyngeal sphincter is maintained in tonic state to prevent gastric reflux from esophagus into pharynx
    c. Lower esophageal sphincter is maintained in tonic state to prevent reflux of stomach contents into the esophagus

B. Neurogenic-based swallowing disorders
1. May be associated with any of several neurological conditions
    a. Stroke

Figure 12.2. Cranial and Cervical Nerves Involved in the Swallowing Process

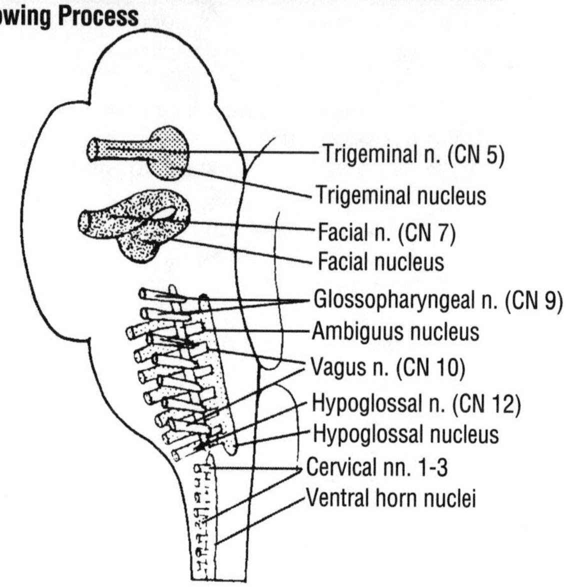

Reprinted with permission of Springer-Verlag New York, Inc., and James F. Bosma, MD, from Bosma, J.F., Donner, M.W., Tanaka, E., & Robertson, D. (1986). Anatomy of the pharynx pertinent to swallowing. *Dysphagia, 1*(1), 29.

    b. Head trauma
    c. Amyotrophic lateral sclerosis
    d. Parkinson's disease
    e. Poliomyelitis
    f. Guillain-Barré syndrome
    g. Multiple sclerosis
    h. Cerebral palsy
2. Implications
    a. Interfere with any phase of swallowing process
    b. Require astute nursing assessment and interventions for phase-specific dysfunctioning
    c. Client with cognitive or behavioral problems will need specialized teaching strategies associated with dysphagia training

II. Nursing Assessment

A. Facial asymmetry
B. Drooling
C. Oral mucosal sensation
D. Reflexive swallowing
E. Cough during or after swallow
F. Oral muscle weakness
1. Lips
2. Tongue
3. Cheek
4. Pharynx

G. Voice quality
H. Elevated temperature
I. Dentition and chewing ability
J. Weight pattern
K. Cognition
L. Level of consciousness

Figure 12.3. Swallowing Mechanism at Rest

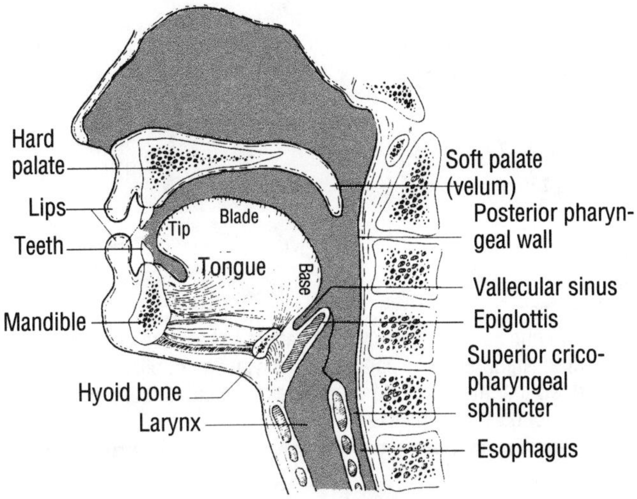

Reprinted with permission of Sister Kenny Institute from Roueche, J.R. (1980). *Dysphagia: An assessment and management program for the adult* (p. 7). Minneapolis: Sister Kenny Institute.

Figure 12.4. Late Oral Phase (Bolus in Swallow Preparatory Position)

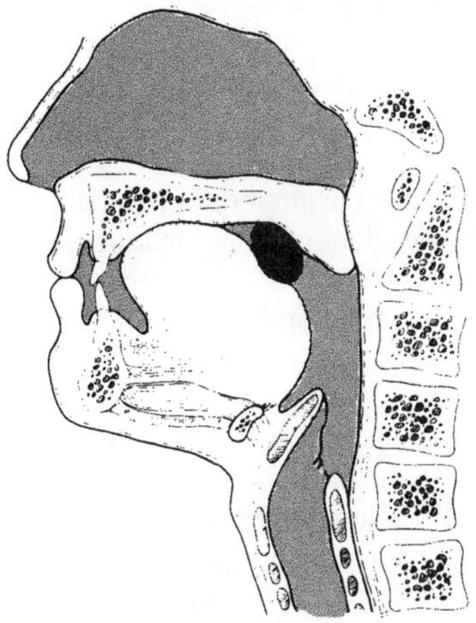

Reprinted with permission of Sister Kenny Institute from Roueche, J.R. (1980). *Dysphagia: An assessment and management program for the adult* (p. 9). Minneapolis: Sister Kenny Institute.

Figure 12.5. Middle Pharyngeal Phase

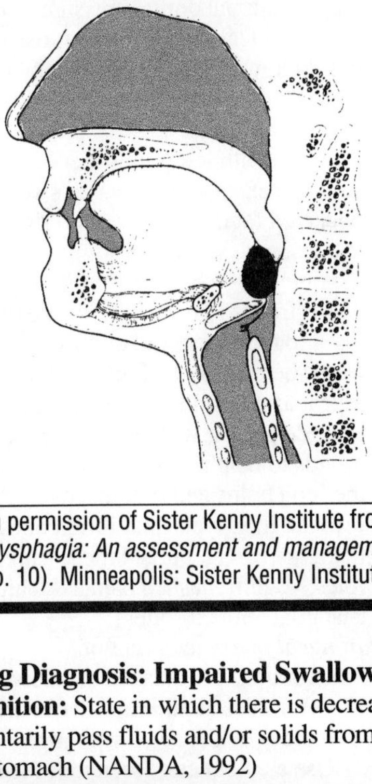

Reprinted with permission of Sister Kenny Institute from Roueche, J.R. (1980). *Dysphagia: An assessment and management program for the adult* (p. 10). Minneapolis: Sister Kenny Institute.

Figure 12.6. Late Pharyngeal Phase

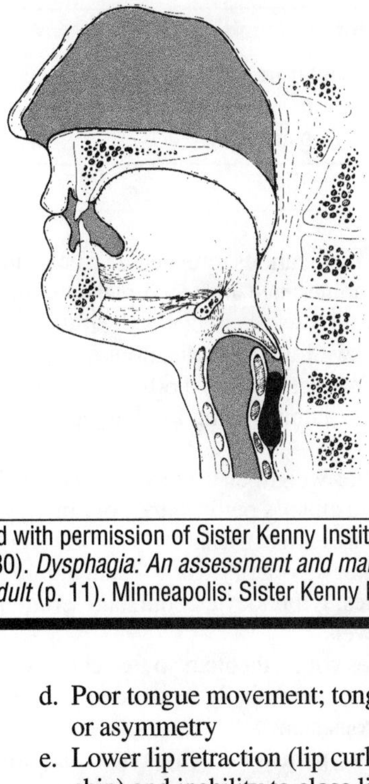

Reprinted with permission of Sister Kenny Institute from Roueche, J.R. (1980). *Dysphagia: An assessment and management program for the adult* (p. 11). Minneapolis: Sister Kenny Institute.

➤ III. Nursing Diagnosis: Impaired Swallowing

A. Definition: State in which there is decreased ability to voluntarily pass fluids and/or solids from the mouth to the stomach (NANDA, 1992)

B. Major defining characteristics

1. Evidence of aspiration
2. *Oral phase*
   a. Presence of drooling or food particles on affected cheek or side of chin
   b. Facial asymmetry
   c. Pocketed food between the teeth and inside the cheek (lateral sulcus)
   d. Poor tongue movement; tongue weakness and/or asymmetry
   e. Lower lip retraction (lip curls down toward chin) and inability to close lips tightly
   f. Soft palate elevation with phonation
   g. Weakened or absent gag reflex
   h. Excessive chewing (can result from perseveration)
   i. Nasal drainage and/or sniffling during eating (due to nasal regurgitation)
   j. Inability to finish a meal within a 30-minute time frame
   k. Oral mucosal ulcerations (from biting self in-

discriminately due to loss of oral sensation)

l. Loss of internal and/or external oral sensation

3. *Pharyngeal phase*
   a. Delayed or absent swallow (inability to visualize or auscultate a swallow)
   b. Coughing while drinking fluids, especially thin liquids
   c. History of aspiratory pneumonia
   d. Report of weight loss, fear of eating, or poor appetite
   e. Wet, gurgly, or nasal voice, particularly during eating
   f. Frequent throat clearing
   g. Report of tickling, burning, or something sticking to the back of the throat (burning is especially noteworthy because it may be caused by medication or food that has become trapped in the valleculae and is eroding the tissue)
4. *Esophageal phase*
   a. Burping, report of indigestion or substernal pain (due to esophageal reflux)
   b. Bad breath or report of bad taste in mouth on awakening
   c. Respiratory symptoms of coughing and/or wheezing
   d. Unusually high incidence of dental cavities

C. Related factors/etiologies

1. Neuromuscular impairment
2. Muscle fatigue
3. Cognitive impairment

D. Interventions

1. *General*
   a. Give medications (crushed or whole) in baby food applesauce and teach patient to turn his or her head toward affected side, if there is difficulty swallowing medications
   b. Help patient sit up at a 60- to 90-degree angle prior to administering food, liquid, or medication orally
   c. Monitor weight on a scheduled weekly basis
   d. Ensure client's performance of oral hygiene measures after meals
   e. Monitor laboratory work—total albumins, electrolytes, lymphocyte count, and serum transferrin levels
   f. Confer with a dietitian so that client's diet becomes progressively more advanced in texture and consistency
   g. Monitor patient for dehydration and offer liquid-dense foods (e.g., ice cream, thick soup) if he or she has difficulty swallowing liquids
   h. Suspect silent aspiration if fever and pneumonia emerge
   i. To stop chewing perseveration, ask patient to take a drink
   j. Encourage oral motor exercises to strengthen tongue and mouth movements
   k. Reinforce recommendations of other members of the dysphagia team (e.g., occupational therapist for visual and/or perceptual problems, physical therapist for positioning, speech therapist for in-depth dysphagia techniques)

Figure 12.7. Adaptation of a Cup for Dysphagic Clients

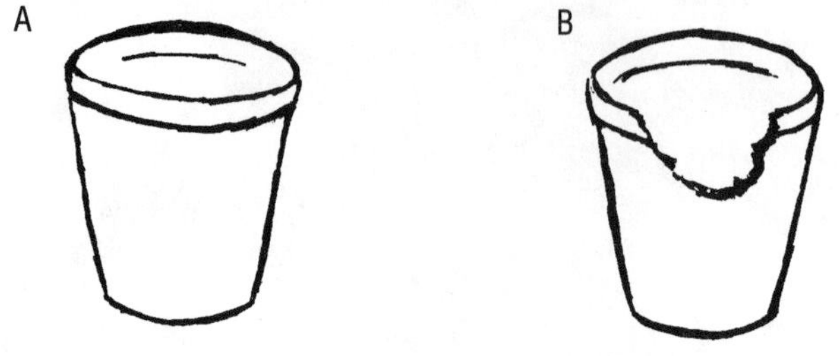

A. Normal styrofoam cup

B. Styrofoam cup with piece torn out to make a "cutout cup": The cutout cup allows the dysphagic patient to keep his or her head in neutral alignment. The patient drinks with lips opposite the cutout part, so that the nose clears the side of the cup and the patient does not have to hyperextend his or her neck.

2. *Oral phase* interventions
   a. Use a mirror and/or give patient verbal cues during meals to promote awareness of drooling of food or liquids on mouth or chin
   b. Apply external digital pressure to patient's cheek to clear pocketed food; teach patient and family how to perform this technique
   c. Obtain orders for team evaluation and dysphagia programming
   d. To those with left-hemispheric lesions, demonstrate an exaggerated tongue sweep to retrieve pocketed food; for those with right-hemispheric lesions, give verbal cues
   e. Do quick stretch (application of quick downward strokes to the affected side of the chin, using a roughly textured cloth such as a washcloth) before meals if lip retraction is present; repeat as needed if it reoccurs during the meal
   f. Provide patient with warm or cool foods and liquids to help him or her differentiate between the food bolus and oral mucosa
   g. Provide food types that form cohesive boluses (e.g., hot cereal, puréed meat with gravy, casseroles, yogurt, mashed bananas, canned fruit, custard, creamed soups)
3. *Pharyngeal phase* interventions
   a. Interventions for delayed swallow reflexes
      1) Offer thick liquids and avoid using straws, if there is evidence of aspiration
      2) Use a cutout cup for liquids (see Figure 12.7)
      3) Teach and have patient consistently do a modified supraglottic swallow
      4) Perform icing techniques (Emick-Herring & Wood, 1990) for those with absent swallow reflexes according to dysphagia team's protocols
   b. Interventions for pharyngeal wall residue
      1) Avoid offering sticky foods (e.g., peanut but-

ter, mashed potatoes without gravy, yeast breads, pancake syrup)
   2) Have patient turn his or her head as far as possible toward affected side when swallowing
   3) Instruct patient to swallow twice per bite, drink a thick liquid after every few bites, and/or clear the throat, if voice takes on gurgling sound during eating
   4) Have patient use a straw if his or her soft palate needs strengthening
4. *Esophageal phase* interventions
   a. Offer 30 cc of a carbonated beverage (such as a soft drink) just before bedtime
   b. Elevate head of bed to at least 30 degrees
   c. Teach patient to sit up for 30 minutes after meals and snacks
   d. If ordered, administer medications that raise esophageal sphincter pressure
   e. Teach patients and family that citrus juices and coffee exacerbate heartburn; also teach that fats, chocolate, alcohol, and nicotine lower esophageal sphincter pressure and, thus, should be avoided

E. Expected outcomes

1. Client exhibits no evidence of aspiration
2. Client demonstrates and initiates compensatory strategies to ensure a safe swallow
3. Client verbalizes comfort and self-assurance in eating in a social situation

Skin Integrity

The development of skin breakdown often interferes with or delays the achievement of rehabilitation goals. Rehabilitation nurses frequently work with clients who exhibit multiple risk factors for the development of skin breakdown. A thorough assessment facilitates the nurse's appropriate and effective decision making. Once the client has been identified as being at risk, early intervention can minimize the long-term sequelae of skin impairment. A proactive response to an identified risk typically requires fewer dollars and less time than reactive treatment of the results of an unmanaged risk. This unit describes the anatomic, physiological, and environmental factors that cumulatively increase the probability of the development of an interruption in skin integrity. The nursing diagnoses included here are high risk for impaired skin integrity and pressure ulcer.

The potential for skin problems is found in many rehabilitation situations. For example, neurologic and orthopedic disabilities can interfere with one's sense of, or response to, pressure. Vascular disease as well as endocrine and metabolic disorders can impair cellular nutrition. Excessive moisture and incontinence promote maceration and can cause chemical irritation. Orthotic and prosthetic devices can impair circulation or cause excessive shear or friction. Effective management of risk factors is based on the pathophysiology of the risk factors. The objective of management is to eliminate or reduce the risk (Kosiak, 1991).

The prevalence of pressure ulcers varies within settings. In 1989 it was estimated that there were more than 2 million pressure ulcers in hospitalized persons (Fowler, 1990). Several subpopulations, such as quadriplegic patients or those who have sustained a femoral fracture, can be at higher risk than the general population (Panel for the Prediction and Prevention of Pressure Ulcers in Adults, 1992).

Risk that remains unmanaged or inappropriately managed can result in pressure ulcers and unnecessary delays in the rehabilitation process. The Panel for the Prediction and Prevention of Pressure Ulcers in Adults (1992) identified factors that increase the risk of developing pressure ulcers. The panel suggests that bed- and chair-bound individuals and those with impaired ability to reposition themselves should be assessed for additional factors that increase the risk of developing pressure ulcers. These factors include immobility, incontinence, impaired nutritional status, and altered level of consciousness. The objectives of intervention should be resolving predisposing factors, reducing and controlling pressure placed on high-risk or impaired areas, preventing the development or recurrence of an ulcer, and supporting the healing of an existing wound.

I. Related Theory and Concepts

A. Physiological factors in skin breakdown

1. Altered metabolic states, such as fever, infection, or diabetes mellitus: Can increase nutrient and oxygen demands and increase or impair use of nutrients at the cellular level
2. Hypoproteinemia, hypoalbuminemia, and anemia
   a. Can impair nutrient availability at the cellular level with a resulting increase in sensitivity to other factors
   b. There is a significant relationship between low serum albumin and pressure ulcer development
3. Inadequate or inappropriate nutrient intake
   a. Contributes to low tissue tolerance, which has an adverse effect on nutrient availability at the cellular level
   b. Due to poor vascularity of adipose tissue, nutrient delivery is impeded; consequently, excessive intake that produces obesity can be as harmful as insufficient intake (Krasner, 1990)
4. Neurological or orthopedic disability
   a. Can impair one's ability to respond to external factors by decreasing sensory feedback that would trigger discomfort and a change in position
   b. Can impair one's ability to shift position to relieve external pressure or respond to other sensory stimuli
   c. Can affect sensation with subsequent injury from bath water and other hot objects
   d. Impaired proprioception and pain sensors can result in undetected trauma and skin tears
5. Systolic and/or diastolic hypotension: Decrease in pressures of sufficient magnitude and duration can contribute to diminished perfusion of tissues under external pressure
6. Smoking: Induces physiological changes in the vascular bed that can impair cellular respiration; this reduces the ability to tolerate and recover from trauma

B. Mechanical factors in skin breakdown

1. External pressure from hard surfaces such as tracheostomy tubes, seats, and support surfaces (e.g., wheelchairs, beds, commodes): Considered to be one of the primary causes of skin breakdown, particularly when it is extended or repeated pressure (Dinsdale, 1973; Kosiak, 1961)
   a. Pressure over a bony prominence induces a wide, three-dimensional pressure gradient
   b. Normal capillary arteriolar limb pressure ranges from 22 to 32 mmHg; sitting pressure over the ischial tuberosities can exceed 300 mmHg
   c. Amount of time needed to produce tissue necrosis is inversely proportional to amount of pressure applied
2. Vascular constriction
   a. Can be due to improper fit of orthotic or prosthetic appliances
   b. When unrelieved, it interferes with cellular nutrition
   c. Also can be produced by chronic edema
3. Moisture from incontinence, wound drainage, exudate from surgical stomas, or an external source
   a. Promotes maceration with subsequent skin damage
   b. Incontinence creates chemical irritation and increases susceptibility to injury from friction, abrasion, and bacterial growth
   c. Drainage from abdominal stomas also can contain digestive juices that can cause chemical damage to skin
4. Friction and shear
   a. Both can interfere with cellular nutrition and impose direct trauma upon the skin
   b. Shear distorts the capillary lumen and can occlude blood flow or reduce amount of pressure required to produce occlusion

C. Psychobehavioral factors in skin breakdown

1. Nonconformance with care recommendations: Can indirectly cause risks from any of the aforementioned physiological or mechanical risk categories *(Author's note:* Nonconformance *is used here intentionally. It reflects the failure to act in conformity with generally accepted beliefs and practices, whereas* noncompliance *means the failure or refusal to yield or agree.)*
2. Client's conflicting healthcare belief systems: Can promote nonconformance
   a. When clinician's recommendations for care conflict with client's underlying beliefs as to etiology of any concurrent or potential health problems, client may disregard professional advice
   b. Conflict might arise between client's beliefs and clinician's recommendations regarding appropriate interventions for existing health problems
3. Socioeconomic supports and resources: Can be involved in the degree of client conformance with care recommendations
   a. Client may opt to divert available resources to areas other than those recommended by the clinician
   b. In some cases, both financial and human resources might not be available or are inadequate for full implementation of all recommended interventions
4. Substance abuse or other concurrent psychological disorders, such as depression, can impair client's ability to conform to recommended practices
5. Intellectual capacity: Can impair ability to comprehend recommendations and can result in inadequate or inappropriate health maintenance behaviors

D. Physiology of wound healing

1. Complex process that has four interdependent phases (Harding, 1990)
   a. Progression through four phases
      1) Different parts of wound can be in different phases at different times
      2) Wound must progress through all four phases before healing can occur
      3) An understanding of the phases and factors that interfere with them is necessary to design an intervention protocol to attempt to ameliorate their effects
   b. Phases
      1) Hemostasis
         a) Vascular supply to wound is stabilized
         b) Damaged blood vessels sealed by clotting to prevent or minimize blood loss
      2) Inflammation
         a) Phagocytes converge on area to begin removal of necrotic debris
         b) Peripheral blood flow might be increased
         c) Increased warmth and redness might be noted during this process
      3) Proliferation
         a) Fibroblasts begin to proliferate and form a collagen matrix in traumatized area
         b) Network of new epithelium is laid and wound margins begin to contract
      4) Maturation: Reconstructed collagen matrix begins to reorganize itself from a chaotic network to a structured matrix of healthy tissue
2. Factors that can have an impact on wound healing at various phases of the process *(Author's note: This is not an all-inclusive listing.)*
   a. Systemic factors
      1) Drug therapy: Especially anti-inflammatory and cytotoxic drugs
      2) Anemia
      3) Malnutrition
         a) Macronutrients (deficiencies in total calories, protein, and carbohydrates)
         b) Micronutrients (deficiencies in vitamins and minerals)
      4) Metabolic dysfunctions such as diabetes or fever
   b. Local factors (Harding, 1990; Torrance, 1983)
      1) Blood supply

Table 12.1. Staging of Pressure Ulcers

Stage I

Nonblanchable erythema of intact skin; the heralding lesion of skin breakdown (Stage I may be difficult to detect in darkly pigmented skin)

Stage II

Partial-thickness skin loss involving epidermis and/or dermis; the ulcer is superficial and presents clinically as an abrasion, blister, or shallow crater

Stage III

Full-thickness skin loss involving damage or necrosis of the subcutaneous tissue that may extend down to, but not through, the underlying fascia; the ulcer presents clinically as a deep crater with or without undermining of adjacent tissue

Stage IV

Full-thickness skin loss with extensive destruction, tissue necrosis, or damage to muscle, bone, or supporting structures (e.g., tendon, joint capsule)

Source Consulted

Panel for the Prediction and Prevention of Pressure Ulcers in Adults. (1992). *Pressure ulcers in adults: Prediction and prevention* (p. 56). Clinical Practice Guideline, Number 3, AHCPR Publication No. 92-0047. Rockville, MD: Agency for Health Care Policy and Research, Public Health Service, U.S. Department of Health and Human Resources.

2) Mechanical stress or trauma
3) Radiation

II. Nursing Assessment

A. Assessment tools (Panel for the Prediction and Prevention of Pressure Ulcers in Adults, 1992, p. 14-15)
1. Numerous risk assessment tools exist; however, only the Braden and Norton scales (original and modified) have been tested extensively
2. The Braden Scale (Bergstrom, Braden, Laguzza, & Holman, 1987) has been evaluated in diverse sites, including medical-surgical units, intensive care units, and nursing homes; the Norton Scale (Norton, McLaren, & Exton-Smith, 1975) has been tested with elderly subjects in hospitals
3. The reported sensitivity and specificity of these risk assessment tools have varied greatly; this variability probably reflects differences in study settings, populations, and outcome measures
4. Use of the Norton and Braden scales ensures systematic evaluation of individual risk factors; overall scores obtained by the tools are the best predictors of risk currently available

B. Areas to be addressed in a complete assessment
1. Medical diagnoses
2. History and chronicity of any concurrent health problems
3. Ability to move independently and change body position
4. Sensory-perceptual ability
5. Level of consciousness
   a. Ability to follow commands
   b. Ability to respond to internal stimuli and then move spontaneously
6. Age: Elderly are at greater risk
7. Nutritional status
8. Temperature (fever)
9. Adequacy of circulation
10. Bladder and bowel control
11. Blood pressure (hypotension)
12. Psychosocial support
13. Emotional status
14. Additional factors specific to an existing or actual pressure ulcer
    a. *Classification of pressure ulcer*: Complete assessment of actual pressure ulcer should be performed on a regular basis (at least weekly) and documented using a grading, or staging, methodology such as the method developed by Darrel Shea (1975) that has been adapted by the International Association of Enterostomal Therapists and recommended by the Panel for the Prediction and Prevention of Pressure Ulcers in Adults (1992) (see Table 12.1)
    b. *Physical parameters of wound*
       1) Size: Measure in centimeters across the largest diameter of the wound and record size
       2) Shape: Draw shape of wound in medical record
       3) Color: Determine if base of wound is red, yellow, or black; this indicates general health of the tissues (red for healthy tissue, yellow for infected tissue, black for necrotic tissue)
       4) Location: Identify anatomic location of wound and associated bony prominence
       5) Heat and/or edema: Look for presence of infection
       6) Surrounding tissue: Ascertain whether it is healthy or if it is likely to slough
       7) Drainage: Describe four aspects
          a) Absence or presence
          b) Color
          c) Odor
          d) Amount

III. Nursing Diagnoses

➤ **A. High risk for skin breakdown**

1. **Definition:** Presence of risk factors for skin ulceration, particularly over bony prominences (Gordon, 1993)

2. **Risk factors**

   a. Physical immobilization
   b. Sensory loss
   c. Presence of shearing forces, friction, pressure
   d. Excretions and/or secretions on skin

Table 12.2. Topical Products for Skin Care

Class	Indications	Comments
Emollients	For dry intact skin, to lubricate surface of the skin	Scant research base to substantiate use
Skin and wound cleansers	To assist in the removal of foreign material in wounds	May be used on intact skin instead of soaps; use in place of povidone-iodine and hydrogen peroxide, which may impair healing
Skin barriers and plasticized coatings	Protective agents to shield skin from shear and moisture, especially from incontinence	Available as gels, sprays, wipes, and roll-ons
Protective skin preparations	To provide protective film over skin	Available in sprays, liquids, gels, and wipes; have high alcohol content; should be used only on healthy skin

e. Failure to change position for time periods greater than patient's skin can tolerate
f. Altered level of consciousness
g. Altered metabolic states
h. Altered nutritional states
i. Altered circulation
j. Hypo- or hyperthermia
k. Decreased fatty tissue
l. Alteration in skin turgor

3. Interventions

a. *General* (includes recommendations of the Panel for the Prediction and Prevention of Pressure Ulcers in Adults, 1992)
   1) Inspect skin at least once per day, paying particular attention to bony prominences
   2) Keep skin clean and dry; avoid hot water and use mild cleansing agent (see Table 12.2)
   3) Avoid massage over bony prominences
   4) Minimize skin exposure to moisture due to incontinence, perspiration, or wound drainage (see Table 12.2)
   5) Minimize injury from friction and shearing
      a) Positioning, transferring, and turning techniques should be carried out with the least amount of friction
      b) Lubricants, protective films, or dressings can be utilized
   6) Ensure adequate hydration, protein, and caloric intake
   7) Enhance mobility and activity status
   8) Teach patient and caregivers preventive interventions
      a) Include rationale for each selected intervention
      b) Verify learning through return demonstration or verbalization
      c) Teach how to evaluate effectiveness of interventions
      d) Teach when to seek professional intervention

b. Interventions for *clients on bedrest*
   1) Turn and reposition at least every 2 hours, based on an assessment of pressure-bearing areas; written schedule should be used
   2) Positioning devices, such as pillows or foam wedges, should be used to keep bony prominences from direct contact with one another; pressure should be totally relieved from heels
   3) When the side-lying position is used, avoid positioning client directly on the trochanter
   4) Limit the amount of time the head of the bed is elevated; maintain head of bed at lowest degree of elevation consistent with medical condition
   5) Clients at risk of developing pressure ulcers should be placed on a pressure-reducing device—such as foam, static air, alternating air, gel, or water mattresses—when lying in bed
   6) Lifting devices, such as a trapeze or bed linen, should be used rather than dragging client

c. Interventions for *clients in chairs or wheelchairs*
   1) Relieve pressure periodically
      a) This is the one consistent intervention that must accompany any treatment plan
      b) Intermittent relief of pressures above the capillary occlusion might prevent pressure-related injury; long-term maintenance of pressure below level of capillary occlusion can have negative effect on cardiovascular tone
   2) Consider using pressure-reducing devices (e.g., foam, gel, air); do not use donut-type devices
   3) Reposition those in a sitting position every hour; those who are able to be so taught should shift their weight every 15 minutes
   4) Try pressure-relieving techniques
      a) Push-ups: Placing hands on armrests and pushing against them to lift buttocks off cushion
      b) Side leans: Placing one arm behind wheelchair handles while leaning toward opposite side of wheelchair
      c) Forward lean: Resting forearms alongside thighs and leaning forward as far as possible

Table 12.3. Pressure Ulcer Products

Dressing Type†	Indications	Comments
Coarse mesh gauze	As a dry dressing for minor abrasions; for wet-to-dry dressings; for wounds with scattered eschar or necrosis; as a topper dressing	Is not indicated for weeping or open wounds because coarse mesh gauze will become entangled in granulating epithelium; for debriding only when used for wet-to-dry procedures
Fine mesh gauze	For draining wounds or stomas; as a protective or topper dressing	Is less likely to adhere to a draining wound
Impregnated saline gauze—(Mesalt®)	For clean draining wounds	Is not recommended for dry wounds; uses fluid from the wound to produce a moist environment
Impregnated charcoal gauze	For draining odiferous wounds; as a cover dressing	Has activated charcoal embedded in dressing for odor control
Nonadherent pad (Alldress®, Release®, Telfa®)	For clean wounds with scant drainage, minor burns; as a cover dressing	Absorbs small amounts of drainage with minimal disruption of the wound bed; protects red granulating wounds
Vaselinated gauze (Adaptic™, Aquaphor®, Vaseline® gauze, Xeroform™)	As a nonadherent dressing for minor to extensive burns	Is widely used for burns and abrasions; Xeroform™ has some antimicrobial properties
Polymeric membrane dressings (Bioclusive™, Comfeel® Transparent, Opraflex®, Opsite*, Tegaderm™)	For abrasions, Stage I or II pressure ulcers	Provide a moist healing environment
Hydrocolloid dressing wafers (Comfeel® products, Duoderm® products, RepliCare™, Restore™ products)	For ulcers at Stages I through IV, vascular ulcers	Are available in various thicknesses; colloid interacts with fluid from the wound to provide a moist environment for wound healing and to promote epithelial migration; may allow for extended time periods between dressing changes; most are self-adhering to healthy tissue; may be contraindicated for infected ulcers
Hydrogel dressings (Carrington™ Hydrogel Wound Dressing, Clear Site®, IntraSite*, Normlgel™, Nu-Gel™)	For ulcers at Stages I through IV, for skin tears	Three types: (a) self-adhering wafer type that has a low water content, can be changed up to once per week, and has small amount of absorption; (b) nonadhering wafer type that has a high percentage of water content and is usually changed daily; (c) a gel that is partially composed of water, has minimal absorption, and helps maintain a moist wound surface
Hydrocolloid and hydrogel flakes and pastes (Bard® Absorption dressing, Comfeel®, DuoDERM®, HydraGran™, RepliCare™)	For ulcers at Stages II and III, draining ulcers, vascular ulcers	Provide a moist environment; are effective for drainage control in deep, draining ulcers; can be used with gauze or other toppers to provide nonocclusive dressing with the benefits of a hydroactive dressing
Alginate sponges and ropes (Algosteril®, Kaltostat® products, Sorbsan™)	For Stage II and III draining ulcers, vascular ulcers	Are highly absorbent for effective drainage control, provide a moist environment with low adherence; not indicated for wounds with scant drainage, as they can desiccate wound bed; might be contraindicated for infected wounds
Polymeric foam dressings (Allevyn* products, Epi-Lock™, Lyofoam® products, Mitraflex™ products)	For ulcers at Stages II through IV, venous ulcers, draining stomas and/or tubes	Have high absorbency and low adherence; some are available with impregnated charcoal for odor control

†*Editor's note: This list of products is not comprehensive, nor does products' listing constitute an endorsement by the editors or the publishers; the products serve only as examples. The comments in the "Indications" column of the table are generalized; please refer to specific manufacturer's instructions for each product's specific action and recommended use.*
* = internationally registered trademark

d) Wheelchair tilts: Second person tilts wheelchair backward so that patient is in a reclining position

4. **Expected outcomes**

a. Client has intact skin
b. Client or caregiver verbalizes risk factors for the development of pressure ulcers
c. Client or caregiver verbalizes and/or demonstrates knowledge of interventions for preventing pressure ulcers

➤ B. **Pressure ulcer** (specify stage in scale for grading pressure ulcers [see Table 12.1])

1. **Definition:** Break in skin integrity, usually over a bony prominence, associated with lying or sitting for prolonged periods (Gordon, 1993)

2. **Major defining characteristics**

a. If redness or darkened skin persists for more than 24 hours, a pressure ulcer might be forming; redness might not be readily apparent in highly pigmented skin; changes in texture of the underlying tissue—such as a "doughy" or mushy feel, localized warmth, or an ashen appearance—might be more obvious
b. Ulceration: Disruption of skin surface, usually over a bony prominence
c. Verbalization of pain, discomfort, or numbness over a bony prominence

3. **Related factors/etiologies**

a. Prolonged pressure
b. Friction or shear injury
c. Immobility
d. Incontinence or moisture from another source
e. Malnutrition
f. Sensorimotor loss
g. Cognitive impairment

4. **Interventions**

a. Interventions for high risk for skin breakdown (see page 86) must be continued while managing an actual pressure ulcer
b. Avoid repetitive stress and trauma to injured tissues—that is, do not continue to apply pressure to a pressure ulcer
c. Address systemic pathophysiology—for example, provide nutritional support, medication evaluation, and treatment of vascular disease and other conditions that can negatively affect cellular metabolism and availability of nutrients
d. The focus of local treatment should be removing local barriers to healing (e.g., removing necrotic tissue, supporting granulation and reepithelization, and preventing infection)
   1) Ensure that dressings are appropriate for the phase of healing (see Table 12.3)
   2) Minimize or eliminate identified causative factors
   3) Assess and record wound characteristics regularly
   4) Keep the area clean
   5) Determine best method for debridement (surgical, mechanical, or chemical) if necrotic tissue is present
   6) Use a dressing that maintains a moist environment for wound (see Table 12.3)
   7) Teach dietary modifications that can promote wound healing—for example, high intake of protein, zinc, vitamin C
e. Teach patient and caregivers appropriate interventions
   1) Include rationale for each intervention
   2) Verify learning through a return demonstration or verbalization, as appropriate
   3) Teach how to evaluate effectiveness of selected interventions
   4) Teach when to seek additional professional intervention

5. **Expected outcomes**

a. Tissue is intact with absence of persistent nonblanching erythema
   1) Intact skin remains intact
   2) Pressure ulcers decrease in size until they are completely closed
   3) Previously damaged areas are supported through wound maturation process and ulceration does not reoccur
b. Client verbalizes risk factors for development of pressure ulcers
c. Client achieves maximum functional level using available resources

Autonomic Dysreflexia

Autonomic dysreflexia is an uninhibited sympathetic response of the nervous system in persons with cervical and thoracic spinal cord injury. It is a neurological emergency that, in the vast majority of cases, is resolved by nursing interventions.

I. Related Pathophysiology

A. Initial autonomic response (see Figure 12.8)
   1. Noxious stimuli from below level of injury stimulate transmission of proprioceptive and pain impulses into dorsal columns and spinothalamic tracts
   2. These ascending tracts synapse with sympathetic neurons in intermediolateral cell columns in gray matter and cause a generalized sympathetic hyperactive response
   3. This sympathetic response results in vasoconstriction of splanchnic bed and peripheral vasculature
   4. This vasoconstriction causes a hypertensive situation and various other signs and symptoms for patient experiencing autonomic dysreflexia (Bell & Hannon, 1986; Dunn, 1991; Erickson, 1980; Hickey, 1986)

B. Autonomic/cardiovascular response to hypertension (Bell & Hannon, 1986; Dunn, 1991; Erickson, 1980; Hickey, 1986)

Figure 12.8. Pathophysiology of Autonomic Dysreflexia

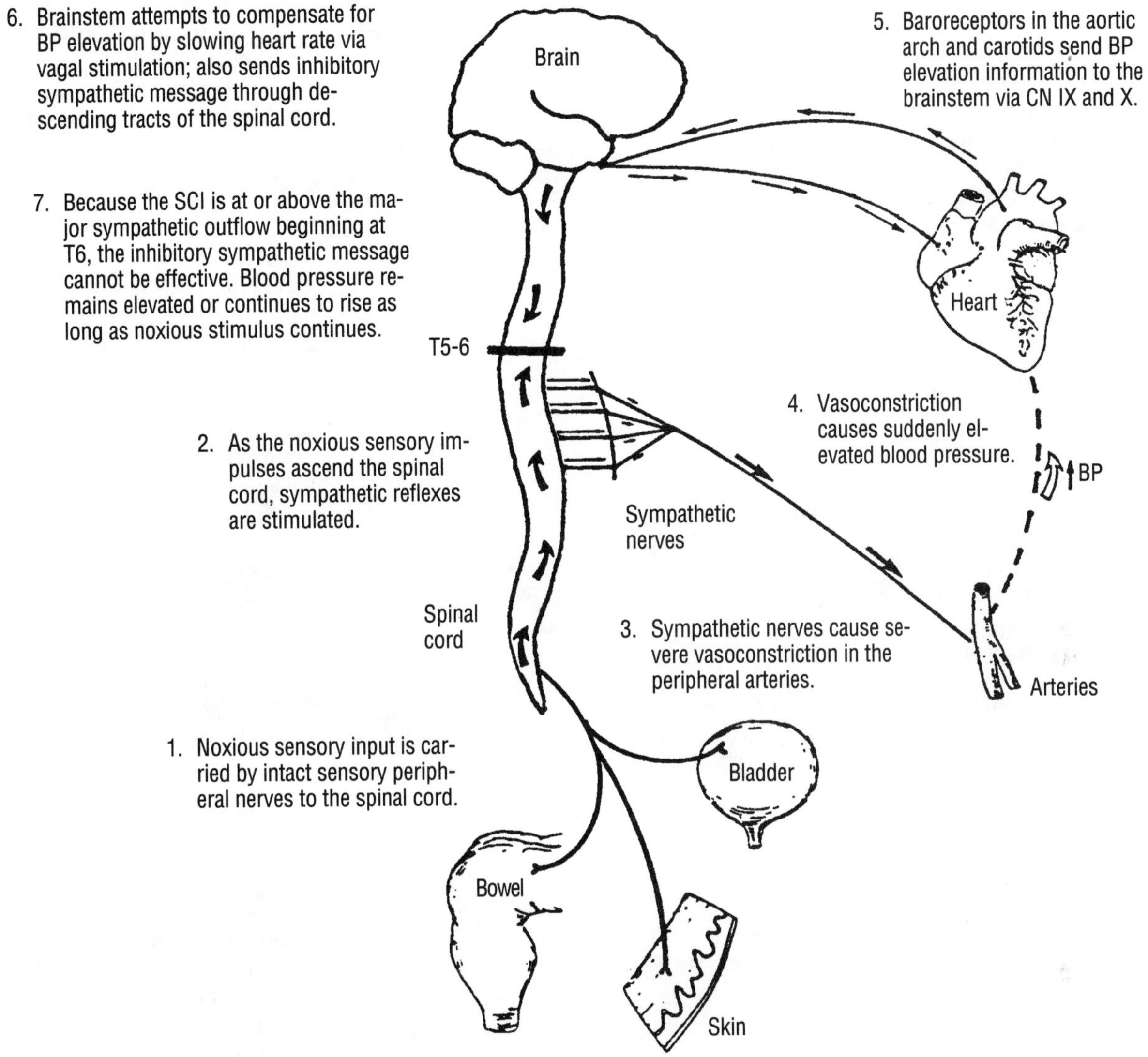

Reprinted with permission of Aspen Publishers, Inc., from Dunn, K.L. (1991). Autonomic dysreflexia: A nursing challenge in the care of a patient with a spinal cord injury. *The Journal of Cardiovascular Nursing, 5*(4), 58. Copyright © 1991 Aspen Publishers, Inc.

1. Hypertension stimulates baroreceptors in carotid sinus and aortic arch via glossopharyngeal and vagus nerves, which, in turn, send messages to vasomotor centers in the brain
2. Parasympathetic stimulation of heart via vagus nerve results in two vasocentral reflexes
   a. Bradycardia
   b. Vasomotor response: In turn, results in the following conditions
      1) Vasodilation above level of injury
      2) Continued vasoconstriction below level of injury

II. Nursing Assessment

A. Autonomic dysreflexia is a medical emergency; there should be established protocols in both rehabilitation facilities and the homes of patients at risk to address these emergencies

B. Assessment should focus on presence of the defining characteristics listed below

➤ III. Nursing Diagnosis: Autonomic Dysreflexia

A. Definition: State in which an individual with a spinal cord injury at T7 or above experiences life-threatening uninhibited sympathetic response of the nervous system to noxious stimulus (NANDA, 1992)

B. Major defining characteristics

1. Sudden paroxysmal hypertension
   a. 20 mmHg over baseline is considered hypertensive; normal blood pressure for persons with SCI can range from 80-90/50-60

   b. Blood pressure can reach as high as 300/160 (Chui & Bhatt, 1983)
2. Severe pounding headache
3. Pallor below level of injury
4. Pilomotor reflex (goose bumps) below level of injury
5. Bradycardia
6. Profuse diaphoresis above level of injury
7. Flushing (usually blotchy) over face and neck
8. Nasal congestion
9. Blurred vision
10. Anxiety or feeling of impending doom
11. Metallic taste in mouth
12. Cardiac irregularities
13. Respiratory distress
14. Nausea
15. Increased spasticity

C. Related factors/etiologies

1. Bladder stimuli: Account for 76% of cases of autonomic dysreflexia (Kewalramani, 1980)
   a. Distension
   b. Detrusor sphincter dyssynergia
   c. Urinary tract infection
   d. Calculi
   e. Catheterization
   f. Cystitis
   g. Epididymitis
2. Bowel stimuli: Account for 19% of the cases of autonomic dysreflexia (Kewalramani, 1980)
   a. Distension
   b. Digital stimulation
   c. Enemas
   d. Suppositories
   e. Hemorrhoids
3. Skin stimuli: Account for much of remaining 5% of cases of autonomic dysreflexia
   a. Pressure over bony prominences
   b. Pressure ulcers
   c. Wounds not related to pressure
   d. Ingrown toenails
   e. Temperature extremes
   f. Sunburn
   g. Tight clothes or leg bag straps
4. Other causes of autonomic dysreflexia
   a. Certain medical procedures
      1) Extracorporeal shock wave lithotripsy
      2) Cystoscopy
      3) Bladder instrumentation or surgery
      4) Bowel instrumentation or surgery
   b. Labor and delivery
   c. Pressure on the penis
   d. Sexual activity
   e. Menstrual cramps
   f. Fractures
   g. Infection
   h. Thrombophlebitis

D. Interventions

1. Monitor vital signs frequently; interval usually accepted in rehabilitation facilities is every 2 to 5 minutes
   a. Heart rate and blood pressure are crucial vital signs to monitor
   b. Someone must stay with client to monitor vital signs and address client's anxiety while another person calls for help
2. Institute immediate measures to decrease blood pressure
   a. Raise head of bed
   b. Remove antiemboli stockings, abdominal binders, and any other restrictive clothing
   c. Lower the legs, if possible
3. Remove trigger stimulus
   a. Bladder stimuli
      1) If client is wearing a catheter, unkink tubing or empty a full drainage bag
      2) If catheter is plugged, irrigate with no more than 30 cc of normal saline
      3) If catheter remains plugged or uncatheterized bladder is distended, replace indwelling catheter or straight catheter using generous amounts of a local anesthetic jelly (e.g., 2% Xylocaine)
      4) Drain bladder slowly to prevent rebound hypertension
      5) If blood pressure is still elevated after these measures and there is a possibility of a urinary tract infection or the patient has undergone recent bladder instrumentation, an anesthetic agent such as Pontocaine hydrochloride® can be instilled into the bladder (do not use Pontocaine hydrochloride if there is blood in the urine)
   b. Bowel stimuli
      1) Check bowel for impaction; if present, gently insert an anesthetic agent (common lubricants are Nupercaine® or Xylocaine®) and gently remove fecal mass
      2) Anesthetic ointment might need to be used prophylactically prior to routine bowel care
   c. Skin stimuli
      1) Remove stimuli such as pressure, tight clothing, and temperature extremes
      2) Topical anesthetics might be helpful in relieving stimulation from pressure ulcers
4. If nursing measures do not control the symptoms, consult with physician immediately and institute pharmacological measures as ordered
   a. Sublingual: Nifedipine (Procardia®) can be used
      1) Nifedipine serves as early pharmacological intervention to stabilize blood pressure while searching for triggering stimulus
      2) To manage autonomic dysreflexia via a sublingual route, the capsule must be ruptured and the contents placed under the tongue
   b. Oral: Phenoxybenzamine (Dibenzyline®), prazosin (Minipress®), or nifedipine (Procardia®) can be used as prophylaxis or for acute management of autonomic dysreflexia
   c. Intravenous: Hydralazine hydrochloride

(Apresoline®) and diazoxide (Hyperstat®), and nitroprusside sodium (Nipride®) are intravenous antihypertensive medications commonly used for acute management of autonomic dysreflexia (Bell & Hannon, 1986; Dunn, 1991; Erickson, 1980; Hickey, 1986)

5. Prevent reoccurrence of autonomic dysreflexia
   a. Provide routine and effective management of bladder and bowel for spinal cord injured persons, especially those prone to autonomic dysreflexia
   b. Institute quality skin management program to include routine assessment and prevention of pressure sores
   c. Administer prophylactic medications (such as anesthetic ointment) as indicated, to prevent episodes of autonomic dysreflexia prior to bowel care
   d. Assist persons at risk for autonomic dysreflexia in obtaining adequate access to health care for routine health maintenance and treatment of complications
6. Educate client and other providers
   a. Educate client and family and those in contact with client in the community (for example, friends, school personnel, coworkers) regarding causes, signs and symptoms, prevention, and treatment of autonomic dysreflexia
   b. Provide client with written information, such as a wallet card, for treating the condition and consulting healthcare practitioners in community
   c. Educate healthcare providers in other specialty areas about all aspects of detection and management of autonomic dysreflexia

E. Expected outcomes

1. Client does not experience dysreflexic episodes; if they occur, client acts appropriately to minimize complications
2. Client verbalizes causes, signs and symptoms, prevention, and treatment of autonomic dysreflexia
3. Client identifies individual trigger stimuli for autonomic dysreflexia
4. Client uses preventive measures for autonomic dysreflexia
5. Client identifies a plan for treating episodes of autonomic dysreflexia and for seeking medical care if initial measures do not relieve the symptoms

References: Nutrition and Metabolism

Axelsson, K., Asplund, K., Norberg, A., & Eriksson, S. (1989). Eating problems and nutritional status during hospital stay of patients with severe stroke. *Journal of the American Dietetic Association, 89*, 1092-1096.

Bivins, B.A., & Fath, J.J. (1990). The patient with acute neurologic injury or disease. In J.L. Rombeua & M.D. Caldwell (Eds.), *Clinical nutrition: Enteral and tube feeding* (2nd ed.) (pp. 250-262). Philadelphia: W.B. Saunders Company.

Blissitt, P.A. (1990). Nutrition in acute spinal cord injury. *Critical Care Nursing Clinics of North America, 2*, 375-384.

Bodinski, L.H. (1987). *The nurse's guide to diet therapy* (2nd ed.). New York: John Wiley & Sons, Inc.

Dietz, W.H., & Bandini, L. (1989). Nutritional assessment of the handicapped child. *Pediatrics in Review, 11*(4), 109-115.

Drinka, P.J., & Goodwin, J.S. (1991). Prevalence and consequences of vitamin deficiency in the nursing home: A critical review. *Journal of the American Geriatric Society, 39*, 1008-1017.

Dudek, S. (1987). *Nutrition handbook for nursing practice.* Philadelphia: J.B. Lippincott.

Godbole, K.B., Berbiglia, V.A., & Goddard, L. (1991). A head-injured patient: Caloric needs, clinical progress and nursing care priorities. *Journal of Neuroscience Nursing, 23*(5), 290-294.

Huang, C.T., DeVivo, M.J., & Stover, S.L. (1990). Anemia in acute phase of spinal cord injury. *Archives of Physical Medicine and Rehabilitation, 71*, 3-7.

Kaufman, H.H., Bretaudiere, J-P., Rowlands, B.J., Stein, D.K., Bernstein, B.A., Wagner, K.A., & Gildenberg, P.L. (1987). General metabolism in head injury. *Neurosurgery, 20*(2), 254-265.

Kearns, P.J., Thompson, J.D., Werner, P.C., Pipp, T.L., & Wilmot, C.B. (1992). Nutritional and metabolic response to acute spinal-cord injury. *Journal of Parenteral and Enteral Nutrition, 16*(1), 11-15.

Kersten, L. (1989). *Comprehensive respiratory nursing: A decision making approach.* Philadelphia: W.B. Saunders Company.

Miller, M.A. (1986). A practical approach to eating and breathing in respiratory failure. *TICN, 1*(4), 61-70.

Moore, R., Najarian, M.P., & Konvolinka, C.W. (1989). Measured energy expenditure in severe head trauma. *The Journal of Trauma, 29*, 1633-1636.

Morely, J.E. (1991). Why do physicians fail to recognize and treat malnutrition in older persons? *Journal of the American Geriatrics Society, 39*, 1139-1140.

Williams, S.R. (1989). *Nutrition and diet therapy* (6th ed.). St. Louis: Times Mirror/Mosby College Publishing.

Wood, P. (1991). Managing dysphagia in patients with traumatic brain injury. *Nutritional News and Views, 2*(1), 3-5.

Yankelson, S. (1990). Traumatic brain injury. In D.J. Gines (Ed.), *Nutrition management in rehabilitation* (pp. 175-184). Rockville, MD: Aspen Publishers, Inc.

Suggested Readings: Nutrition and Metabolism

Bosma, J.F., Donner, M.W., Tanaka, E., & Robertson, D. (1986). Anatomy of the pharynx pertinent to swallowing. *Dysphagia, 1*(1), 23-33.

Buelow, J.M., & Jamieson, D. (1990). Potential for altered nutritional status in the stroke patient. *Rehabilitation Nursing, 15*, 260-263.

Kay, S.P., Moreland, J.R., & Schmitter, E. (1987, April). Nutritional status and wound healing in lower extremity amputations. *Clinical Orthopaedics and Related Research*, pp. 253-256.

North American Nursing Diagnosis Association. (1992). *NANDA nursing diagnoses: Definitions and classification 1992.* St. Louis: Author.

Panush, R.S. (1991). American College of Rheumatology position statement: Diet and arthritis. *Rheumatic Disease Clinics of North America, 17*, 443-444.

Roueche, J.R. (1980). *Dysphagia: An assessment and management program for the adult.* Minneapolis: Sister Kenny Institute.

References: Fluid Volume Deficit and Excess

Bindler, R.M., & Howry, L.B. (1991). *Pediatric drugs and nursing implications.* Norwalk: Appleton & Lange.

Dolan, J.T. (1991). *Critical care nursing: Clinical management through the nursing process.* Philadelphia: F.A. Davis Company.

Goldberger, E. (1986). *A primer of water, electrolytes and acid-base syndrome* (7th ed.). Philadelphia: Lea & Febiger.

Gordon, M. (1993). *Manual of nursing diagnosis: 1993-1994.* St. Louis: Mosby-Year Book, Inc.

Groer, M.W. (1981). Volume disturbances. In T.A. Manning (Ed.), *Physiology and pathophysiology of the body fluids* (pp. 132-157). St. Louis: The C.V. Mosby Company.

Horne, M.M., Heitz, U.E., & Swearingen, P.L. (1991). *Fluid, electrolyte, and acid base balance: A case study approach.* St. Louis: Mosby-Year Book, Inc.

Kositzke, J.A. (1990). A question of balance: Dehydration in the elderly. *Journal of Gerontological Nursing, 16*(5), 4-11.

Reedy, D.F. (1988). How can you prevent dehydration? *Geriatric Nursing, 9*(4), 224-226.

Stroot, V.R., Lee, C.A.B., & Barrett, C.A. (1984). *Fluids and electrolytes: A practical approach* (3rd ed.). Philadelphia: F.A. Davis Company.

Suggested Readings: Fluid Volume Deficit and Excess

Aaronson, L., & Seaman, L.P. (1989). Managing hypernatremia in fluid deficient elderly. *Journal of Gerontological Nursing, 15*(7), 29-34.

◆Gershan, J.A. (1990). Fluid volume deficit: Validating the indicators. *Heart & Lung: Journal of Critical Care, 19*(2), 152-156.

Kokko, J.P., & Tannen, R.L. (1990). *Fluid and electrolytes* (2nd ed.). Philadelphia: W.B. Saunders Company.

McFarland, G., & McFarlane, E. (1989). *Nursing diagnosis and interventions: Planning for patient care.* St. Louis: The C.V. Mosby Company.

Saba, M.T., & Magolan, J.M. (1991). Understanding cerebral edema: Implications for oncology nurses. *Oncology Nursing Forum, 18*, 499-505.

◆Sergent, E., Strauss, C., Jaffe, M., Majewsky, E., & Mitchell, C.A. (1991). Diagnostic content validity of the diagnostic category fluid volume excess: A construct replication. In R.M. Carroll-Johnson (Ed.), *Classification of nursing diagnosis: Proceedings of the North American Nursing Diagnosis Association.* Philadelphia: J.B. Lippincott Company.

Wandel, J.C. (1990). The use of postural vital signs in the assessment of fluid volume status. *Journal of Professional Nursing, 6*(1), 46-54.

Yucha, C., & Suddaby, P. (1991). David could have died of thirst: Yet he never felt thirsty. *Nursing 91, 21*(7), 42-43, 45.

References: Impaired Swallowing

Bosma, J.F., Donner, M.W., Tanaka, E., & Robertson, D. (1986). Anatomy of the pharynx pertinent to swallowing. *Dysphagia, 1*(1), 23-33.

Emick-Herring, B., & Wood, P. (1990). A team approach to neurologically based swallowing disorders. *Rehabilitation Nursing, 15*, 126-132.

North American Nursing Diagnosis Association (NANDA). (1992). *NANDA nursing diagnoses: Definitions and classification 1992.* St. Louis: Author.

Roueche, J.R. (1980). *Dysphagia: An assessment and management program for the adult.* Minneapolis: Sister Kenny Institute.

Suggested Readings: Impaired Swallowing

◆DeVita, M.A., & Spierer-Rundback, L. (1990). Swallowing disorders in patients with prolonged orotracheal intubation or tracheostomy tubes. *Critical Care Medicine, 18*, 1328-1330.

Dittmar, S. (1989). *Rehabilitation nursing: Process and application.* St. Louis: The C.V. Mosby Company.

Ellis, F.H. (1986). Hiatus hernia. *Clinical Symposia, 38*(5), 8.

Gordon, M. (1991). *Manual of nursing diagnosis 1991-1992.* St. Louis: Mosby-Year Book, Inc.

Logemann, J.A. (1986). Treatment for aspiration related to dysphagia: An overview. *Dysphagia 1*, 34-38.

Rubin-Terrado, M., & Linkenheld, D. (1991). Don't choke on this: A swallowing assessment. *Geriatric Nursing, 12*(6), 288-291.

◆Sorin, R., Somers, S., Austin, W., & Bester, S. (1988). The influence of videofluoroscopy on the management of the dysphagic patient. *Dysphagia 2*(3), 127-135.

Wood, P. (1991). Managing dysphagia in patients with traumatic brain injury. *Nutritional News and Views, 2*(1), 3-5.

References: Skin Integrity

Bergstrom, N., Braden, B.J., Laguzza, A., & Holman, V. (1987). The Braden Scale for Predicting Pressure Sore Risk. *Nursing Research, 36*, 205-210.

Dinsdale, S.M. (1973). Decubitus ulcers in swine: Light and electron microscopy study of pathogenesis. *Archives of Physical Medicine and Rehabilitation, 54*, 51-56.

Fowler, E. (1990). Chronic wounds: An overview. In D. Krasner (Ed.), *Chronic wound care: A clinical source book for healthcare professionals* (pp. 12-18). King of Prussia, PA: Health Management Publications, Inc.

Gordon, M. (1993). *Manual of nursing diagnosis (1993-1994).* St. Louis: Mosby-Year Book, Inc.

Harding, K.G. (1990). Wound care: Putting theory into clinical practice. *Wounds, 2*(1), 21-32.

Kosiak, M. (1961). Etiology of decubitus ulcers. *Archives of Physical Medicine and Rehabilitation, 42*, 19-29.

Kosiak, M. (1991). Prevention and rehabilitation of pressure ulcers. *Decubitus, 4*(2), 60-68.

◆Krasner, D. (Ed.). (1990). *Chronic wound care: A clinical source book for healthcare professionals.* King of Prussia, PA: Health Management Publications, Inc.

Norton, D., McLaren, R., & Exton-Smith, A.N. (1975). *An investigation of geriatric nursing problems in hospital.* London, England: Churchill Livingstone.

Panel for the Prediction and Prevention of Pressure Ulcers in Adults. (1992). *Pressure ulcers in adults: Prediction and prevention.* Clinical Practice Guideline, Number 3, AHCPR Publication No. 92-0047. Rockville, MD: Agency for Health Care Policy and Research, Public Health Service, U.S. Department of Health and Human Resources.

Shea, D. (1975, October). Pressure sores: Classification and management. *Clinical Orthopedics and Related Research,* pp. 89-100.

Torrance, C. (1983). *Pressure sores: Ætiology, treatment and prevention.* London, England: Croom Helm Ltd.

Suggested Readings: Skin Integrity

Alterescu, V., & Alterescu, K. (1988). Etiology and treatment of pressure ulcers. *Decubitus, 1*(1), 28-35.

Alvarez, D., Rozint, J., & Wiseman, D. (1989). Moist environment for healing: Matching the dressing to the wound. *Wounds, 1*, 35-51.

Bergstrom, N., Braden, B.J., Laguzza, A., & Holman, V. (1987). The Braden Scale for predicting pressure sore risk. *Nursing Research, 36*(4), 205-210.

Braden, B. (1990). Innovations to prevent and treat pressure ulcers. *Geriatric Nursing, 11*(4), 182-186.

Bryant, R. (1987). Wound repair: A review. *Journal of Enterostomal Therapy, 14*(6), 262-266.

◆Carlson, C.E., & King, R.B. (1990). Prevention of pressure sores. In J.J. Fitzpatrick, R.L. Taunton, & J.Q. Benoliel (Eds.), *Annual Review of Nursing Research, Volume 8* (pp. 35-46). New York: Springer Publishing Co.

Cassell, B. (1986). Treating pressure sores stage by stage. *RN, 49*(1), 36-40.

Ebersole, P., & Hess, P. (1985). *Toward healthy aging: Human needs and nursing response.* St. Louis: The C.V. Mosby Company.

Eriksson, E. (1980). Etiology: Microcirculatory effects of pressure. In M.B. Constantian (Ed.), *Pressure ulcers—Principles and tech-*

niques of management (pp. 7-14). Boston: Little, Brown & Company.

Fowler, E. (1987). Equipment and products used in management and treatment of pressure ulcers. *Nursing Clinics of North America, 22*, 449-461.

Gosnell, D.J. (1973). An assessment tool to identify pressure sores. *Nursing Research, 22*(1), 55-59.

Kosiak, M. (1959). Etiology and pathology of ischemic ulcers. *Archives of Physical Medicine and Rehabilitation, 40*, 62-69.

Maklebust, J., & Sieggreen, M. (1991). *Pressure ulcers: Guidelines for prevention and nursing management.* West Dundee, IL: S-N Publications.

◆Merbitz, C.M., King, R.B., Bleiberg, J., & Grip, J.C. (1985). Wheelchair push-ups: Measuring pressure relief frequency. *Archives of Physical Medicine and Rehabilitation, 66*, 433-438.

Roach, L.B. (1982). Color changes in dark skins. *Nursing, 11*, 19-22.

◆Williams, A. (1972). A study of factors contributing to skin breakdown. *Nursing Research, 21*(3), 238-243.

References: Autonomic Dysreflexia

Bell, J., & Hannon, K. (1986). Pathophysiology involved in autonomic dysreflexia. *Journal of Neuroscience Nursing, 18*(2), 86-88.

Chui, L., & Bhatt, K. (1983). Autonomic dysreflexia. *Rehabilitation Nursing, 8*(2), 83-85, 89.

Dunn, K.L. (1991). Autonomic dysreflexia: A nursing challenge in the care of the patient with a spinal cord injury. *The Journal of Cardiovascular Nursing, 5*(4), 57-64.

Erickson, R.P. (1980). Autonomic dysreflexia: Pathophysiology and medical management. *Archives of Physical Medicine and Rehabilitation, 61*, 431-440.

Hickey, J.V. (1986). *The clinical practice of neurological and neurosurgical nursing.* Philadelphia: J.B. Lippincott Company.

Kewalramani, L.S. (1980). Autonomic dysreflexia in traumatic myelopathy. *American Journal of Physical Medicine, 59*(1), 1-21.

North American Nursing Diagnosis Association (NANDA). (1992). *NANDA nursing diagnoses: Definitions and classification 1992-1993.* St. Louis: Author.

Suggested Readings: Autonomic Dysreflexia

◆Barton, C.H., Khonsari, F., Vaziri, N.D., Byrne, C., Gordon, S., & Friis, R. (1985). The effect of modified transurethral sphincterotomy on autonomic dysreflexia. *Journal of Urology, 135*(1), 83-85.

Bloch, R.F. (1986). Autonomic dysfunction. In J. Butler & C. Eckhart (Eds.), *Management of spinal cord injuries* (pp. 149-163). Baltimore: Williams and Wilkins.

Charbonneau-Smith, R. (1990). Autonomic dysreflexia: A nurse's challenge. *Axon, 12*(2), 36-39.

◆Craig, D.I. (1990). The adaptation to pregnancy of spinal cord injured women. *Rehabilitation Nursing, 15*, 6-9.

◆Fagius, J., & Karhuvaara, S. (1989). Sympathetic activity and blood pressure increases with bladder distention in humans. *Hypertension, 14*, 511-517.

Finocchiaro, D.N., & Herzfeld, S. T. (1990). Understanding autonomic dysreflexia. *American Journal of Nursing, 90*(19), 56-59.

◆Givre, S., & Freed, H.A. (1989). Autonomic dysreflexia: A potentially fatal complication of somatic stress in quadriplegics. *The Journal of Emergency Medicine, 7*, 461-463.

Guttman, L., & Whitteridge, D. (1947). Effects of bladder distention on autonomic mechanisms after spinal cord injuries. *Brain, 70*, 361-404.

◆Hall, P.A., & Young, J.V. (1983). Autonomic hyperreflexia in spinal cord injured patients: Trigger mechanism, dressing changes of pressure sores. *Journal of Trauma, 23*, 1074-1075.

Hanak, M. (1983). *Spinal cord injury.* New York: Springer Publishing Company.

Head, H., & Riddock, G. (1917). Autonomic bladder, excessive sweating and some reflex conditions in gross injuries of the spinal cord. *Brain, 46*, 188-263.

Johnson, B., & Thomason, R. (1975) Autonomic hyperreflexia: A review. *Military Medicine, 140*, 345-349.

Katz, V.L., Thorp, J.M., & Cefalo, R.C. (1990). Epidural analgesia and autonomic dysreflexia: A case report. *American Journal of Obstetrics and Gynecology, 162*, 471-472.

◆Krum, H., Howes, L.G., Brown, D.J., & Louis, W.J. (1989). Blood pressure variability in tetraplegic patients with autonomic hyperreflexia. *Paraplegia, 27*(4), 284-288.

◆Kumar, V.N., & Mullican, C.N. (1989). Ovarian cysts and autonomic dysreflexia. *Archives of Physical Medicine and Rehabilitation, 70*, 547-548.

◆Longo, W.E., Ballantyne, G.H., & Modlin, I.M. (1990). Colorectal disease in spinal cord patients. *Diseases of the Colon and Rectum, 3*, 131-134.

McGuire, T.J., & Kumar, V.N. (1986). Autonomic dysreflexia in the spinal cord injured. *Postgraduate Medicine, 80*(2), 81-89.

◆Naftchi, N.E. (1990). Mechanisms of autonomic dysreflexia: Contributions of catecholamine and peptide neurotransmitters. *Annals of the New York Academy of Science, 579*, 133-148.

◆Raeder, J.C., & Gisvold, S.E. (1986). Perioperative autonomic hyperreflexia in high spinal cord lesions: A case report. *Acta Anaesthesiology Scandinavia, 30*, 672-673.

◆Steinberger, R.E., Ohl, D.A., Bennett, C.J., McCabe, M., & Wang, S.C. (1990). Nifedipine pretreatment for autonomic dysreflexia during electroejaculation. *Urology, 36*(3), 228-231.

Wanner, M.B., Rageth, C.J., & Zach, G.A. (1987). Pregnancy and autonomic hyperreflexia in patients with spinal cord lesions. *Paraplegia, 25*, 482-490.

◆Yarkony, G.M., Katz, R.T., & Wu, Y. (1986). Seizures secondary to autonomic dysreflexia. *Archives of Physical Medicine and Rehabilitation, 67*, 834-835.

Zedjlik, C.P. (1992). *Management of spinal cord injury* (2nd ed.). Boston: Jones & Bartlett Publishers.

◆indicates a research-based work

CHAPTER 13

Elimination Pattern

The management of elimination problems is an area of continuing concern for rehabilitation nurses. Alteration in elimination patterns can create feelings of powerlessness, dependency, and loss of control in the client. Loss of control of bowel and urinary elimination can lead to embarrassment, shame, and isolation, and in turn, limits the client's involvement in vocational, social, and other aspects of daily living. Incontinence is the most common reason for a client to limit activity or to leave a social situation and has been noted to be a restrictive factor in sexual satisfaction for both the individual and his or her partner. With dependent clients, loss of bladder and bowel control is a common catalyst for the caretaker's consideration of alternative placement such as in an extended-care facility. A managed and successful outcome supports a client's reintegration into the community. Nursing interventions focus on helping the individual achieve a predictable and effective elimination plan, minimizing complications, and restoring an acceptable level of activity and socialization.

According to the Urinary Incontinence Guideline Panel (1992), urinary incontinence affects 10 million people annually. A conservative estimate of the direct cost of this problem is $10 billion per year. The indirect costs incurred by individuals and their families can be immeasurable.

Nursing has a major role to play in treating bladder and bowel conditions. Although some aspects of management require collaboration with the physician, there is a growing body of nursing research demonstrating the beneficial impact of nursing intervention strategies on incontinence. This is highlighted in the practice guidelines on urinary incontinence published by the Agency for Health Care Policy and Research (Urinary Incontinence Guideline Panel, 1992). Nursing research, although limited in the area of bowel incontinence, has increasingly addressed the related etiology, management, and outcomes of this nursing diagnosis.

There are several types of urinary incontinence: urge, stress, overflow, and functional. In rehabilitation, nurses most commonly see patients with bladder or bowel dysfunction related to neurologic damage. The etiology of the problem is significant, as rehabilitation nurses need to understand the causes and manifestations of different types of neurogenic bladder and bowel conditions. The broader diagnostic statement of urinary incontinence, with Lapides and Diokno's (1976) classification of neurogenic bladder, is included in this chapter with the nursing diagnoses of colonic constipation, incontinence related to neurogenic bowel, urinary retention, and high risk for urinary tract infection.

Bowel Elimination

I. Related Theory and Concepts

A. Normal mechanisms promoting fecal continence

1. Function of the ileum, cecum, and colon
   a. Promote active absorption of water and sodium
   b. Trigger secretion of certain substances essential to stool formation
      1) Mucus
      2) Potassium
      3) Bicarbonate
2. Colon performs secretory and absorptive functions and is responsible for moving stool toward rectum
3. Rectal compliance and capacity are critical factors in maintaining bowel continence; in turn, there are several important factors related to these
   a. Reverse colon gradient activity that occurs from distal to proximal: Inhibits progression of feces—that is, there is a mechanism in the colon to retain stool until voluntary defecation is initiated
   b. Anal canal and rectal pressures: Responsible for maintaining continence; however, internal sphincter is major controller of continence
   c. Other structures of importance in maintaining continence during activities that increase intra-abdominal pressure, thereby preventing stool leakage and emptying
      1) Angulation of the rectosigmoid
      2) Spiral valves of Houston
      3) Rectal flap
      4) Anal flutter valve
   d. Striated musculature dominant in the anal canal and pelvic floor
      1) Helps maintain continence
      2) Provides sling-like support to posterior rectal wall and causes sphincter-like action between rectum and anus
      3) Striated muscles
         a) Puborectal
         b) Pubococcygeal
         c) Iliococcygeal
         d) Coccygeal
   e. Weight and volume of stool
      1) Liquid stool has rapid transit time and is poorly absorbed in colon due to its liquid state; this is critical, because stool consistency is one predictor of continence
      2) Some individuals may be able to retain solid fecal material rectally, but may be inconti-

nent of liquid fecal material

f. Internal and external anal sphincters
   1) Innervated by sacral roots 2, 3, and 4 (S2, S3, S4)
   2) Internal sphincter is supplied by motor fibers from hypogastric nerve and parasympathetic system
   3) With rectal distension, reflex relaxation of internal sphincter occurs; external sphincter tone increases to prevent bowel emptying
   4) Afferent impulses stimulate cerebral recognition of anal contents and need to empty stool or need to defecate

B. Influence of autonomic and somatic nervous systems on fecal continence

1. In the intact system, cortical recognition of stimuli will initiate or inhibit defecation mechanisms
2. Defecation process
   a. With distension of colon, rectal stretch receptors stimulate inferior hypogastric plexus and inferior mesenteric plexus; impulses enter spinal cord, ascend to cortex, and initiate awareness of colonic and rectal distension
   b. Peristalsis of colon propels feces to rectum, which initiates a reflex rectal contraction mediated by pelvic splanchnic nerves originating from S2, S3, and S4
   c. Rectal reflexes relax internal sphincter and contract external sphincter so that stool can be expelled
   d. Voluntary defecation begins with closure of the glottis, followed by descent of diaphragm and contraction of abdominal muscles; this provides increased intra-abdominal pressure, which promotes movement of stool
   e. Pelvic musculature relaxes simultaneously with internal and external anal sphincters until complete emptying occurs
   f. Following rectal emptying, pelvic floor rises and anal sphincters return to their tonic state of contraction

C. Neurogenic bowel conditions

1. Occur commonly as a result of one of three types of conditions
   a. Central nervous system vascular disorders (e.g., stroke)
   b. Traumatic injury (e.g., intracranial bleeding, traumatic brain injury, or spinal cord injury)
   c. Neurological diseases (e.g., multiple sclerosis, Parkinson's disease)
2. Such conditions can cause partial or complete loss of innervation of gastrointestinal tract, resulting in incontinence and/or constipation
3. Neurogenic bowel is influenced by alterations in mobility, activity, cognition, diet, and medications
4. Neurogenic bowel alterations typically are categorized into three classifications: uninhibited, reflex, and areflexic
   a. Uninhibited neurogenic bowel (see Figure 13.1)
      1) Results from damage to upper motor neurons; typically seen after stroke, traumatic

Figure 13.1. Uninhibited Neurogenic Bowel

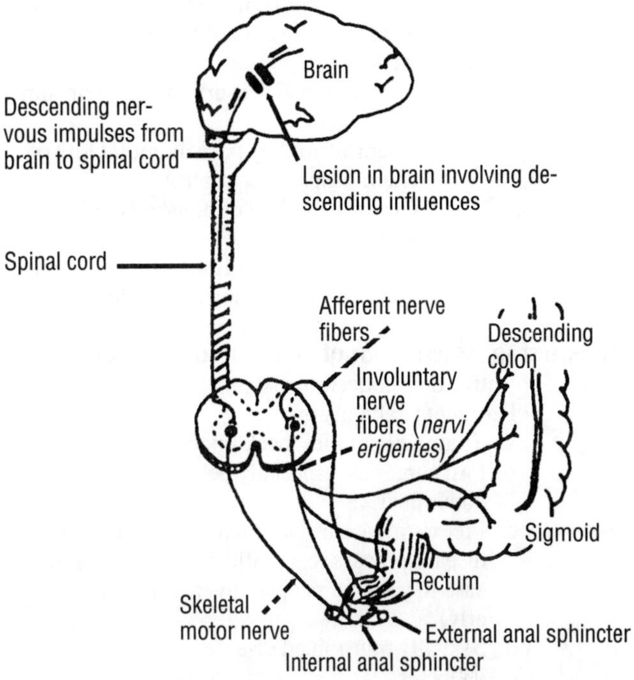

brain injury, multiple sclerosis, and trauma
      2) Internal and external sphincters are intact or hypertonic
      3) Saddle sensation usually is preserved
      4) Bulbocavernosus (BC) reflex is varied or increased
      5) Sacral reflex is intact
      6) Defecation is involuntary and sudden
   b. Reflex neurogenic bowel (also called *upper motor neuron* [UMN] *paralysis* or *spastic bowel paralysis*)
      1) Results from complete or incomplete spinal cord trauma or any central nervous system pathology above T12 or L1
      2) Defined as partial or complete loss of cortical control of defecation process with partial or complete loss of voluntary sphincter activity, resulting in reflex bowel emptying
      3) Defecation is purely reflexive due to total or partial absence of cortical control
      4) Partial or total sensory loss in perineum and rectum
      5) Partial or total loss of external sphincter control
      6) Diminished or absent saddle sensation
      7) Increased bulbocavernosus reflex and anal reflexes
   c. Areflexic neurogenic bowel (also called *autonomous neurogenic bowel, lower motor neuron* [LMN] *paralysis*, or *flaccid bowel paralysis*)
      1) Results from complete or incomplete lower

motor neuron trauma or any central nervous system pathology at or below T12
2) Results from partial or complete destruction of the sacral reflex arc of S2, S3, and S4
3) Characteristics
a) Partial or total sensory loss in perineum and rectum
b) Characterized by partial or total loss of external sphincter control
c) Characterized by diminished or absent saddle sensation
d) Characterized by diminished or absent bulbocavernosus and anal reflexes

II. Nursing Assessment of Bowel and Bladder

A. Subjective data collection
1. Pertinent health history
a. Traumatic injuries, back injuries
b. Past surgeries, especially pelvic, urologic, or abdominal
c. Preexisting gastrointestinal, metabolic, or other disease process (e.g., inflammatory bowel disease in younger people, diverticulitis in the elderly)
d. Sexually transmitted disease
e. Diabetes
f. Dementia
g. Use of medications that influence bowel activity
1) Diuretics
2) Antacids
3) Nonsteroidal and anti-inflammatory agents
4) Anticholinergics
5) Antidepressants
6) Antibiotics
7) Laxatives and enemas
h. Use of medications that can influence urinary continence
1) Diuretics
2) Sedatives and hypnotics
3) Anticholinergics
4) Beta blockers
5) Antidepressants
i. Mental status
1) Level of consciousness
2) Orientation and memory
3) Cognitive status (including ability to learn)
j. Drug reactions and side effects
k. In women, number of children and type of deliveries
2. Continence history
a. Premorbid pattern of elimination (what was "normal")
b. Chief complaint (symptoms)
c. Presence or absence of awareness of need to defecate or void
d. Frequency and quantity of stool and/or urine
1) Color, consistency
2) Ability to start urinary stream; force of stream
3) Dribbling of urine after voiding
e. Quantity of fluid intake and types of fluids ingested; use of caffeine or artificial sweeteners
f. Nutritional intake (for bowel incontinence), including 24-hour intake of bulk, carbohydrates, fats, and minerals
g. Times when incontinent episodes occur (day versus night, especially for urinary incontinence)
h. Client's method of handling incontinence
i. Voiding record
1) Frequency and quantity voided during episodes of incontinence
2) Patient's mental status at time of incontinence and/or other precipitant of incontinence
3) Activities that seem to trigger urinary incontinence (coughing, sneezing, laughing, lifting)
3. Psychosocial status
a. Impact of incontinence on emotional status
b. Vocational and/or avocational status and future plans to determine most effective routine (e.g., a morning program may not be practical for a student or for someone who must be at work early)

B. Objective assessment
1. Physical examination
a. Abdominal examination
1) Auscultate for bowel sounds for presence or absence of hyper- or hypomotility
2) Palpate for distension, tenderness, and masses
3) Percuss abdomen to determine distension and presence or absence of stool
b. Genital, perianal, and peritoneal inspection
1) Swelling
2) Redness, rash
3) Discharge
c. Rectal examination
1) Fecal impaction
2) Internal and external sphincter tone
3) Internal and external hemorrhoids
4) Guiac (if indicated)
d. Neurological examination (depending on primary diagnosis—for example, spinal cord injury)
1) Test for saddle sensation: Critical determinant of neurological integrity of sacral nerve roots 2, 3, 4; sacral nerve roots determine sensation and sphincter function; test by pinprick or light touch
2) Test for bulbocavernosus reflex: Indicates an intact reflex on sensory and motor components of S2, S3, S4; squeezing of the glans penis or clitoris (sensory input) should elicit tightening of the external anal sphincter and contraction (motor response) of bulbocavernosus and ischiocavernosus muscles
3) Anal reflex, or anal wink: another indication of intact sacral nerve roots wherein a pinprick to one or both sides of external anal

sphincter results in tightening of the sphincter (a contracture known as *anal wink*)

C. Functional ability
1. Ability to use bathroom, commode, chair, or assistive devices
2. Toileting ability: Ability to remove clothing and perform necessary hygiene

D. Evaluation of laboratory and diagnostic tests

III. Nursing Diagnoses

➤ A. Colonic constipation

1. **Definition:** Pattern of elimination characterized by hard, dry stool resulting from delay in passage of food residue (NANDA, 1992)

2. **Major defining characteristics**

a. Decreased frequency
b. Hard, dry stool
c. Straining, bleeding
d. Painful defecation
e. Abdominal distension, pain, cramping
f. Headache (may be a sign of autonomic dysreflexia—see Chapter 12)
g. Decreased appetite, nausea
h. Increased spasticity in individuals with neurogenic impairments
i. Rectal pressure, pain

3. **Related factors/etiologies**

a. Change in or less than adequate physical activity; impaired mobility
b. Change in or less than adequate intake of fluids or dietary fiber
c. Sensorimotor disorders
d. Postoperative complications
e. Side effects of medication regimen
f. Slowed peristalsis from disorder of central nervous system or autonomic nervous system

4. **Interventions**

a. Increase fluid intake as tolerated and monitor intake and output
b. Increase bulk and fiber in diet
c. Provide for colonic and rectal emptying through use of stimulants or irritant cathartics, bulk-forming agents (to be taken at least 6 to 8 hours prior to expected and/or desired emptying) (see Table 13.1); use low-volume enemas or suppositories alone or in conjunction with oral medications for complete emptying
d. Promote use of stool softeners or bulk formers with adequate fluids and food intake to establish bowel routine until regularity is achieved
e. Promote habitual toilet routine (after meals or coffee) at convenient, uninterrupted, consistent time
f. Use commode or toilet rather than bedpan
g. Integrate anticipated and current activity levels when establishing program and assessing effectiveness of program
h. Instruct client and family about symptoms of developing impaction and about the risks associated with it
i. Reinforce need to limit routine use of laxatives and enemas

5. **Expected outcomes**

a. Client achieves regular and, when possible, routine bowel evacuation
b. Client identifies and avoids factors that contribute to development of constipation
c. Client demonstrates ability to recognize when to seek medical attention for constipation
d. Client verbalizes knowledge about relationship between diet, activity, and constipation

➤ B. Incontinence related to neurogenic bowel

1. Uninhibited neurogenic bowel

a. **Definition:** Impaired cortical awareness of urge to defecate, characterized by urgency and involuntary stools

b. **Major defining characteristics**

1) Defecation is sudden, with or without urgency
2) Hard stool with smearing is common
3) Internal and external sphincters intact or hypertonic
4) Saddle sensation is usually preserved
5) Bulbocavernosus reflex is varied or increased
6) Sacral reflex is intact

c. **Related factor/etiology**

1) Damage to upper motor neuron
2) Typically seen after stroke, traumatic brain injury, multiple sclerosis, and trauma

d. **Interventions**

1) Initiate bowel program that includes adequate bulk and fiber
2) Avoid overly spiced and gas-forming foods such as broccoli, cauliflower, apples, grapes, seeded fruits and vegetables, or any food that has previously caused problems for client
3) Encourage client to use adaptive clothing to ease donning and doffing for toileting
4) Encourage client to decrease and gradually eliminate bowel medications and establish diet and consistent routine as primary modalities of bowel program
   a) Evaluate impact of bowel medications (softness, bulk, firmness)
   b) Wean client from one medication at a time to better assess impact each may have on routine—for example, discontinue an irritating cathartic but continue with a liquid suppository such as a bisacodyl enema
   c) Use only one type of intervention at a time whenever possible—for example, initiation of intermittent catheterization

Table 13.1. Types of Medications Used in a Bowel Program

The nurse should perform an ongoing assessment of the effect of bowel medications on desired bowel program outcomes.

Drug Class	Purpose	Considerations
Bulk formers	Typically contain cellulose derivatives that swell in the intestinal fluid, promote bowel motility, and facilitate movement of the fecal matter toward the anal canal	• Must be taken with adequate fluids according to instructions on the package insert; use to minimize the risk of esophageal or intestinal obstruction • Should be used cautiously in individuals who are on fluid restriction for any reason (e.g., those with cardiac problems or renal failure and those on an intermittent catheterization program)
Emollients	Surfactants increase the wetting efficiency of intestinal water, thereby softening the fecal mass; useful when the Valsalva maneuver must be avoided	• Should be used judiciously • Stool that is too soft can result in impaction because fecal mass might not be easily evacuated • Review package inserts to determine whether the emollient could be toxic to the liver if used chronically, as some emollients can be • Adequate fluid intake is required to promote drug action
Saline and osmotic products (oral, rectal)	Used to increase osmotic pressure in the intestinal lumen; this increases stool water content, softens stool, and stimulates bowel motility through osmotic activity	• Drugs given orally must be used cautiously in individuals with electrolyte disturbances • If magnesium products are used chronically, toxicity can result • Use judiciously when initiating a bowel routine; eventually wean the client from products by incorporating digital stimulation into the program
Stimulants (oral, rectal) (e.g., irritant cathartics)	Used to increase peristalsis, probably by direct action on colonic sensory endings; onset of action is 6 to 10 hours when taken by mouth, but liquid or solid suppositories have an onset within 15 to 60 minutes	• Many clients do not consider these over-the-counter (OTC) products to be drugs; many will use OTC drugs with prescribed drugs that interfere with prescribed bowel routine • Plan oral administration of drugs 6 to 8 hours before expected or planned evacuation • Action of liquid or solid suppository will be enhanced if suppository is placed directly against the rectal mucosal wall and not within the stool settled in the rectal vault

will limit fluid intake and can lead to change in stool consistency or cause an impaction

5) Use a small bisacodyl enema or a suppository to stimulate rectal emptying
   a) Apply directly along rectal mucosa
   b) Assess time between insertion and emptying
   c) Repeat once and reassess if there are no results
6) Investigate cause of fecal smears to rule out constipation and impaction
7) Use alternative modalities such as biofeedback, if they are indicated, to enhance sphincter tone and thereby increase continence
8) Ensure adequate hydration, which varies by individual
9) Incorporate consistent exercise and activity into daily routine

e. Expected outcomes

1) Patient achieves predictable, regular bowel program and at least three planned evacua-

tions per week
2) Patient has decreased incidence of involuntary bowel movements
3) Patient has adequate nutrition, hydration, and activity to maintain a bowel program and prevent constipation
4) Patient verbalizes early signs of constipation, impaction, and, when applicable, autonomic dysreflexia (see Chapter 12)
5) When indicated, patient demonstrates knowledge of digital stimulation, suppository insertion, and application of an abdominal binder
6) When appropriate, patient verbalizes and/or demonstrates appropriate selection of continence products that provide personal comfort and control
7) Patient verbalizes knowledge of situations and/or complications requiring medical attention

2. **Reflex neurogenic bowel**
   a. **Definition:** Partial or complete loss of cortical control of defecation process with partial or complete loss of voluntary sphincter activity resulting in reflex bowel emptying (also called *upper motor neuron paralysis* or *spastic bowel paralysis*)

   b. **Major defining characteristics**
      1) Defecation is involuntary; there is sudden, mass emptying when rectal vault becomes full (due to sacral reflex)
      2) Partial or total sensory loss in perineum and/or rectum
      3) Partial or total loss of external sphincter control
      4) Diminished or absent saddle sensation
      5) Increased bulbocavernosus reflex and anal reflexes

   c. **Related factor/etiology**
      1) Damage to UMN at spinal level
      2) Typically seen after spinal cord injury

   d. **Interventions**
      1) Use irritant cathartics, bulk formers (see Table 13.1), and stool softeners appropriately timed to facilitate routine results; administer irritant cathartics at least 6 hours before planned program evacuation
      2) Insert suppository or liquid suppository while patient is lying on his or her side; transfer client to toilet or commode approximately 15 to 20 minutes after insertion to facilitate complete emptying of stool
      3) Use upright posture and support for trunk as well as upper and lower extremities during routine
      4) Use circular digital stimulation to facilitate reflex contraction of colon and rectum to enhance emptying; use adequate lubricant, anesthetic ointment (if client is prone to dysreflexia), and universal precautions
      5) Discontinue digital stimulation if rectal bleeding or dysreflexia occurs and apply anesthetic, if ordered; always inspect rectal area for external or internal hemorrhoids; modify stimulation accordingly, by either decreasing the frequency or avoiding use of stimulus until hemorrhoids are repaired
      6) Establish realistic routine that allows for client's level of independence, extent and amount of assistance client requires, and client's daily life schedule (including work and school activities)
      7) Ensure consistent and adequate amounts of fiber and fluid each day
      8) Reassess program if any changes in health, activity, nutritional level, or life schedule occur

   e. **Expected outcomes** (see outcomes listed for "Uninhibited neurogenic bowel" on page 98)

3. **Areflexic neurogenic bowel**
   a. **Definition:** Involuntary defecation is experienced due to partial or total absence of rectal compliance and/or sphincter control

   b. **Major defining characteristics**
      1) Hard, formed stool requiring disimpaction
      2) Stool leakage with activity and/or stress
      3) Partial or total sensory loss in rectum and perineum
      4) Partial or total loss of external sphincter control
      5) Diminished or absent saddle sensation
      6) Diminished or absent bulbocavernosus and anal reflexes
      7) Decreased or absent sensory awareness or urge to defecate

   c. **Related factors/etiologies**
      1) Sensory or motor loss of sacral nerve root
      2) Injury to the lumbosacral core and spinal roots (LMN), trauma, or postoperative complications

   d. **Interventions**
      1) Maintain adequate nutrition and hydration for stool consistency
      2) Maintain consistent routine
      3) Add bulk formers to therapeutic regimen
      4) Evacuate stool from distal colon and rectum with a liquid suppository and other suppositories
      5) Establish routine based on premorbid bowel habits
      6) Instruct patient and caregiver regarding signs and symptoms of potential gastrointestinal complications (e.g., nausea, loss of appetite, vomiting, bloating, distension)
      7) Use an abdominal binder and or abdominal

massage (right to left, up, around, and down) to facilitate emptying during bowel routine
8) Note that in very rare situations, patients might opt for ostomy as a means of control

e. **Expected outcomes** (see outcomes listed for "Uninhibited neurogenic bowel" on page 98)

Bladder Elimination

I. Related Theory and Concepts

A. Normal anatomy/physiology of lower urinary tract

1. Bladder
   a. Muscular organ that functions as a reservoir for urine
   b. Detrusor muscle is the main bladder body and is composed of smooth muscle
   c. Trigone muscle is an interlacing network of smooth muscle forming posterior base of the bladder and continuing into proximal urethra
   d. Detrusor muscle allows for bladder wall expansion while maintaining a fairly constant low pressure as bladder fills with urine
2. Urethra
   a. Passageway for urine expulsion
   b. Internal sphincter (bladder neck) remains compressed in a resting state to prevent urine leakage when there is low or moderate pressure in the bladder
   c. Maintenance of constant tension throughout the urethra depends on fibroelasticity and thickness of urethral wall
3. External sphincter: Striated skeletal muscle that surrounds distal portion of the urethra; serves as a last line of defense for maintaining continence

B. Neurological control of lower urinary tract

1. Central nervous system
   a. Frontal cerebral cortex facilitates or inhibits pontine micturition center
   b. Pontine micturition center, which is located in the brainstem, facilitates impulses to bladder
   c. Spinal cord tracts (see Chapter 5 for further information)
      1) Spinothalamic tracts (sensory, ascending): Carry pain and temperature messages from lower urinary tract to cerebral centers
      2) Posterior columns (sensory, ascending): Carry sensations of fullness and desire to void to cerebral centers
      3) Reticulospinal tract (motor, descending): Transmits inhibitory messages from the pons to the detrusor
      4) Corticospinal tract (motor, descending): Carries messages from cerebral centers to pudendal nucleus in sacral micturition center to provide voluntary control over external sphincter
2. Peripheral nervous system
   a. Parasympathetic innervation through the pelvic nerve provides motor stimulation to bladder and facilitates detrusor contraction
   b. Sympathetic innervation through hypogastric nerve facilitates bladder storage by inhibiting detrusor contractility while maintaining contraction of bladder neck and proximal urethra
   c. Somatic innervation through pudendal nerve facilitates voluntary contraction of external sphincter

C. Normal micturition reflex

1. Filling phase
   a. Bladder slowly fills with urine and maintains low intravesical pressure with increasing volume; continence is maintained as long as pressure within bladder is lower than urethral pressure
   b. As volume of urine increases, sensory receptors in bladder wall are stimulated to transmit sensation of fullness to sacral cord reflex center (S2, S3, S4) via pelvic nerve (the first urge to void occurs when the urine level is around 150-200 cc; a marked sensation of fullness occurs at 300-400 cc)
   c. Sensory messages are sent from spinal cord to higher centers in cerebral cortex through spinothalamic tract and posterior columns
2. Postponement phase
   a. Inhibitory centers in frontal lobe can override micturition reflex by voluntarily contracting the external sphincter via pudendal nerve
   b. Postponement becomes more difficult as volume increases, which causes sensory receptors to bombard the sacral reflex center, and as bladder pressure increases and approaches the level of urethral pressure; detrusor muscle begins rhythmic contractions, causing notable discomfort
3. Emptying phase
   a. Messages of fullness and urge to void are processed in frontal lobe and motor messages are sent through the corticoregulatory tract to sacral reflex center (S2, S3, S4)
   b. Peripheral nervous system relays these messages via parasympathetic and somatic fibers thereby stimulating detrusor contraction, external sphincter relaxation, and consequent bladder emptying
   c. External sphincter must relax as detrusor contracts to allow for complete bladder emptying

D. Effects of neurological lesions on micturition

1. Any disruption of sensory or motor pathways in the central or peripheral nervous systems that have input to bladder will cause a disruption in micturition cycle
2. Disruption in central nervous system above sacral reflex center generally causes a hyperreflexic bladder and is considered an upper motor neuron injury (for additional information, see Chapter 5)
3. Disruption at sacral reflex center or in peripheral nervous system causes an areflexic bladder and is considered a lower motor neuron injury (for addi-

Figure 13.2. Uninhibited Neurogenic Bladder

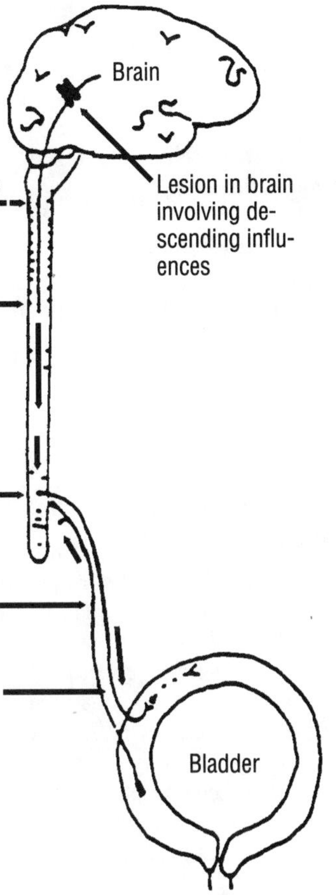

Figure 13.3. Reflex Neurogenic Bladder

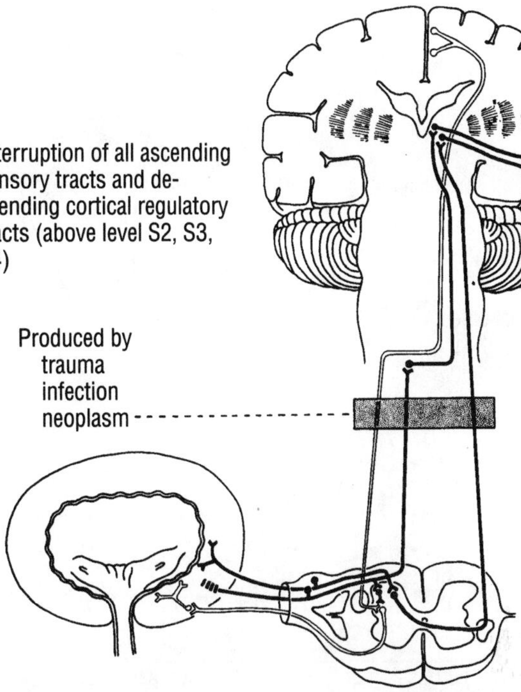

Reprinted with permission of W.B. Saunders Company from Lapides, J., & Diokno, A.C. (1976). Urine transport, storage, and micturition. In J. Lapides (Ed.), *Fundamentals of urology* (p. 218). Philadelphia: W.B. Saunders Company.

tional information, see Chapter 5)

E. Classification of neurogenic bladders

1. Characteristics of uninhibited neurogenic bladder, which occurs in patients with lesions in the brain and pontine center (from stroke, traumatic brain injury, multiple sclerosis, and brain tumor) (see Figure 13.2)
   a. Failure of inhibitory fibers of corticoregulatory tract to suppress involuntary detrusor contractions
   b. Strong uncontrolled voiding contractions of smooth muscle in bladder wall
   c. Urgency, frequency, nocturia resulting in urge incontinence
   d. Reduced bladder capacity with little or no residual urine
   e. Intact saddle sensation and bulbocavernosus reflex
2. Characteristics of reflex neurogenic bladder, which occurs in patients who have spinal cord lesions above T12-L1 or who have experienced an interruption of blood supply to the cord secondary to trauma, tumors, infection, vascular infarction, or multiple sclerosis (see Figure 13.3)
   a. Disruption of both the sensory and motor nerve tracts above sacral segments 2, 3, and 4 (upper motor neuron damage)
   b. Loss of control from higher brain centers resulting in uninhibited, involuntary detrusor contractions and uncontrolled voiding; spinal reflex arc takes over control of micturition
   c. Decreased bladder capacity with high urine residuals
   d. Inability of external sphincter to relax in coordination with detrusor contraction (this is called *detrusor external sphincter dyssynergia*); this results in increased bladder pressure with emptying and large amount of residual urine
   e. Impaired or absent saddle sensation and a hyperactive bulbocavernosus reflex
3. Characteristics of autonomous neurogenic bladder (or areflexic neurogenic bladder), which occurs in patients with spinal cord lesions at or below T12-L1 or with other conditions, such as spina bifida, meningocele, and herniated intervertebral disc, that damage the lower motor neurons (see Figure 13.4)
   a. Disruption of the sensory and motor branches of the sacral spinal reflex arc S2, S3, and S4 (lower motor neuron damage)
   b. Decreased sensation of fullness, weak or absent detrusor contractions, increased bladder capacity with high residual urine

Figure 13.4. Autonomous Neurogenic Bladder

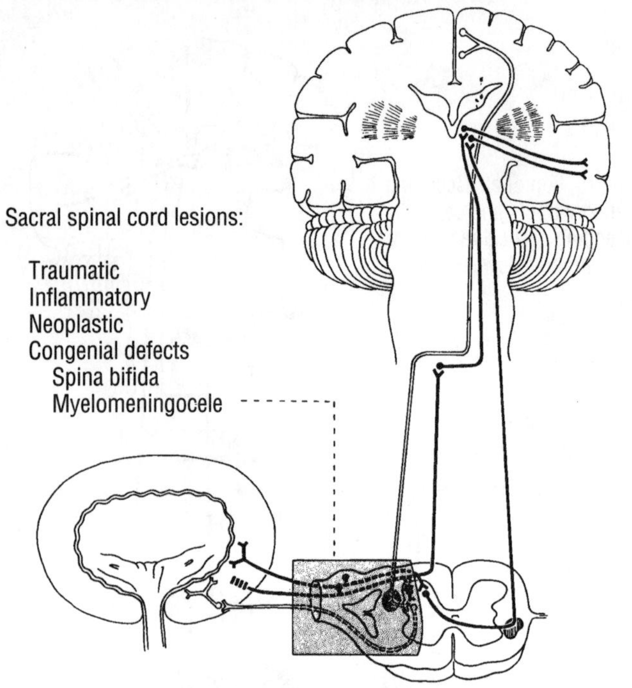

Reprinted with permission of W.B. Saunders Company from Lapides, J., & Diokno, A.C. (1976). Urine transport, storage, and micturition. In J. Lapides (Ed.), *Fundamentals of urology* (p. 222). Philadelphia: W.B. Saunders Company.

c. Loss of voluntary voiding except with straining; overflow incontinence is common
d. Impaired or absent saddle sensation and absent bulbocavernosus reflex

4. Characteristics of motor paralytic neurogenic bladder, which occurs in patients with poliomyelitis, herniated disc, trauma, or tumors
   a. Disruption of motor branches (ventral roots) of sacral reflex center (S2, S3, S4) or damage to anterior horn cells of spinal cord
   b. Partial or complete motor loss of bladder function; intact sensory nerves
   c. Difficulty with starting a stream, decreased force of urinary stream, interrupted stream, or a need to strain to void
   d. Increased bladder capacity with high residual urine; overflow incontinence is common
   e. Intact saddle sensation; absent bulbocavernosus reflex
5. Characteristics of sensory paralytic neurogenic bladder, which occurs in patients with disruption of sensory segment of reflex arc secondary to diabetic neuropathy, tabes dorsalis, syringomyelia, and multiple sclerosis
   a. Disruption of sensory branches (dorsal roots) of the sacral reflex center S2, S3, and S4 or in pathways that carry sensory messages to cerebral cortex
   b. Decreased or absent sensations of pain, temperature, and/or fullness in the bladder
   c. Infrequent voiding with large output; increased bladder capacity with overflow incontinence is also common
   d. Variable saddle sensation and bulbocavernosus reflex according to progression of the disease

II. Nursing Assessment (see Nursing Assessment on pages 96-97)

III. Nursing Diagnoses

➤ A. Urinary incontinence

1. **Definition:** Involuntary loss of urine sufficient to be a problem (Urinary Incontinence Guideline Panel, 1992)
2. **Major defining characteristic:** Uncontrollable loss of urine
3. **Related factors/etiologies**
   a. Neurological impairment
   b. Sensorimotor impairment
   c. Decreased bladder capacity
   d. Bladder spasm and/or irritation of bladder wall stretch receptors
   e. Environmental barriers
   f. Sensory deficits (vision, hearing)
   g. Mobility deficits
   h. Neuropathies (e.g., lack of sensory awareness of bladder fullness)
   i. Cognitive deficits
4. **Interventions**
   a. Reduce or eliminate factors contributing to incontinence, if possible
      1) Urinary tract infection
      2) Medications that can exacerbate incontinence
         a) Diuretics
         b) Sedatives, hypnotics, tranquilizers
         c) Anticholinergics
         d) Antihypertensives
         e) Antiarrhythmics
         f) Over-the-counter cold medications
      3) Environmental barriers
         a) Remove obstacles in path to bathroom and ensure adequate lighting, especially for elderly patients
         b) Assess bathroom size, height of toilet, and need for raised toilet seat, grab bars, or other adaptive equipment
         c) Consider use of bedside commode for nighttime use
         d) Ensure that there is an adequate signal system for requesting assistance
   b. Maintain adequate hydration
      1) Increase fluid intake to approximately 2,000-3,000 cc/day unless contraindicated
      2) Ensure that consistent amounts of fluids are given throughout the day and consider need to decrease fluid intake in the early evening

3) Decrease and/or eliminate intake of fluids with diuretic, dehydrating, or irritating effects on bladder
   a) Caffeinated drinks
      (1) Tea
      (2) Coffee
      (3) Colas
   b) Grapefruit juice
   c) Drinks containing aspartame
4) If patient is on a bladder management program, document fluid intake and involve the patient in keeping his or her own record, if possible

c. Ensure adequate bowel elimination (see pages 97-100)

d. Promote individual's personal integrity, self-esteem, and privacy
1) Encourage patient to share feelings about incontinence and determine its effects on his or her social patterns
2) Encourage socialization
   a) Encourage temporary use of pads, briefs, or external catheters if fear of embarrassment is preventing socialization
   b) Encourage and help patient to maintain grooming and personal hygiene

e. Maintain skin integrity
1) Monitor skin for reddened and sore areas
2) Perform perineal hygiene at least twice a day and after every episode of incontinence; instruct patient and family on proper technique
3) Use moisture barrier creams or films as appropriate

f. **Establish a bladder program:** Incorporate management strategies appropriate for the specific type of neurogenic bladder
1) Teach about and administer *medications* as ordered by the physician and monitor the patient's response
   a) Cholinergics stimulate cholinergic receptors of the bladder wall, causing detrusor contraction and thus facilitating bladder emptying (contraindicated with bladder outlet obstruction)
   b) Anticholinergics inhibit the action of acetylcholine; this inhibits bladder contraction and assists in increasing bladder capacity
   c) Antispasmodics and anticholinergics directly depress the smooth muscle of the bladder, produce local anesthesia, and increase bladder capacity
   d) Alpha-adrenergics stimulate alpha-adrenergic receptors of bladder outlet, causing contraction of smooth muscle and increased urethral pressure
   e) Alpha-adrenergic blockers block alpha-adrenergic receptors, reducing urethral resistance and facilitating bladder emptying
   f) Skeletal muscle relaxants decrease contractility of skeletal muscle, including spasticity of external sphincter
2) Implement bladder management techniques
   a) *Intermittent catheterization* (procedures vary among institutions)
      (1) Empty bladder at regular intervals
      (2) Start with straight catheterization at regular intervals of 2 to 4 hours as ordered by physician
      (3) Monitor fluid intake patterns in relation to catheterized amounts and adjust intake patterns accordingly
      (4) Incorporate bladder-triggering techniques to facilitate bladder emptying before catheterizations
         (a) Suprapubic stimulation (for those with upper motor neuron lesions): Stimulation of sacral-lumbar dermatomes by manually tapping the suprapubic area, pulling pubic hairs, or stroking the medial thighs
         (b) Instructing patient in use of Valsalva maneuver (for those with lower motor neuron lesions)
            - Lean forward on thighs
            - Contract abdominal muscles, if possible, and strain or bear down
            - Hold the strain or one's breath until urine flow stops
         (c) Credé maneuver (appropriate only for those with lower motor neuron lesions): Manual expression of bladder by placing hands flat (or in fists) just below umbilical area and pressing firmly down and in toward pelvic arch; this is repeated until no more urine can be expelled
      (5) Increase intervals between catheterizations as residual urine decreases and spontaneous voiding increases
      (6) Stop intermittent catheterization under the following circumstances according to institutional guidelines
         (a) When adequate amount of urine is voided
         (b) When residual urine volume is in the range of 100-150 cc or less
         (c) When genitourinary tract is free of pathological changes or infection
      (7) Teach patient and family sterile and/or clean catheterization techniques for home and long-term use
   b) *Indwelling catheterization*
      (1) Use only as a last resort
      (2) Select the smallest size catheter that will drain adequately (12F, 14F, 16F for adults)

(3) Use catheters with nonstick surface to reduce urethritis, stone formation, and encrustation
(4) Use aseptic technique at time of insertion
(5) Maintain smallest feasible balloon size to prevent leakage; if leakage occurs, decrease catheter size and/or balloon size
(6) Maintain closed-system drainage as much as possible
(7) Irrigate catheter only if an obstruction is suspected
(8) Determine need for a change of catheter by rolling the catheter between fingers and feeling for grit
(9) Meatal care is controversial and is not endorsed by Centers for Disease Control (Wong, 1983)
(10) Retract the foreskin of uncircumcised males, clean around glans penis, and replace foreskin
(11) Tape female catheter to thigh when patient is sitting or supine; tape male catheter to thigh when patient is sitting and to abdomen when supine
(12) Teach patient and family proper management of indwelling catheter, including when to change it and how to clean tubing and drainage bags

c) *Behavioral strategies*
(1) Use timed voiding (toileting the patient at regular 2- to 3-hour intervals) for patients with uninhibited or sensory paralytic neurogenic bladders who have impaired memory or advanced dementia
(2) Use prompted voiding (which teaches the person to take responsibility for toileting and/or wetness) for patients with uninhibited neurogenic bladder and cognitive impairment
(a) Check the patient at regular set intervals and ask whether he or she is wet or dry
(b) Physically check the patient and give feedback on accuracy of patient's response
(c) Give verbal or nonverbal approval if patient is dry and corrective feedback if he or she is wet
(d) Prompt patient to request toileting assistance and give assistance when patient requests it
(3) Use habit training (individualizing a toileting schedule to patient's voiding pattern) for patients with uninhibited neurogenic bladder
(a) Assess baseline continence and incontinence patterns
(b) Establish toileting schedule to anticipate and prevent incontinence
(c) Progressively increase toileting time intervals as continence is achieved
(4) Use bladder training with patients with uninhibited neurogenic bladder who have adequate comprehension and motivation
(a) Educate them on physiology and pathophysiology of lower urinary tract
(b) Do baseline assessment of voiding and incontinence patterns for 3 to 7 days prior to initiating program
(c) Establish an initial toileting schedule according to baseline assessment patterns (except for nighttime, because nocturia is resolved as daytime frequency is resolved)
(d) Gradually increase time between toileting with encouragement to practice inhibiting urge sensation and postponing voiding (e.g., ask patient to take two to three deep breaths)
(5) Use pelvic muscle exercises for patients with uninhibited neurogenic bladder who have adequate comprehension and memory and are motivated to participate; pelvic muscle exercises are generally used in conjunction with a bladder training program
(a) Educate patients and help them identify the pubococcygeal muscle and explain purpose of exercises
(b) Have patients follow through with exercises on a regular basis (three sets of 15 per day)
(c) Have patients lie, sit, or stand with knees slightly apart during exercises
(d) Have patients slowly and firmly contract pelvic muscles holding the contraction for 5 to 10 seconds, then relax muscles

d) Use of continence products (e.g., pads, briefs, underpads, external catheters, leg bags): As appropriate

5. Expected outcomes

a. Client achieves an acceptable level of continence

b. Client and family follow a bladder management program consistent with lifestyle
c. Client verbalizes knowledge of medications related to a bladder management program
d. Client demonstrates, as applicable, the ability to take care of indwelling catheters, straight catheters, and external urinary collection devices and perineal/periurethral skin

➤ B. Urinary retention

1. **Definition:** Condition in which individual experiences incomplete emptying of bladder (NANDA, 1992)

2. Major defining characteristics

a. Bladder distension
b. Frequent voiding in small amounts or absence of urine output
c. Sensation of bladder fullness
d. Dribbling
e. Residual urine
f. Dysuria
g. Overflow incontinence

3. Related factors/etiologies

a. High urethral pressure (caused by a weak detrusor)
b. Inhibition of reflex arc
c. Strong external sphincter
d. Blockage of urine

4. Interventions

a. Initiate a bladder management program with a combination of the following techniques depending on cause of retention
   1) Institute timed voiding schedule with intermittent catheterization for postvoid residual (for use with patients who have mild-to-moderate outlet obstruction)
   2) Institute double voiding: Patient is taught to void, wait a few minutes, and then void again (for use with patients who have mild-to-moderate outlet obstruction)
   3) Ensure that fluid intake is distributed throughout the waking hours; decrease or curtail fluids early in the evening
   4) Ensure intake of at least 2,000 cc of fluids in a 24-hour period (if not contraindicated)
   5) Institute an intermittent catheterization program (see page 103)
   6) Use mechanical methods to empty bladder (see triggering techniques on page 103)
   7) Teach about and administer medications (cholinergics or alpha-adrenergic blocking agents) as ordered by physician; monitor patient's response; assess for increased retention, hypotension, and/or dizziness
   8) Use an indwelling Foley catheter if other interventions are inadequate
b. Teach the patient measures for managing acute urinary retention, the symptoms of which include abrupt cessation of micturition followed by increased suprapubic discomfort as bladder fills
   1) Relax and sit in a tub of warm water or stand in a warm shower and attempt to void
   2) Drink warm liquids, such as tea
   3) Seek help from a physician or an emergency care facility if the procedures listed above fail
   4) Teach patient with prostatic outlet obstruction to avoid factors that can precipitate an episode of acute urinary retention
      a) Consumption of large amounts of alcohol
      b) Use of over-the-counter cold medicines or diet pills that contribute to closure of the bladder neck
      c) Use of any antidepressant or anticholinergic medications (physician should always be consulted before these are taken)

5. Expected outcomes

a. Client achieves complete bladder emptying by using appropriate bladder management techniques
b. Client verbalizes signs and symptoms of urinary retention and actions to take when it occurs
c. Client verbalizes signs and symptoms of urinary tract infection and the actions to take should these occur
d. Client verbalizes knowledge of prescribed medications and their side effects

➤ C. High risk for urinary tract infection

1. **Definition:** State in which an individual's urinary tract is at risk of being invaded by pathogenic agents (NANDA, 1992)

2. Risk factors and/or etiologies

a. Urinary retention
b. Indwelling catheter
c. Urinary calculi
d. Neurogenic bladder
e. Poor personal hygiene
f. Any surgery or trauma to the genitourinary tract
g. Bladder diversion or urinary ostomies
h. History of cystitis

3. Interventions

a. Ensure adequate fluid intake (at least 2,500-3,500 cc per day, unless contraindicated)
b. Encourage intake of fluids that will acidify urine
   1) Cranberry juice
   2) Apple juice
   3) Grape juice
c. Eliminate residual urine by facilitating urine outflow through various techniques (see page 103)
   1) Double voiding
   2) Valsalva maneuver
   3) Suprapubic tapping

4) Credé maneuver (use only if there is lower motor neuron damage and there is no evidence or history of reflux)
5) Intermittent catheterization

d. Monitor residual urine
e. Maintain sterile technique with intermittent catheterization while patient is hospitalized
f. Implement measures to prevent or reduce incidence of infection specific to genitourinary tract
   1) Washing hands thoroughly
   2) Using an aseptic technique
   3) Avoiding use of an indwelling catheter
   4) Maintaining closed drainage systems when indwelling catheters are necessary
   5) Administering anti-infective medications
g. Instruct patient on signs and symptoms of urinary tract infection
h. Teach patient how to prevent and/or reduce infection

4. Expected outcomes

a. Client is free of symptoms of urinary tract infection
b. Client verbalizes signs and symptoms of urinary tract infection and follows measures to prevent and/or reduce infection

References

Lapides, J., & Diokno, A.C. (1976). Urine transport, storage, and micturition. In J. Lapides (Ed.), *Fundamentals of urology* (pp. 190-231). Philadelphia: W.B. Saunders Company.

North American Nursing Diagnosis Association. (1992). *NANDA Nursing diagnoses: Definitions and classification 1992-1993.* St. Louis: Author.

Urinary Incontinence Guideline Panel. (1992). *Urinary incontinence in adults: Clinical practice guideline* (AHCPR Publication No. 92-0038). Rockville, MD: Agency for Health Care Policy and Research, Public Health Service, U.S. Department of Health and Human Services.

Wong, E.S. (1983). Guidelines for prevention of catheter-associated urinary tract infections. *American Journal of Infection Control, 11*(1), 28-36.

Suggested Readings

Aaronson, M.J., Freed, M.M., & Burakoff, R. (1985). Colonic myoelectric activity in persons with spinal cord injury. *Digestive Disorders in Science, 30*(4), 295-300.

Anichini, M.A., Mulrow, M., & Griggs, W.P. (1985). *Alterations in urine elimination: Incontinence.* Chicago: Rehabilitation Institute of Chicago.

Burgio, K.L., & Burgio, L.D. (1986). Behavioral therapies for urinary incontinence in the elderly. *Clinics in Geriatric Medicine, 2*, 809-827.

Carnevali, D.L., & Patrick, M.P. (Eds.). (1979). *Nursing management for the elderly.* Philadelphia: J.B. Lippincott Company.

Carpenito, L.J. (1989). *Nursing diagnosis: Application to clinical practice* (3rd ed.) (pp. 688-693). Philadelphia: J.B. Lippincott Company.

Carpenito, L.J. (1991). *Nursing care plans and documentation* (pp. 637-638). Philadelphia: J.B. Lippincott Company.

◆Cerulli, M.A., Nikoomanesh, P., & Schuster, M.M. (1979). Progress in biofeedback conditioning for fecal incontinence. *Gastroenterology, 76*, 742-746.

◆Cornell, S.A., Campion, L., Bacero, S., Frazier, J., Kjellstrom, M., & Purdy, S. (1973). Comparison of three bowel management programs during rehabilitation of spinal cord injured patients. *Nursing Research, 22*, 321-328.

Creason, N.S., Grybowski, J.A., Burgener, S., Whippo, C., Yeo, S., & Richardson, B. (1989). Prompted voiding therapy for urinary incontinence in aged female nursing home residents. *Journal of Advanced Nursing, 14*(2), 120-126.

Davis, F.A. (1989). *Taber's cyclopedia medical dictionary.* Philadelphia: F.A. Davis Company.

Dittmar, S. (1989). Bladder elimination. In S. Dittmar (Ed.), *Rehabilitation nursing* (pp. 150-195). St. Louis: The C.V. Mosby Company.

Dittmar, S. (1989). *Rehabilitation nursing: Process and application.* St. Louis: The C.V. Mosby Company.

Dittmar, S., Grossman, D.A., Sandler, R.S., McKee, D.C., & Lovits, A.J. (1982). Bowel patterns among subjects not seeking health care: Use of a questionnaire to identify a population with bowel dysfunction. *Gastroenterology, 83*, 529.

Doughty, D.B. (1991). *Urinary and fecal incontinence: Nursing management.* St. Louis: Mosby-Year Book, Inc.

Gordon, M. (1991). *Manual of nursing diagnosis: 1991-1992.* St. Louis: Mosby-Year Book, Inc.

Gore, G.M., Mintzer, R.A., & Calenoff, L. (1981). Gastrointestinal complications of spinal cord injury. *Spine, 6*, 538-544.

Gray, M., & Dougherty, M.C. (1987). Urinary incontinence—Pathophysiology and treatment. *Journal of Enterostomal Therapy, 14*(4), 152-162.

Henry, M.M. (1987). Pathogenesis and management of fecal incontinence in the adult. *Gastroenterology, 16*(1), 37.

Ingersoll, R.N. (1985). Abdominal pathology in spinal cord injured persons. *Journal of Neurosurgical Nursing, 17*, 344-348.

Jeter, K.F., Faller, N., & Norton, C. (1990). *Nursing for continence.* Philadelphia: W.B. Saunders Company.

Kegel, A.H. (1948, July-December). Progressive resistance exercises in the restoration of the perineal muscles. *American Journal of Obstetrics and Gynecology,* pp. 238-248.

Krane, R., & Siroky, B. (1979). *Clinical neuro-urology.* Boston: Little, Brown & Company.

Malseed, R.T. (1982). *Drug therapy and nursing considerations. Pharmacology* (pp. 467-471). Philadelphia: J.B. Lippincott Company.

McCormick, K.A., Scheve, A.A., & Leahy, E. (1988). Nursing management of urinary incontinence in geriatric inpatients. *Nursing Clinics of North America, 23*(1), 231-263.

McFarland, G., & McFarlane, E. (1989). *Nursing diagnosis and intervention: Planning for patient care.* St. Louis: The C.V. Mosby Company.

Middaugh, S.J., Whitehead, W.E., Burgio, K.L., & Engel, B.T. (1989). Biofeedback in treatment of urinary incontinence in stroke patients. *Biofeedback and Self-Regulation, 14*(1), 3-19.

Mumma, C.M. (Ed.). (1987). *Rehabilitation nursing: Concepts and practice—A core curriculum* (2nd ed.). Evanston, IL: Rehabilitation Nursing Foundation.

Ohry, A., Shemesh, Y., & Rozin, R. (1985). Are chronic spinal cord injured patients (SCIP) prone to premature aging? *Medical Hypotheses, 11*, 467-469.

Perkash, I. (1982). Management of neurogenic dysfunction of the bladder and bowel. *Krusen's handbook of physical medicine & rehabilitation* (3rd ed.) (p. 724). Philadelphia: W.B. Saunders Company.

Petrilli, C.O., Traugher, B., & Schnelle, J.F. (1988). Behavioral management in the inpatient geriatric population. *Nursing Clinics of North America, 23*(1), 265-277.

Piotrowski, M.M. (1980). Functioning of the normal and neurogenic bladder: Programmed instruction. *ARN Journal, 5*(2), 13-20.

Read, N.W., Al-Janabi, M.N., Holgate, A.M., Barger, D.C., & Edwards, C.A. (1986). Simultaneous measurement of gastric emptying, small bowel residence and colonic filling of a solid meal by the use of gamma camera. *Gut, 27*, 300-308.

Richardson, K., Campbell, M.A., Brown, M.R., Masiulis, B., & Liptak, G.S. (1985). Biofeedback therapy for managing bowel incontinence caused by meningomyelocele. *The American Journal of Maternal/Child Nursing, 10*, 388.

Sawin, K.J. (1990). The AHCPR effectiveness initiatives: Opportunities for rehabilitation nursing. *Rehabilitation Nursing, 15*, 264-266.

Staas, W.E., Jr., & Cioschi, H.S. (1989). Neurogenic bowel dysfunction. *Physical and Rehabilitation Medicine, 1*(1), 11-21.

Staas, W.E., Jr., & LaMantia, J.G. (1984). Bowel function and control. In A. Ruskin (Ed.), *Current therapy in physiatry* (pp. 405-410). Philadelphia: W.B. Saunders Company.

Vantrappen, G., Janssens, J., Coremans, G., & Jian, R. (1986). Gastrointestinal motility disorders. *Digest Disorders in Science, 31*(9 Suppl.), 55-255.

Voith, A.M. (1986). A conceptual framework for nursing diagnosis: Alterations in urinary elimination. *Rehabilitation Nursing, 11*(1), 18-21.

Voith, A.M. (1988). Alteration in urinary elimination: Concepts, research, and practice. *Rehabilitation Nursing, 13*, 122-131.

Wald, A. (1986). Fecal incontinence: Effective nonsurgical treatments. *Postgraduate Medicine, 80*(3), 123-130.

◆Wald, A. (1981). Use of biofeedback in treatment of fecal incontinence in patients with meningomyelocele. *Pediatrics, 68*(1), 45-49.

Zedjlik, C. (1992). *Management of spinal cord injury* (2nd ed.). Boston: Jones and Bartlett Publishers.

Suggested Resources

Pires, M., & Lockhart-Pretti, P. (Speakers). (1992). *Nursing management of neurogenic incontinence* (Cassette recording and booklet). Skokie, IL: The Rehabilitation Nursing Foundation of the Association of Rehabilitation Nurses.

Pires, M., Lockhart-Pretti, P., Newman, D.K., & Smith, D.J. (1991). *CONTINENCE: Every nurse's responsibility—Part I: An overview* (Videotape and companion booklet). Skokie, IL: The Rehabilitation Nursing Foundation of the Association of Rehabilitation Nurses.

Pires, M., Lockhart-Pretti, P., Newman, D.K., & Smith, D.J. (1991). *CONTINENCE: Every nurse's responsibility—Part II: Specialized nursing management* (Videotape and companion booklet). Skokie, IL: The Rehabilitation Nursing Foundation of the Association of Rehabilitation Nurses.

Smith, D.J., & Newman, D.K. (Speakers). (1992). *Behavioral management of incontinence* (Cassette recording and booklet). Skokie, IL: The Rehabilitation Nursing Foundation of the Association of Rehabilitation Nurses.

◆ indicates a research-based work

CHAPTER 14

Activity–Exercise Pattern

The activity–exercise pattern is broad, complex, and basic to the field of rehabilitation. Inherent in this pattern are activities relating to functional ability, improvement in which is a primary goal for most rehabilitation clients. Concepts in this chapter range from self-care, mobility, and home maintenance management to the physiological problems of disuse and immobility and respiratory dysfunction and to the psychosocial area of leisure and recreation (diversional activity).

Although rehabilitation nurses frequently work with other team members, the involvement of nurses in assisting clients with self-care and mobility activities is highlighted by two recent surveys of ARN members. In a study by Sawin and Heard (1992), impaired physical mobility and self-care deficits ranked first and second among the top 10 most frequently cited nursing diagnoses. In another survey by Gordon (1993b), mobility and self-care deficits were reported to be highly prevalent diagnoses made by rehabilitation nurses.

Preventing complications resulting from prolonged immobility is a continuing responsibility for nurses and other caregivers. The difficulty of preventing complications increases for those with clients whose respiratory status has been compromised and who, additionally, might be dependent on ventilators. It is imperative that rehabilitation nurses teach clients and caregivers how to prevent or minimize the potential complications of immobility.

For clients returning to the community, the ability to manage the home is a functional activity essential to reintegration. Work simplification techniques, environmental adaptations, and assistive devices are available to increase the functional independence of the homemaker with impaired physical mobility.

The lives of people with disabilities are not complete without activities to fill their leisure time. Participation and interest in diversional activities depend on the client's age and functional ability, as well as on the availability of leisure and recreational activities. Rehabilitation nurses in all settings must be cognizant of their clients' needs for leisure activities and of the resources available to them.

Self-Care, Mobility, and Home Maintenance Management

I. Related Theory and Concepts

A. Concepts related to disability

1. Nagi (1976), an early pioneer in disability theories, defined three major consequences of disease
   a. Impairment due to physiological abnormality
   b. Functional limitation
   c. Disability, or an "inability or limitations in performing social roles and activities such as in relation to work, family or to independent living" (p. 441)
2. Wood (1980) expanded Nagi's work to include the concept of *handicap* as the limitation of role function that is normal for that person
3. In 1991, the Committee on a National Agenda for the Prevention of Disabilities of the Institute of Medicine's Division of Health Promotion proposed a framework that builds upon the World Health Organization (WHO) classifications; framework includes deleting the term *handicap* and the Nagi framework and adds the concepts of *risk factors* and *quality of life* to a model describing the disability process (Pope & Tarlov, 1991)

B. Nursing theories and concepts (see Chapter 3 for additional information)

1. Orem's Self-Care Theory
   a. "Self-care is integral to rehabilitation" (Orem, 1985, p. 35)
   b. Self-care has two phases
      1) Investigative/decision-making: Patient has control and input regarding activity
      2) Production: Patient performs activity
   c. Research supports assertion that persons with disabilities are able to control their care even though they might be unable to perform it (Doyle & Stern, 1992)
2. Roy's Adaptation Theory (Roy, 1980)
   a. Nursing demonstrates a concern for the person as a total being in areas of health and illness
   b. The nurse supports and assists client and/or family in achieving a response and adaptation to environmental stimuli

C. Development of functional ability: Hierarchical relationships of self-care activities

1. Katz and Akpom (1976) noted that sociobiological activities (e.g., feeding, continence, transfer, toileting, bathing, and dressing) are hierarchically related to each other; that is, they are developed and demonstrated in a specific sequence from less to more complex
2. Some of these activities—particularly dressing, bathing, and toileting—are heavily influenced by cultural norms; nevertheless, during recovery, dis-

abled persons were noted to pass through successive stages similar to the phases of development for functional ability in children

a. Return of or development of independence in feeding activities and continence
b. Recovery of or development of ability to transfer and manage toileting
c. Recovery of or development of ability to dress and bathe

3. Rehabilitation nurses can observe similar phenomena as they assess patients for their level of functional ability—for example, a patient who cannot feed himself or herself is unlikely to be independent in bathing and dressing because bathing and dressing are more complex tasks than feeding

D. Concepts and definitions related to mobility

1. Impaired physical mobility
   a. Term suggests that the patient has decreased ability or an inability to purposefully change the position of his or her body without assistance
   b. Nursing goals are to promote patient's ability to move (McFarland & McFarlane, 1989)
   c. Physical mobility has four aspects of significance to rehabilitation nurses—bed mobility, transfers, wheelchair mobility, and ambulation
      1) *Bed mobility*: The most basic stage of mobility
         a) Without aids: Includes turning from side to side, redistributing pressure, moving up in bed, moving to side of bed, bridging (lifting hips off bed while in supine position), and sitting up in bed
         b) With aids: Use of siderails, overhead frame, and trapeze can be helpful
      2) *Transfers*: The second stage of functional mobility, includes skills used to move between wheelchair and bed, toilet, bath bench, shower chair, standard seating, and seat in a motor vehicle
         a) Dependent transfer: Nurse uses total lift, pivot transfer, or mechanical lift device
         b) Partially dependent: Nurse and patient perform hemiplegic, paraplegic, or sliding board transfers
            (1) Hemiplegic transfer
               (a) Wheelchair is placed on unaffected side
               (b) Armrest is removed
               (c) Patient stands and places unaffected hand on armrest while moving unaffected foot toward chair
               (d) Patient lowers self into chair
            (2) Paraplegic transfer (also useful for bilateral amputee)
               (a) Chair is placed perpendicularly to bed at the middle of bed
               (b) Patient's trunk and legs are positioned to line up with chair
               (c) Patient's hips and legs are pushed back from bed while he or she grasps the armrests with arms
            (3) Sliding board transfer
               (a) Wheelchair is placed alongside bed
               (b) Armrest is removed
               (c) Sliding board is placed under patient's buttocks
               (d) Client pulls self toward far armrest of chair by using upper extremity
               (e) Hips and legs slide along into chair
      3) *Wheelchair mobility* (Britell & McFarland, 1988): Can be primary mode of locomotion or used in addition to ambulation for energy conservation
         a) Wheelchair types are diverse; prescription for them is based on individual patient needs, including energy expenditure; physiological, cosmetic, and psychological factors; and occupational and recreational factors
         b) Wheelchairs are manually or electrically powered with rechargeable batteries
         c) Control systems for electrical wheelchairs
            (1) Joystick: Operates by hands or arms or by feet, chin, or tongue
            (2) Pneumatic switches: Operate by mouth using "sip and puff" techniques
            (3) Voice-actuated controls: Use voice recognition and actuation technology
      4) *Ambulation*
         a) Requires sitting and standing balance
         b) May require assistive equipment such as crutches, cane, walker, orthoses, and prostheses
         c) Abnormal gait patterns (Hickey, 1992)
            (1) Hemiplegic
               (a) Noted with stroke; unilateral involvement
               (b) Characteristics: Arm is semiflexed with elbow held close to waist; fingers flexed and wristdrop noted; extended spastic, stiff leg is swung in a semicircle when walking; foot is inverted; footdrop noted
            (2) Ataxic/cerebellar gait
               (a) Noted with cerebellar tumor, multiple sclerosis, Friedreich's ataxia
               (b) Characteristics: Wide-based, staggering, lurching, and uncoordinated
            (3) Parkinsonian
               (a) Defect in basal ganglia
               (b) Characteristics: Loss of automatic arm swinging; arms semi-

flexed and adducted; legs rigid and flexed; head and body flexed forward; gait is slow and shuffling; once walking, person may propel himself or herself forward with increased momentum

(4) Spastic
  (a) Involves corticospinal tract
  (b) Characteristic: Shuffling with the legs stiff

(5) Steppage
  (a) Due to lesion of the lower motor neurons, anterior horn cell, or cauda equina
  (b) Characteristics: Associated with footdrop and flaccidity of leg; to compensate, leg is lifted high to clear the foot from floor, resulting in slapping of foot as the toes touch floor

2. Physical factors related to mobility
   a. Range of motion (ROM)
      1) Definition: Full range of movement that a joint can normally perform
      2) Passive ROM exercises are carried out when patient is unable to perform active ROM
         a) Method: One hand is placed above the joint to provide support and the other gently moves the joint
         b) Rationale: Passive ROM exercises help to prevent contractures
   b. Strength: Ability of muscle to produce or resist a physical force; mobility, exercises, and adequate nutrition help to maintain strength that is necessary for functional ability
   c. Balance: Ability to sit and stand erectly; affected by orthostatic hypotension, hemiplegia, and paralysis
   d. Endurance: Ability to produce work over time or the ability to persist in or maintain an effort
   e. Tone: Normal state of balanced tension in the muscle
      1) Hypotonicity (flaccidity): Decreased tone; muscle is weak, soft, and flabby
      2) Hypertonicity (spasticity): Increased tone with resistance of muscle to passive lengthening
      3) Rigidity: Constant state of resistance
   f. Proprioception: Sensation related to stimulus originating from within the body regarding spatial position and muscular activity; helps to identify location of body parts in space
3. Impaired physical mobility versus broader concept of mobility
   a. Impaired physical mobility is limited to the physical realm
   b. Concept of mobility, however, is broader and extends to emotional, cognitive, physical, and social dimensions that interact with one another
   c. Ouellet and Rush (1992) provide a synthesis of selected literature on mobility and suggest that this broader concept is more consistent with nursing's holistic philosophy

E. Concepts and theories related to home maintenance management
1. "Living in a private home is believed to provide a higher quality of life than institutional care because it supports independence and individuality" (McFarland & McFarlane, 1989, p. 399)
2. Importance of homemaking was established in 1954 when the Federal Rehabilitation Law was interpreted to include homemakers (Leslie, 1990)
3. Management is a process by which energy can be saved; home maintenance management is the economy of human resources, accomplished by planning of work and evaluation of various tasks
4. Management involves not only the patient but also the entire family and the use of their skills, income, and possessions as well as their scheduling of tasks and supervision of work done by others
5. Development of home maintenance skills contributes to self-concept and initiative (Leslie, 1990)
6. Kahana (1982) model explores compatibility between individual needs and environmental factors; when individual needs and environmental factors are congruent, function will be optimal

II. Nursing Assessment

A. General assessment
1. Physical factors
   a. Are ROM, strength, balance, endurance, tone, and proprioception adequate for functional activities?
   b. Does pain interfere with functional ability?
   c. Are visual and/or auditory capabilities adequate for functional ability?
   d. Is the status of physical mobility—including bed mobility, transfers, wheelchair mobility, and/or ambulation—adequate?
2. Cognitive factors
   a. What is the status of orientation level?
   b. How great is the client's attention span?
   c. What is the status of the client's memory?
   d. What communicative ability is present?
   e. Is there adequate safety awareness?
3. Psychological factors
   a. Is patient motivated to perform functional activities?
   b. Is anxiety, fear, decreased self-concept, or depression present?
4. Environmental factors: Are there adequate and accessible equipment, lighting, and privacy?

B. Task-specific assessment
1. Can client feed herself or himself?
2. Can client bathe herself or himself?
3. Can client dress herself or himself?
4. Can client toilet herself or himself?
5. Can client move in bed?
6. Can client transfer herself or himself?
7. Can client propel wheelchair?
8. Can client ambulate?
9. Can client perform tasks involved in home mainte-

Figure 14.1. Scale for Assessing Clients' Functional Levels for Self-Care and Mobility

Level 0: Is independent in activity

Level I: Requires use of equipment or device

Level II: Requires help (assistance, supervision, teaching) from another person(s)

Level III: Requires help from another person(s) as well as equipment and devices

Level IV: Is dependent and does not participate in activity

Reprinted with permission of North American Nursing Diagnosis Association from North American Nursing Diagnosis Association. (1992). *NANDA nursing diagnoses: Definitions and classification 1992-1993* (p. 54). St. Louis: Author.

Figure 14.2. Index of Functional Ability for Long-Term Care

0 = Independent
1 = Requires use of equipment/assistive device
2 = Requires help from another person for supervision, assistance, or teaching
- 2.2 Supervision or contact guarding
- 2.4 Minimal assistance: Patient does 75% of the work
- 2.6 Moderate assistance: Patient does 50% of the work
- 2.8 Maximum assistance: Patient does 25% of the work

3 = Requires help from another person *plus* equipment/assistive device
- 3.2 Supervision or contact guarding in addition to equipment/assistive device
- 3.4 Minimal assistance in addition to equipment/assistive device
- 3.6 Moderate assistance in addition to equipment/assistive device
- 3.8 Maximum assistance in addition to equipment/assistive device

4 = Dependent: Does not participate in activity

Reprinted with permission of A. McCourt from McCourt, A. (1987). Implementation of nursing diagnosis through integration with quality assurance. *Nursing Clinics of North America, 22,* 903.

nance management?

C. Scoring functional assessments
   1. Many instruments are available for scoring or grading functional ability (see Chapter 24)
   2. Self-care deficit and mobility deficit nursing diagnoses can be graded using an incremental scale (see Figure 14.1)
      a. Each self-care or mobility nursing diagnosis should be assigned a specific level following diagnosis
      b. Different levels require different nursing interventions
   3. For clients whose recovery in functional activities is slower but shows continual improvement, a more sensitive scale using smaller increments can be helpful (see Figure 14.2)

D. Specific areas of assessment for home maintenance management
   1. Physical facilities in the home
      a. Utilities: Availability of water, heat, lighting
      b. Communication systems: Accessible telephones, intercoms
      c. Safety features
         1) Accessible exits, fire alarms
         2) Awareness of local agencies to contact in emergencies: Police, fire department, health-care agency
   2. Ability to perform household chores
      a. Food preparation
      b. Housekeeping
      c. Laundry
      d. Transportation
   3. Availability of caregiver in family system and/or private sector
   4. Level of financial resources

III. Nursing Diagnoses

A. Self-care deficits

1. Related factors/etiologies for *all* self-care deficits
   a. Decreased activity tolerance
   b. Pain and/or discomfort
   c. Uncompensated perceptual and/or cognitive impairment
   d. Uncompensated neuromuscular impairment
   e. Uncompensated musculoskeletal impairment
   f. Anxiety and/or depression
   g. Lack of motivation
   h. Developmental delay
   i. Inability or unwillingness of caregiver to promote mastery of skill

➤ **2. Self-feeding deficit**
   a. Definition: Impaired ability to perform or complete feeding activities for oneself (NANDA, 1992)

   b. Major defining characteristic: Inability to bring food from receptacle to mouth

   c. Related factors/etiologies (see above)

   d. Interventions
      1) Provide safety for the individual with swallowing problems—for example, use Fowler's position when eating, ensure appropriate food consistency
      2) Provide comfortable and pleasant eating environment
      3) Allow sufficient time for eating
      4) Provide supervision and assistance needed for relearning or adaptation
      5) Provide adaptive devices
         a) Plate guard
         b) Suction device or nonskid mat under plate or bowl
         c) Wrist or hand splints with universal cuff or clamp to hold utensils
         d) Swivel utensils

e) Long drinking tube or straw
6) Assist with setup of food tray
a) Open containers
b) Cut up food and arrange for easy access
c) Select easy-to-eat finger foods
7) Provide instructions regarding rationale for and appropriate use of adaptive devices
8) Consult occupational therapist about adaptive equipment and additional assistance if needed

e. Expected outcomes

1) Client is independent or demonstrates improved ability to feed self
2) Client demonstrates ability to make use of adaptive equipment
3) Client demonstrates safe eating habits

➤ **3. Self-bathing/hygiene deficit**

a. Definition: Impaired ability to perform or complete bathing and/or hygiene activities for oneself (NANDA, 1992)

b. Major defining characteristics

1) Inability to bathe body or parts of body; inability to handle soap and washcloth
2) Inability to obtain or get to water source; inability to get in and out of bathtub or shower
3) Inability to regulate water temperature or flow
4) Inability to dry self—that is, to manipulate and use towel

c. Related factors/etiologies (see page 111)

d. Interventions

1) Provide privacy while bathing
2) Help client use shower or tub as soon as possible after onset of disability
3) Arrange a bathing routine that is consistent and corresponds with client's premorbid routine
4) Place all bathing equipment within easy reach
5) Provide safe environment
a) Rubber mats
b) Grab bars
c) Tub or shower seat
6) Teach client how to use adaptive devices
a) Shower chair or bench
b) Long-handled sponge
c) Washing mitt
d) Adapted toothbrush
e) Razor holder
7) Arrange rest periods between self-care activities
8) Consult with home caregiver and members of other disciplines (e.g., occupational therapist) to integrate care into community setting
9) Determine if patients in wheelchairs have access to and sufficient space for bathing
10) Teach client how to maintain safe bathing environment

e. Expected outcomes

1) Client performs bathing activities at optimal level of independence
2) Client demonstrates ability to use adaptive equipment
3) Client maintains safe bathing practices

➤ **4. Self-dressing and/or grooming deficit**

a. Definition: Impaired ability to perform or complete dressing and grooming activities for oneself (NANDA, 1992)

b. Major defining characteristics

1) Impaired ability to put on (don) and take off (doff) clothing
2) Impaired ability to obtain or replace articles of clothing
3) Impaired ability to fasten clothing
4) Inability to maintain satisfactory appearance

c. Related factors/etiologies (see page 111)

d. Interventions

1) Provide privacy during dressing
2) Encourage wearing of own clothing
3) Encourage choice of clothing that is loose-fitting and easy to put on—for example, clothing with wide sleeves and pant legs and front fasteners
4) Avoid fabrics, such as stiff denim or polyester, which do not absorb moisture
5) If the client has sensory impairment, avoid clothing that might produce pressure points from hard seams and tight, constricting closures
6) Lay clothes out in order in which they are needed for dressing
7) Allow sufficient time for dressing
8) Promote independence in dressing through continued practice with assistance or cueing
9) If client has paresis, paralysis, or another form of immobility, begin by dressing the affected side or parts of the body first
10) Begin client's self-dressing activities in bed first if fatigue, balance, or medical problems are present; when client is stable, encourage dressing while client is out of bed
11) Provide visual and/or verbal cues
12) Demonstrate use of adaptive equipment to facilitate independent dressing—for example, longhandled shoehorn, button hook, stocking aids, zipper pull; consult with an occupational therapist or other resource persons when indicated

e. Expected outcomes

1) Patient demonstrates increased ability to dress self
2) Patient shows increased interest in wearing own clothes

3) Patient demonstrates ability to cope with having assistance in performing dressing tasks

➤ 5. **Self-toileting deficit**

a. **Definition:** Impaired ability to perform or complete toileting activities for oneself (NANDA, 1992)

b. **Major defining characteristics**

1) Impaired ability to get to toilet or commode
2) Impaired ability to sit on or rise from toilet or commode
3) Impaired ability to manipulate clothing for toileting
4) Impaired ability to carry out adequate toilet hygiene
5) Impaired ability to flush toilet or empty commode

c. **Related factors/etiologies** (see page 111)

d. **Interventions**

1) Maintain bowel and bladder record to determine evacuation pattern
2) Individualize toileting program
3) Maintain regular, consistent schedule
4) Allow sufficient time for toileting
5) Provide privacy
6) Provide assistance and cueing
7) Consult occupational therapist regarding adaptive devices, if they are indicated
8) Consult with physical therapist for individualized transfer techniques and/or equipment, if they are indicated
9) Provide a safe and clear access to toilet area with a night light as necessary
10) Ensure the availability of a call system on the nursing unit and in the community setting, if indicated
11) Provide client education

e. **Expected outcomes**

1) Client demonstrates optimal independence in self-toileting
2) Client uses adaptive devices appropriately
3) Client copes with inability to use toilet independently
4) Client describes rationale for regular toileting routine

➤ B. **Impaired physical mobility**

1. **Definition:** A state in which the individual experiences or is at risk of experiencing limitation of ability for independent physical movement within the environment

2. **Major defining characteristics**

a. Inability to move purposefully within the physical environment; includes activities such as bed mobility, transfers, ambulation, and wheelchair mobility
b. Imposed restrictions on movement, including mechanical or medical protocol restrictions

3. **Related factors/etiologies**

a. Uncompensated neuromuscular impairment
b. Uncompensated perceptual and/or cognitive impairment
c. Uncompensated musculoskeletal impairments
d. Restrictive or suppressive therapeutic regimens
   1) Bedrest
   2) Halo or skeletal traction
   3) Body cast
e. Decreased activity tolerance
f. Anxiety and/or depression
g. Discomfort and/or pain

4. **Interventions**

a. Provide supervision, assistance, and teaching
b. Promote client's use of equipment and assistive devices
c. Instruct client in activities and exercise that promote increased function
d. Assist client in bed to maintain proper body alignment by using siderails and overhead trapeze
e. Encourage transfer mobility
f. Encourage increased participation in activity and self-care
g. Teach energy conservation techniques
h. Provide adequate rest periods between activities
i. Educate client regarding relationship between physical condition and ability to be active
j. Teach client appropriate safety measures for various tasks
   1) Bed mobility
   2) Transfer techniques
   3) Wheelchair mobility
   4) Ambulation
k. Adapt environment to maximize client's independence consistent with highest level of function achieved

5. **Expected outcomes**

a. Client demonstrates optimal independence in mobility skills
b. Client performs safe transfers
c. Client uses safety measures to minimize potential for injury
d. Client demonstrates energy conservation measures when performing activities related to mobility

➤ C. **Impaired home maintenance management**

1. **Definition:** Inability to independently maintain a safe, growth-promoting immediate environment

2. **Major defining characteristics**

a. Expression of difficulty by individual and/or household members regarding satisfactory maintenance of their home
b. Unavailability of support systems
c. Unkempt home environment
d. Repeated infestations or infections

e. Overtaxed family systems (e.g., caregiver stress syndrome)
f. Poor hygienic practices
g. Financial debts

3. Related factors/etiologies

a. Insufficient finances
b. Lack of knowledge
c. Inadequate support systems
d. Insufficient family organization and planning
e. Inadequate dwelling and/or furnishings
f. Chronic disability
g. Cognitive, motor, or sensory deficit(s)

4. Interventions

a. Determine adequacy of environment and need for home modification (May, 1993)
b. Identify, rectify, or compensate for safety problems
c. Teach patient and/or family caregivers to contact community resources (e.g., homemaker services) for assistance
d. Secure assistance for external household maintenance—for example, lawn care, gardening, home repairs
e. Develop safety backup system within community for emergencies: Establish contacts with local police and fire departments, neighbors, and healthcare system
f. Teach work simplification techniques (Leslie, 1990)
   1) Using fixed workstations
   2) Letting gravity work—that is, use laundry chutes, refuse chutes, and gravity-fed flour bin
   3) Sitting to perform tasks whenever possible
   4) Choosing household appliances because of their ease of operation
g. Teach specific food preparation techniques (Dudek, 1987)
   1) Keeping utensils that are used most often within easy reach; placing duplicates in strategic locations
   2) Wearing apron with several pockets to keep small utensils handy
   3) Hanging pots and pans on wall rack to avoid bending and stretching
   4) Using lazy Susans and pull-out shelves
   5) Taking advantage of "good" days by making extra portions to be frozen for later use
   6) Using one-dish meals and convenience foods
   7) Investing in labor-saving appliances (e.g., food processor, blender, electric knife, can opener)
   8) Using lightweight cooking utensils and bowls (e.g., aluminum, plastic)
   9) Using nonstick cookware and soaking dishes immediately after use to reduce cleanup
   10) Using paper products when possible
   11) Tying a looped rope around appliance handles and cabinet doors and opening them by slipping forearm through the loop and pulling
   12) Opening pull-top cans with a knife or screwdriver inserted through the metal ring
   13) Using cookware that has two handles
   14) Using tongs rather than a fork to release food
   15) Boiling foods in wire mesh basket inserted in pot; when food is done, simply removing the basket rather than lifting the whole pot
   16) Using sponge mitt rather than handheld sponge for cleanup

5. Expected outcomes

a. Client demonstrates ability to maintain safe and growth-promoting home environment
b. Client obtains appropriate community services
c. Client expresses satisfaction with home situation
d. Client uses adaptive equipment and supplies appropriately (Austill-Clausen, 1993)
e. Client completes home modifications

Disuse Phenomenon

In 1967, Edith V. Olson wrote a definitive article about immobility and disuse, entitled "The Hazards of Immobility," that was published in *American Journal of Nursing*. Her remarks are as applicable today as they were then: "The effect of immobility on the human organism to which motion is synonymous with life is a problem as old as time and as timely as space exploration. Knowledge of the physiologic and psychologic alterations which result from the confinement of [hu]man[s], whether to bed or the astronaut's couch, is advancing rapidly. That such alterations can be drastic in their effect, even on healthy persons, has been known for some time" (p. 779). "Nursing of the future must not be partner to disability induced by dependent immobility. It must, instead, be a catalyst in the prevention of one of the nation's major health problems—immobilization disability" (p. 797).

I. Related Theories and Concepts

A. Disuse phenomena involve the entire body's response to immobilization
B. Goal of nursing is to prevent or minimize deterioration of bodily functions and systems
C. Healthy function of the body depends, in part, on minimum level of activity
   1. Most body systems, whether healthy or ill, are adversely affected when individuals are immobilized
   2. Adverse effects begin to occur in body systems within 24 hours of onset of immobility
   3. Research continues to support evidence for pathologic consequences of disuse
      a. National Aeronautics and Space Administration (NASA) research (Nicogossian & Parker, 1982) produced evidence of the many physiological problems resulting from weightlessness that were similar to those resulting from disuse and prolonged immobility

b. For development of the nursing diagnosis of disuse syndrome, Esposito, Tracey, and McCourt (1989) conducted a survey among nurses working with spinal cord injured patients and with pediatric patients who had long-term neurological impairments; the results supported concern about potential as well as actual complications of disuse and prolonged immobility

D. Pathophysiological manifestations of the consequences of prolonged immobilization or disuse in body systems
1. Integumentary system
a. Complications: Skin breakdown, pressure sores
b. Consequences of immobilization: Pressure over bony prominences, particularly extended or repetitive pressure associated with lying or sitting in one position
2. Gastrointestinal system
a. Complications: Constipation, impaction
b. Consequences of immobilization
1) Interference with normal position for evacuation (that is, sitting or squatting)
2) Decrease in peristalsis and normal bowel function
3. Urinary system
a. Complications: Urinary retention, infection, calculi, reflux
b. Consequences of immobilization
1) Decreased voiding sensation and inadequate emptying of bladder
2) Prolonged retention that can lead to infection, calculi formation, and urinary reflux
4. Respiratory system
a. Complications: Stasis of pulmonary secretions, pneumonia
b. Consequences of immobilization
1) Increased difficulty in coughing and clearing of secretions
2) Pooling of secretions and decreased oxygenation
3) Eventually, pneumonia
5. Cardiovascular system: Vascular system depends on activity to promote muscle contraction and venous return
a. Complications: Thrombus formation, pulmonary embolus, orthostatic hypotension
b. Consequences of immobilization
1) Venous stasis and increased risk for thrombus formation and pulmonary embolus
2) Reduced venous return and pooling of blood in lower extremities and dizziness, which leads to drop in blood pressure when person moves from supine position to upright position
6. Musculoskeletal system
a. Complications: Decreased range of motion, contracture, decreased strength, muscle atrophy, bone demineralization, osteoporosis
b. Consequences of immobilization
1) Shortening of muscle fibers around joints, which results in limited range of motion and possible contractures
2) Decrease in size and strength of muscles, which promotes lack of use and further compounds atrophy
3) Lack of weight-bearing, which decreases bone formation, which, in turn, results in increased risk for osteoporosis and fracture
7. Psychosocial equilibrium
a. Complications: Powerlessness, sensory deprivation
b. Consequences of immobilization
1) Loss of independence, which can lead to feelings of powerlessness
2) Reduced environmental stimuli and social interaction, which might lead to sensory deprivation

II. Nursing Assessment: Evaluation of Presence of Following Factors

A. Extensive paralysis
B. Immobilization
1. Prescribed
2. By mechanical means (e.g., traction)
C. Severe pain preventing unassisted turning
D. Unconsciousness

➤ III. Nursing Diagnosis: Disuse Syndrome

A. **Definition:** A state in which an individual is at risk for the complications of prescribed or unavoidable immobilization

B. **Major defining characteristic:** Prolonged immobilization

C. Related factors/etiologies

1. Paralysis
2. Mechanical immobilization
3. Prescribed immobilization
4. Pain
5. Altered level of consciousness

D. Interventions

1. Reposition at regularly scheduled intervals
2. Use pressure-reducing devices
3. Maintain adequate nutrition and hydration
4. Maintain effective bowel program
5. Maintain effective bladder program
6. Ensure adequate pulmonary hygiene (e.g., coughing, deep breathing)
7. Promote venous return in lower extremities by elevating lower extremities
8. Perform range-of-motion exercises
9. Promote optimal independence in self-care and mobility activities
10. Promote client's involvement in preventive measures

E. Expected outcomes

1. Client maintains intact skin
2. Client maintains regular bowel movements
3. Client maintains adequate urinary elimination, ab-

sence of infection
4. Client has regular respirations, adequate oxygenation, effective airway clearance
5. Client has no evidence of thrombophlebitis
6. Client maintains adequate muscle mass and strength for activities
7. Client maintains normal range of joint motion; displays no evidence of contractures
8. Client verbalizes feelings of empowerment and control

Respiratory Function

In the rehabilitation population, respiratory impairment is noted in patients with neuromuscular disorders, neurological injury, decreased energy, or premorbid history of respiratory conditions such as chronic obstructive pulmonary disease. Because adequate respiratory function is essential for life, knowledge of respiratory function and care is a critically important aspect of rehabilitation nursing.

I. Physiology and Pathophysiology Related to Respiratory Function

A. General physiology (Wilson & Thompson, 1990)
1. Respiratory function is a process of gas exchange in the lungs
2. Oxygen is diffused into the blood at the same time carbon dioxide is removed from the blood
3. Respiratory tract is divided into upper and lower airways
   a. Upper airway
      1) Components
         a) Nasal cavity
         b) Sinuses
         c) Pharynx
         d) Larynx
         e) Trachea
      2) Function
         a) Humidifies and warms air
         b) Filters foreign particles
   b. Lower airway
      1) Components
         a) Bronchi
         b) Bronchioles
         c) Lungs
         d) Alveoli
      2) Function: Foreign particles become trapped in mucus, which is secreted by cells lining the airway; hairlike processors, or cilia, move mucus toward mouth to be expelled
4. Pulmonary circulation
   a. Respiratory and circulatory systems work closely to transport gases to and from lungs
   b. Lungs receive blood from pulmonary and bronchial circulation
      1) Pulmonary
         a) Blood from body passes through heart and enters pulmonary arteries
         b) This deoxygenated blood reaches pulmonary capillaries, where gas exchange takes place
         c) Blood that is rich in oxygen leaves lungs through pulmonary veins, returns to heart, and is eventually pumped to rest of body
      2) Bronchial: This supply originates from aorta or subclavian artery and supplies blood to lungs through three bronchial arteries
5. Respiratory muscles
   a. Inspiratory muscles
      1) Diaphragm: The most important muscle for breathing; innervated by phrenic nerve, which arises from fourth cervical nerve
      2) External intercostal muscles
      3) Accessory muscles, which include the trapezius and scalenes
   b. Expiratory muscles
      1) Internal intercostal muscles
      2) Abdominal muscles
   c. Accessory muscles: Muscles other than the diaphragm used to inhale and exhale—for example, those used by patients with chronic obstructive pulmonary disease or acute respiratory distress
6. Respiratory centers in the brainstem, peripheral chemoreceptors, and certain cranial nerves affect respiratory function

B. General pathophysiology (Dettenmeier, 1992)
1. Pathology of respiratory function can be divided into obstructive and restrictive disease
   a. Obstructive: Block or obstruction in normal flow of air through respiratory system
      1) Includes emphysema and chronic bronchitis
      2) Asthma included when airway hyperactivity is noted
      3) Cigarette smoking is most common cause
      4) Can affect endurance, strength, physical mobility, and functional abilities
      5) Long-term oxygen therapy might be indicated
   b. Restrictive: Restriction of lung expansion due to muscle weakness resulting in decreased lung volume and capacity
      1) Related to certain disorders noted in the rehabilitation population
         a) Progressive neuromuscular disease—for example, Guillain-Barré syndrome, amyotrophic lateral sclerosis, and poliomyelitis
         b) Traumatic spinal cord injuries
            (1) Injury below L1: No impairment
            (2) Injury between T6 and L1: Limited ability to exhale forcibly
            (3) Thoracic injuries: Limited expiration and inspiration
            (4) Cervical injury between C5 and C6: Diaphragm intact but expiratory muscles paralyzed
            (5) Cervical injury at C3 and above: Requires total ventilatory support
         c) Long-term ventilation (Traver, 1991)
            (1) Ventilator selection depends on indi-

vidual requirements

(2) Home ventilators are small and lightweight with an internal battery backup system as well as an external battery supply

(3) Alarm systems for patient disconnection, varying pressures, and machine failure are included

2. Infectious processes of the lung can result in exudate that impairs gas exchange; exudates form mucous plugs that can affect ventilatory flow
3. Anxiety and pain can affect respiratory function

II. Nursing Assessment (Morton, 1991)

A. Note respiratory disease or neurological impairment that would have an impact on the respiratory system

B. Perform physical examination by inspection, palpation, percussion, and auscultation

C. Perform functional assessment of client's abilities

1. Ability to conserve energy while performing activities of daily living
2. Ability to perform pulmonary hygiene activities
3. Ability to handle secretions after removal from airway
4. Ability to handle any specialized equipment needed for respiration, such as suction catheters, humidification equipment, tracheotomy tubes, and mechanical ventilator

III. Nursing Diagnoses

➤ A. Ineffective breathing pattern

1. **Definition:** Respirations inadequate to maintain sufficient oxygen supply for cellular requirements (Gordon, 1993a)

2. Major defining characteristics

a. Use of accessory muscles, flaring of nostrils, and altered chest excursion

b. Dyspnea, cough, pursed lip breathing, prolonged expiratory phase, tachypnea, cyanosis, change in depth of respirations

c. Reports of decreased energy, presence of anxiety

d. Abnormal arterial blood gas, tachycardia

3. Related factors/etiologies

a. Neuromuscular and/or musculoskeletal impairment

b. Fatigue and/or decreased energy

c. Perceptual and/or cognitive impairment

d. Anxiety

e. Pain

f. Inflammatory process

4. Interventions

a. Position client to maximize ventilations

b. Assist client with coughing and deep-breathing exercises

c. Teach pursed-lip and abdominal-diaphragmatic breathing techniques

d. Teach relaxation techniques, such as guided imagery and meditation, to reduce anxiety

e. Suction, as needed, to clear airways and stimulate cough

f. Perform chest physiotherapy

g. Help client minimize energy demands

1) Teach proper positioning and body mechanics

2) Teach client ways to combine activities

3) Teach client to pace activities to allow adequate rest between periods of exertion

h. Administer medications, as prescribed, to improve airflow

i. Teach client to avoid airway irritants such as cigarette smoke, smog, aerosols, and various products that produce fumes

j. Teach client to avoid respiratory infections

k. Teach client how to care for oxygen, tracheostomy, and mechanical ventilator

l. Provide information regarding strategies for residential and/or community living

1) Notify police and fire departments and ambulance service about existence of client's home ventilatory program in case there are medical emergencies and to ensure power facilities

2) Recommend installation of security system in home to provide immediate contact with fire and police departments and ambulance service for emergency services

3) Coordinate continuous home services by home respiratory therapist, pulmonologist (who will make house calls), and durable medical equipment companies

4) Teach family members about emergency respiratory care—for example, tracheostomy care, bagging; have backup battery source or generator available at all times in case there is a power failure

5. Expected outcomes

a. Client demonstrates adequate oxygenation measured by physical examination, pulse oximetry, and arterial blood gas

b. Client reports comfortable breathing

c. Client exhibits conservation skills when performing activities of daily living

d. Client manages long-term oxygen therapy, tracheostomy, and/or mechanical ventilator

➤ B. Ineffective airway clearance

1. **Definition:** Inability to effectively clear secretions or obstructions from the respiratory tract (Gordon, 1993a)

2. Major defining characteristics

a. Abnormal breath sounds

b. Reduced vital capacity

c. Cough, change in rate and depth of respiration

d. Dyspnea, tachypnea, cyanosis

e. Anxiety, apprehension, or fatigue

f. Change in quality or quantity of mucus

3. Related factors/etiologies

a. Neuromuscular and/or musculoskeletal impairment
b. Fatigue and/or decreased energy
c. Perceptual and/or cognitive impairment
d. Infection
e. Smoking

4. Interventions

a. Keep client in Fowler's or semi-Fowler's position
b. Teach effective coughing techniques—for example, deep-breathing exercises—and/or use of incentive spirometer
c. Teach client how to dispose of secretions
d. Suction, as needed, to clear airways and stimulate cough; teach client to suction himself or herself; consult respiratory therapist or other professional resources regarding setting up home care
e. Provide patient with adequate hydration
f. Perform chest physiotherapy
g. Help client minimize energy demands
   1) Teach proper positioning techniques and body mechanics
   2) Teach ways to combine activities
   3) Teach pacing of activities to allow adequate rest between periods of exertion
h. Encourage smoking cessation
i. Inform client about environmental factors
   1) Importance of adequate humidity
   2) Importance of avoiding contact with smoke, smog, aerosols, and various products that produce fumes
j. Administer medications as ordered

5. Expected outcomes

a. Client maintains patent airway
b. Client produces a small amount of thin white or clear odorless sputum
c. Client performs or directs assistive coughing and pulmonary hygiene techniques
d. Client demonstrates adequate ventilation and tissue oxygenation

Diversional Activity

Diversional activities of play, leisure, and sports are critical for achieving a balance in life and successful adaptation to disability (Peterson & Gunn, 1984). Individuals with disabling conditions are susceptible to diversional activity deficit because participation in premorbid activities might require modification or might be impossible. This diagnosis might be overlooked by rehabilitation nurses, some of whom perceive diversional activity as the domain of occupational or recreational therapists. Addressing this problem is essential to the quality of life of people with disabilities.

I. Related Theories and Concepts

A. General
   1. Leisure experiences are at their best when activities are freely chosen and intrinsically motivated (Iso-Ahola, 1980)
   2. Leisure experiences are determined by individual's use of time, environmental opportunities, functional abilities, and personal interests
   3. Functional ability defines what we are capable of doing and what energy we have to do it
   4. Many sports and recreational activities participated in before injury can be adapted for participation after injury (see Adams & McCubbin, 1991, for specific examples)
   5. Research supports therapeutic benefits of pet, music, and reminiscence therapy in the elderly population (Maas, Buckwalter, & Hardy, 1991)

B. Benefits
   1. Opportunities for resocialization
   2. Opportunities to practice with adaptive equipment
   3. Incorporation of newly learned skills
   4. Participation in sports as an expression of well-being with secondary gain of increased positive self-image, which often results in improved interpersonal relations
   5. Constructive and meaningful use of leisure time that decreases depression

C. Barriers to diversional activities (McFarland & McFarlane, 1989)
   1. Lack of exposure and orientation
   2. Strong work ethic that views leisure as undesirable
   3. Limited finances, lack of transportation, social isolation, and fear of crime
   4. Lack of resources or space in rehabilitation settings

D. Pediatric considerations
   1. Theories related to play
      a. Freud (1946) described play as a coping mechanism that allows a child to escape to a fantasy world to act out anxieties
      b. Piaget (1962) saw play as a tool to assimilate the world and linked it to intellectual growth and cognitive development
      c. Erikson (1964) defined play as a positive and constructive form of human behavior that helps the child act out identities and sexual roles
   2. Purposes of diversional activity and/or play
      a. To learn about environment of objects, relationships, and space
      b. To practice developmental tasks
      c. To promote feelings of success and accomplishment
      d. To provide opportunities for recreation

II. Nursing Assessment

A. Assess premorbid patterns
   1. Amount of time available for diversional activities
   2. Types of diversional activities in which client participated
   3. Satisfaction with the time allotted for and type of diversional activities performed

B. Compare current status and premorbid diversional activity patterns

1. Feasibility of client's using adaptive equipment to continue premorbid types of diversional activities
2. Possibility of substituting other types of diversional activities

C. Watch for signs and symptoms of inadequate diversional activity
1. Yawning and statements of boredom
2. Napping throughout the day
3. Appearing disinterested, exhibiting a flat affect

D. Consider special factors in pediatric cases (Pratt & Allen, 1989)
1. Child's play development and behaviors, including favorite toys and playmates, prior to onset of disability
2. Parents' perceptions of activity
3. Child's developmental play level
4. Barriers to diversional activity

➤ III. Nursing Diagnosis: Diversional Activity Deficit

A. Definition: Decreased engagement in recreational or leisure activities (Gordon, 1993a)

B. Major defining characteristics

1. Nonverbal and verbal expressions of apathy, depression, restlessness, and hostility
2. Verbal expression of desire for additional activity
3. Immobility due to hospitalization and/or rehabilitation
4. Poor physical conditioning

C. Related factors/etiologies

1. In adults
   a. Limited ability to enter the community due to inadequate transportation, finances, social supports, hospitalization, or isolation
   b. Limited functional ability related to sensory, motor, and/or perceptual impairments
   c. Limited capacity related to lack of time
   d. Inability to form new relationships
   e. Lack of physical endurance needed for activity
   f. Lack of barrier-free environments for activities
2. In children
   a. Immobility and isolation from playmates
   b. Lack of developmentally appropriate toys and play situations
   c. Lack of physically challenged playmates for competitive play

D. Interventions

1. For adults
   a. Focus on capabilities, not limitations
   b. Facilitate social interaction by consulting volunteers and through recreational therapies (e.g., art, movement, music, and pet therapies)
   c. Provide materials of interest (e.g., books, magazines, puzzles, crafts)
   d. Consult occupational therapist for adaptive equipment and devices to facilitate participation in previous leisure interests (e.g., card playing, hobbies)
   e. Refer to recreational therapist or community resources for information on recreational and/or leisure activities and sports programs for people with disabilities
2. For children
   a. Bring playmates and peer groups together in hospital and/or provide list of groups and barrier-free environments in the community
   b. Provide developmentally appropriate and adaptive toys for children
   c. Schedule specific time in hospital treatment day for organized play and free play with appropriate toys and adaptive equipment
   d. Establish level of physical fitness and a program to increase endurance for competitive sports and play
   e. Teach family care providers how to use adaptive toys and equipment for competitive sports and play
   f. Encourage play as a means of learning and treatment during therapy schedule

E. Expected outcomes

1. Client participates in a satisfying diversional activity
2. Client verbalizes relief from boredom or anticipation of upcoming activity
3. Client develops a plan for the use of leisure time in the community environment
4. Client establishes daily time for diversional and free play
5. Client demonstrates use of adaptive toys and equipment for competitive sports and play

References

Adams, R.C., & McCubbin, J.A. (1991). *Games, sports, and exercises for the physically disabled.* Philadelphia: Lea & Febiger.

Austill-Clausen, R. (1993). Adaptive equipment for the home. In B.J. May (Ed.), *Home health and rehabilitation: Concepts of care* (pp. 193-216). Philadelphia: F.A. Davis Company.

Britell, C.W., & McFarland, S.R. (1988). Adaptive systems and devices for the disabled. In J.A. DeLisa (Ed.), *Rehabilitation medicine: Principles and practice* (pp. 372-387). Philadelphia: J.B. Lippincott Company.

Dettenmeier, P.A. (1992). *Pulmonary nursing care.* St. Louis: Mosby-Year Book, Inc.

◆Doyle, D.L., & Stern, P.N. (1992). Negotiating self-care in rehabilitation nursing. *Rehabilitation Nursing, 17,* 319-321, 326.

Dudek, S.G. (1987). *Nutrition handbook for nursing practice.* Philadelphia: J.B. Lippincott Company.

Erikson, E.H. (1964). *Childhood and society* (2nd ed.). New York: W.W. Norton.

Esposito, M.C., Tracey, C., & McCourt, A. (1989). Nursing diagnosis: Potential for disuse syndrome. In R.L.M. Carroll-Johnson (Ed.), *Classification of nursing diagnoses: Proceedings of the Eighth Conference, North American Nursing Diagnosis Association* (pp. 464-468). Philadelphia: J.B. Lippincott Company.

Freud, A. (1946). *The ego and mechanisms of defense.* New York: International Universities Press.

Gordon, M. (1993a). *Manual of nursing diagnosis: 1993-1994.* St. Louis: Mosby-Year Book, Inc.

Gordon, M. (1993b). *Rehabilitation nursing diagnosis survey: High-incidence nursing diagnoses in rehabilitation nursing* (preliminary report). Unpublished raw data.

Hickey, J.V. (1992). *The clinical practice of neurological and neurosurgical nursing* (3rd ed.). Philadelphia: J.B. Lippincott Company.
Iso-Ahola, S.E. (1980). *The social psychology of leisure and recreation.* Dubuque, IA: William C. Brown.
Kahana, E. (1982). A congruence model of person-environment interaction. In M.P. Lawton, P.G. Windley, & T.O. Byerts (Eds.), *Aging and the environment: Theoretical approaches* (pp. 97-121). New York: Springer-Verlag.
Katz, S., & Akpom, A. (1976). A measure of primary sociobiological functions. *International Journal of Health Sciences, 6*, 493-506.
Leslie, L.R. (1990). Training in homemaking activities. In F.J. Kottke & J.F. Lehmann (Eds.), *Krusen's handbook of physical medicine and rehabilitation* (4th ed.) (pp. 571-579). Philadelphia: W.B. Saunders Company.
Maas, M., Buckwalter, K., & Hardy, M.A. (1991). *Nursing diagnoses and interventions for the elderly.* Redwood City, CA: Addison-Wesley Nursing.
May, B.J. (1993). *Home health and rehabilitation: Concepts of care.* Philadelphia: F.A. Davis Company/Publishers.
McCourt, A. (1987). Implementation of nursing diagnosis through integration with quality assurance. *Nursing Clinics of North America, 22*, 899-904.
McFarland, G.K., & McFarlane, E.A. (1989). *Nursing diagnosis and interventions: Planning for patient care.* St. Louis: The C.V. Mosby Company.
Morton, P.G. (1991). *Health assessment in nursing* (2nd ed.). Springhouse, PA: Springhouse Corporation.
Nagi, S.Z. (1976). Epidemiology of disability among adults in the United States. *Milbank Memorial Fund Quarterly, 54*, 439-467.
Nicogossian, A.E., & Parker, J.G. (1982). *Space physiology and medicine (NASA—447).* Washington, DC: National Aeronautics and Space Administration.
North American Nursing Diagnosis Association. (1992). *NANDA nursing diagnoses: Definitions and classification 1992-1993.* St. Louis: Author.
Olson, E.V. (1967). The hazards of immobility. *American Journal of Nursing, 67*, 779-797.
Orem, D. (1985). A concept of self-care for the rehabilitation client. *Rehabilitation Nursing, 10*(3), 33-36.
Ouellet, L., & Rush, K.L. (1992). A synthesis of selected literature on mobility: A basis for studying impaired mobility. *Nursing Diagnosis, 3*(2), 72-75.
Peterson, C.A., & Gunn, S.L. (Eds.). (1984). *Therapeutic recreation program design: Principles and procedures* (2nd ed.). Englewood Cliffs, NJ: Prentice-Hall, Inc.
Piaget, J. (1962). *Play, dreams and imitation in childhood.* New York: W.W. Norton.
Pope, A.M., & Tarlov, A.R. (Eds.). (1991). *Disability in America: Toward a national agenda for prevention.* Washington, DC: National Academy Press.
Pratt, P.N., & Allen, A.S. (1989). *Occupational therapy for children* (2nd ed.). St. Louis: The C.V. Mosby Company.
Roy, C. (1980). The Roy adaptation model. In J. Riehl & C. Roy (Eds.), *Conceptual models for nursing practice* (2nd ed.) (p. 179-189). New York: Appleton-Century-Crofts.
Sawin, K.J., & Heard, L. (1992). Nursing diagnoses used most frequently in rehabilitation nursing practice. *Rehabilitation Nursing, 17*, 256-262.
Traver, G.A. (1991). *Respiratory care: A clinical approach.* Rockville, MD: Aspen Publishers, Inc.
Wilson, S.F., & Thompson, J.M. (1990). *Respiratory disorders.* St. Louis: Mosby-Year Book, Inc.
Wood, P.H.N. (1980). The language of disablement: A glossary relating to disease and its consequences. *International Rehabilitation Medicine, 2*, 86-92.

Suggested Readings

Baird, S.E. (1985). Development of a nursing assessment tool to diagnose altered body image in immobilized patients. *Orthopedic Nursing, 4*(1), 47-54.
◆Brukwitzki, G., Holmgren, C., & Maibusch, R. (1992). Validation of the defining characteristics of the nursing diagnosis: Ineffective airway clearance. In R.M. Carroll-Johnson (Ed.), *Classification of nursing diagnoses: Proceedings of the 9th Conference of the North American Nursing Diagnosis Association* (pp. 243-244). Philadelphia: J.B. Lippincott Company.
Bulau, J.M. (1989). *Quality assurance policies and procedures for home health care.* Rockville, MD: Aspen Publishers, Inc.
Caley, J., Dirksen, M., Engalla, M., & Hennrich, M.L. (1980). The Orem self-care nursing model. In J. Riehl & C. Roy (Eds.), *Conceptual models for nursing practice* (2nd ed.) (pp. 302-314). New York: Appleton-Century-Crofts.
Carpenito, L.J. (1991). *Nursing care plans and documentation.* Philadelphia: J.B. Lippincott Company.
Carpenito, L.J. (1991). *Nursing diagnosis: Application to clinical practice* (4th ed.). Philadelphia: J.B. Lippincott Company.
Chiotelis, S., & Zimmerman, M. (1988). Principles of occupational therapy. In J. Goodgold (Ed.), *Rehabilitation medicine* (pp. 727-758). St. Louis: The C.V. Mosby Company.
Christian, B.J. (1982). Immobilization: Psychosocial aspects. In C.M. Norris (Ed.), *Concept clarification in nursing* (pp. 341-356). Rockville, MD: Aspen Publishers, Inc.
Clydesdale, T.T., & Fahs, I.J. (1990). Social dimensions to functional gain in pediatric patients. *Archives of Physical Medicine and Rehabilitation, 71*, 469-472.
Coley, I.L. (1978). *Pediatric assessment of self-care activities.* St. Louis: The C.V. Mosby Company.
Compton, D.M. (Ed.). (1989). *Issues in therapeutic recreation: A profession in transition.* Champaign, IL: Sagamore Publishing.
Cossmyer, V.L. (1989, June). Using physiology in the nursing diagnosis process. *Journal of Advanced Medical Surgical Nursing*, pp. 1-10.
Craft, M.D., & Denehy, J.A. (1990). *Nursing interventions for infants and children.* Philadelphia: W.B. Saunders Company.
◆Fedorich, D., & Littleton, M. (1990). Chest physiotherapy: Evaluating the effectiveness. *Dimensions in Critical Care Nursing, 9*(2), 68-74.
Finnie, N.R. (1975). *Handling the young cerebral palsied child at home.* New York: E.P. Dutton, Inc.
Gordon, M. (1987). *Nursing diagnosis: Process and application* (2nd ed.). New York: McGraw-Hill Book Company.
Grey, M., & Hayman, L. (1987). Assessing stress in children: Research and clinical implications. *Journal of Pediatric Nursing, 8*, 316-327.
Haler, E.M., & Bell, K.R. (1990). Rehabilitation's relationship to inactivity. In F.J. Kottke & J.F. Lehmann (Eds.), *Krusen's handbook of physical medicine and rehabilitation* (4th ed.) (pp. 1113-1133). Philadelphia: W.B. Saunders Company.
Harper, C.M., & Lyles, Y.M. (1988). Physiology and complications of bed rest. *Journal of the American Geriatric Society, 36*, 1047-1054.
Hickey, J.V. (1992). *The clinical practice of neurological and neurosurgical nursing* (3rd ed.). Philadelphia: J.B. Lippincott Company.
Iacovitti, P.A. (1992). Effects of hospitalization on children and families. In P.T. Castiglia & R.E. Harbin (Eds.), *Child health care: Process and practice* (pp. 367-387). Philadelphia: J.B. Lippincott Company.
Jones, M.L. (1985). *Home care for the chronically ill or disabled child.* New York: Harper & Row Publishers.
Kalafatich, A.J. (1982). Immobilization in adolescents. In C.M. Norris (Ed.), *Concept clarification in nursing* (pp. 333-340). Rockville, MD: Aspen Publishers, Inc.

Keating, S.B., & Kelman, G.B. (1988). *Home health care nursing: Concepts and practice.* Philadelphia: J.B. Lippincott Company.

Kersten, L.D. (1989). *Comprehensive respiratory nursing: A decision making approach.* Philadelphia: W.B. Saunders Company.

Lee, J., & Fowler, M.D. (1986). Merely child's play? Developmental work and playthings. *Journal of Pediatric Nursing, 1*(4), 260-270.

Lentz, M. (1981). Selected aspects of deconditioning secondary to immobilization. *Nursing Clinics of North America, 16,* 729-737.

Levy, L. (1989). Activity adaptation in rehabilitation of the physically and cognitively disabled aged. *Topics in Geriatric Rehabilitation, 4*(4), 45-52.

Lyke, E.M. (1992). *Assessing for nursing diagnosis: A human needs approach.* Philadelphia: J.B. Lippincott Company.

Massion, J. (1992). Movement, posture and equilibrium. *Progress in Neurobiology, 38*(1), 35-53.

Moody-Szymanski, E.A., & Scherer, K.A. (1989). Breathing. In S. Dittmar (Ed.), *Rehabilitation nursing: Process and application* (pp. 82-119). St. Louis: The C.V. Mosby Company.

Morton, P.G. (1991). *Health assessment in nursing* (2nd ed.). Springhouse, PA: Springhouse Corporation.

Mumma, C.M. (Ed.). (1987). *Rehabilitation nursing: Concepts and practice—A core curriculum* (2nd ed.). Evanston, IL: Rehabilitation Nursing Foundation.

Nelson, D., & Peterson, C. (1989). Enhancing therapeutic exercise through purposeful activity: A theoretic analysis. *Topics in Geriatric Rehabilitation, 4*(4), 45-52.

O'Neil, R.H. (1981). Problems associated with disuse syndromes—including the integument. In I.L. Beland & J.Y. Passes (Eds.), *Clinical nursing: Pathophysiological and psychosocial approaches* (4th ed.) (pp. 1107-1123). New York: MacMillan Publishing Company, Inc.

Orem, D. (1971). *Nursing concepts in practice.* New York: McGraw-Hill Book Company.

Phipps, M., & Kelly-Hayes, M. (1991). Rehabilitation of older adults. In E.M. Baines (Ed.), *Perspectives on gerontological nursing* (pp. 357-372). Newbury Park, CA: Sage Publications, Inc.

Pratt, P., & Allen, A. (1989). *Occupational therapy for children* (2nd ed.). St. Louis: The C.V. Mosby Company.

Re Johnson, J., & Cedrone, S. (1990). Enabling disabled travelers. *Rehabilitation Nursing, 15,* 92-94.

Riehl, J., & Roy, C. (1980). *Conceptual models for nursing practice* (2nd ed.). New York: Appleton-Century-Crofts.

Rubin, M. (1988). The physiology of bed rest. *American Journal of Nursing, 88*(1), 50-56.

◆Selekman, J. (1983). The development of body image in the child: A learned response. *Topics in Clinical Nursing, 5*(1), 13-21.

Selikson, S., Damus, K., & Hammerman, D. (1988). Risk factors associated with immobility. *Journal of the American Geriatric Society, 6,* 707-712.

◆Smith, A., & Aston, S. (1989). The use of activity in rehabilitation of elders with vision impairments. *Topics in Geriatric Rehabilitation, 4*(4), 45-52.

◆Steller, K., Geake, T., Taylor, V., Grant, R., & Hall, B. (1990). Acute lobar atelectases: A comparison of two chest physiotherapy regimens. *Chest, 98,* 1336-1340.

Taylor, S.G. (1991). The structure of nursing diagnosis from Orem's theory. *Nursing Science Quarterly, 4*(1), 24-32.

Traver, G.A., Mitchell, J.T., & Flodavist-Priestly, G. (1991). *Respiratory care: A clinical approach.* Rockville, MD: Aspen Publishers, Inc.

Weinberg, L.K. (1989). Potential for disuse syndrome. In G.K. McFarland & E.A. McFarlane (Eds.), *Nursing diagnosis and intervention: Planning for patient care* (pp. 361-372). St. Louis: The C.V. Mosby Company.

Winslow, E.H. (1985). Cardiovascular consequences of bed rest. *Heart and Lung, 14*(3), 236-246.

◆ indicates a research-based work

CHAPTER 15

Sleep–Rest Pattern

Rehabilitation nurses are frequently in a position to identify persons at high risk for sleep pattern disturbances, to provide a spectrum of effective interventions, and to make appropriate referrals for the diagnosis and treatment of sleep disorders. This chapter describes patterns of sleep and rest, including sleep routines and satisfaction with the quantity and quality of restorative sleep, over a 24-hour period. The sleep-rest pattern is of importance to rehabilitation nursing clients for many reasons. Many disabling conditions and chronic diseases are associated with sequelae that can impair sleep and rest. At the same time, the physical endurance required for participation in an active rehabilitation program and the lifestyle changes resulting from the disability increase the need for high-quality sleep for physical and mental restoration.

Clients with stroke, arthritis, traumatic brain injury, spinal cord injury, pulmonary disorders, Alzheimer's disease, multiple sclerosis, Parkinson's disease, and postpolio syndrome all experience varying degrees of interference with previous sleep-rest patterns. An inability to effectively manage sleep-rest problems that arise as a result of disability interferes with the ability to maximize self-care and functional independence.

As individuals age, there are significant predictable changes in sleep-rest patterns. Managing disturbances in sleep patterns in older people is essential to provide and maintain quality of life and to foster independence. It is estimated that nearly two-thirds of people over 65 years of age have at least one chronic illness that interferes with sleep patterns. Children with disabilities also have special needs regarding effective sleep and rest.

Significant recent advances have increased the understanding of normal sleep and the effects of ineffective sleep on performance and behavior. Increasingly, the impact of decreased daytime alertness and loss of vigilance as a result of sleep disorders is being recognized as a medical and social problem of unexpected magnitude (Culebras, 1992b). In rehabilitation clients, unrecognized and/or unmanaged sleep disturbances can result in falls, injuries, behavior and performance problems, and institutionalization—all of which are potentially preventable.

Paradoxically, however, sleep problems continue to be underreported by clients and underestimated by healthcare professionals. Research studies indicate that both physicians and nurses infrequently assess and/or diagnose actual disturbances in sleep patterns (Beyerman, 1987; Haponik, 1992). When sleep problems are recognized, lack of knowledge regarding current therapeutic management techniques often results in ineffective treatment.

I. Related Theory and Concepts

A. Sleep as a behavior

1. Sleep
   a. Definition: Patterned physiological phenomenon characterized by an altered state of awareness
   b. Individuals who are sleeping experience profound relaxation and significant decreases in physical and cognitive activities (Chenelly, 1989)
2. Sleeping and waking are processes that depend on interactions between antagonistic areas of the brain
3. Sleep is thought to be linked to the actions of the reticular activating system (RAS) and neurotransmitters (Biddle & Oaster, 1990)
   a. Acetylcholine
   b. Norepinephrine
   c. Serotonin
   d. Dopamine
   e. Histamine
   f. Adenosine
   g. Gaba-aminobutyric acid (GABA)
4. Sleep is synchronized with the light-dark cycle of the environment in conjunction with physiological circadian rhythms
5. Normal sleep is divided into non-rapid eyeball movement (NREM) and rapid eyeball movement (REM) phases
   a. NREM sleep (Biddle & Oaster, 1990)
      1) Stage I
         a) Person becomes drowsy with increasing muscle relaxation
         b) Transitional stage between wakefulness and sleep
         c) Usually accounts for 5% to 10% of total sleep
      2) Stage II
         a) Muscle relaxation intensifies
         b) Cerebral activity decreases
         c) Individual still is easily aroused
         d) Normally accounts for 50% to 55% of total sleep
      3) Stage III
         a) Vital signs are lowered
         b) Gastrointestinal function decreases
         c) Venous dilation occurs
         d) Accounts for 10% to 20% of total sleep
      4) Stage IV

a) Person is in a deep sleep pattern
b) Body functions decrease markedly
c) Accounts for 10% to 20% of total sleep time and is associated with physical repair and restoration

5) In young adults, approximately 90 minutes elapse between onset of Stage I sleep and completion of Stage IV sleep; sleeper then drifts back to Stage I and enters REM sleep

b. REM sleep
   1) Normally accounts for 20% to 25% of total sleep time
   2) Most dreaming occurs in REM sleep
   3) Thought to be necessary for mental restoration and adaptation to stress (Chenelly, 1989)
c. To achieve high-quality restorative sleep, most individuals complete several sleep cycles of 70 to 100 minutes during each sleeping period
d. Sleep patterns are highly individualized and are altered by several factors
   1) Age
   2) Health status
   3) Lifestyle
   4) Stress
   5) Activity
e. Client's perception of sleep disturbance
   1) Problems related to taking an excessive amount of time to fall asleep (sleep latency)
   2) Problems related to staying asleep (sleep maintenance)
   3) Problems related to early awakening or perceptions of inadequate quantity and quality of sleep

B. Classification of sleep disorders

1. A revision of the sleep disorder classification in 1990 reflects significant progress in the scientific study of sleep and sleep disorders (Culebras, 1992b)
2. There are four major classifications (Thorby, 1990)
   a. Dyssomnias: Primary sleep disorders, derived from either intrinsic or extrinsic causes and problems related to disruptions in circadian rhythm
      1) Intrinsic
         a) Psychophysiological insomnia
         b) Narcolepsy
         c) Hypoventilation syndrome
         d) Periodic limb movement disorder (nocturnal myoclonus)
         e) Obstructive, central, and mixed apnea syndromes
      2) Extrinsic
         a) Inadequate sleep hygiene
         b) Environmental sleep disorder
         c) Insufficient sleep syndrome
      3) Circadian rhythm sleep disorders
         a) Disorder due to traveling to another time zone
         b) Disorder due to shift work
   b. Parasomnias: Undesirable physical phenomena that occur predominantly during sleep
      1) Sleepwalking
      2) Nightmares and night terrors
      3) Sudden infant death syndrome (SIDS)
   c. Sleep disorders due to medical and/or psychiatric problems
      1) Medical disorders
         a) Chronic obstructive pulmonary disease
         b) Sleep-related gastroesophageal reflux
         c) Peptic ulcer disease
         d) Neurological problems
            (1) Dementia
            (2) Parkinson's disease
            (3) Sleep-related epilepsy
      2) Psychiatric disorders
         a) Psychoses
         b) Anxiety
         c) Panic
         d) Alcoholism
         e) Depression
   d. Proposed disorders for future diagnostic development

C. Incidence of sleep problems

1. U.S. demographic studies place incidence of insomnia between 30% and 35% for all adults within a given year (Rosekind, 1992)
2. Sleep problems, in spite of this high incidence, are thought to be widely underreported by clients and underdiagnosed by healthcare professionals
3. New classifications of sleep disorders have been expanded to describe daytime consequences of poor sleep quality and to connect inadequate restorative sleep and rest with accidents (Rosekind, 1992)
4. People with disabilities face a barrage of physical and psychological problems that could disrupt sleep patterns; therefore, the possibility of sleep pattern disturbance should be considered in any client with a physical disability, especially when he or she is in an unfamiliar environment (Chenelly, 1989)
5. Fragmentation of sleep due to brief arousals affects clients who are awakened because of health-related procedures, position changes, or pain (Roehrs & Roth, 1989)

D. Healthcare professionals' perception of sleep problems

1. Perception of sleep problems by physicians: A study of geriatricians indicated that they had difficulty recognizing and treating sleep problems (Haponik, 1992)
   a. Comprehensive sleep history was not obtained from 50% of clients
   b. Physicians might attribute complaints about sleep to normal changes in sleep associated with aging
   c. Primary sleep disorders, such as sleep apnea, often were not evaluated or diagnosed
   d. Few physicians routinely used nonpharmacologic sleep treatment strategies in practice

2. Perception of sleep problems by nurses
   a. Study by Beyerman (1987) of etiologies of disturbances in sleep patterns showed that sleep problems could be altered significantly if nurses decreased amount of stimuli in the environment
   b. Despite the frequency of sleep-pattern disturbances, nurses seldom use the nursing diagnosis of *sleep pattern disturbance*
   c. Study by Pulling (1991) showed a positive correlation between critical care nurses' knowledge about sleep and their initiation of sleep-promoting nursing interventions

E. Sleep issues across the life span

1. Pediatric: Young (preschool-aged) children are affected greatly by separation from parents when hospitalized; study by White, Williams, Alexander, Powell-Cope, and Conlon (1990) suggests that using a recorded bedtime story focused on a theme of child/parent reunion and done by a stranger decreased the time of sleep onset in hospitalized children
2. Geriatric
   a. Sleep is shortened and less consolidated as a function of normal aging (Bonnet & Arand, 1989)
   b. Requirement for total amount of sleep does not change with age; however, circadian rhythm is altered, resulting in decreased sleep regulation (Monane, 1992)
   c. Sleep is redistributed over a 24-hour period; although elderly may spend less time in nocturnal sleep, daytime napping is increased to compensate for loss of nighttime sleep
   d. Many elderly people report problems with frequent awakenings, inability to return to sleep after arousal, and early morning awakening (Monane, 1992)
   e. Lighter stages of sleep, especially Stage I sleep, are normally increased in older persons, with significant decreases in Stage III and Stage IV sleep; this is why the elderly often report feeling less rested after appearing to have slept soundly
   f. It is helpful for older persons to be taught about normal sleep patterns of aging
   g. Masked depression and residual effects of medications taken by elderly persons also should be considered as etiological factors of sleep problems
   h. Sleep apnea: Excessive daytime somnolence seen with apnea and daytime napping can be incorrectly assumed to be normal consequence of aging (Schwartz & Smith, 1989)
      1) Definition: Sleep apnea, a relatively common disorder in elderly people, is characterized by recurrent apneas associated with oxyhemoglobin desaturation and arousal from sleep
      2) Differentiation of apneas
         a) Central apnea: Characterized by complete absence of respiratory muscle efforts; referral to a sleep disorder center is required (Schwartz & Smith, 1989)
         b) Obstructive apnea: Characterized by presence of continued thoracoabdominal respiratory effort against occluded pharyngeal airway; various treatment approaches can be used
            (1) Weight reduction of 10% to 15%
            (2) Avoidance of use of hypnotics and alcohol, both of which increase apnea frequency and increase the severity of oxyhemoglobin desaturation
            (3) Use of nasal continuous positive airway pressure (CPAP) to eliminate apneic episodes by maintaining upper airway patency
         c) Mixed apneas: Have both obstructive and central components

F. Sleep problems related to specific disabling disorders

1. Stroke
   a. Within a few days after a major hemispheric stroke, reversal of sleep-wake cycle, characterized by daytime lethargy and wakefulness at night, occurs (Culebras, 1992a)
   b. As recovery from stroke progresses, clients exhibit normal REM sleep and increasing amounts of slow-wave sleep
2. Rheumatological disorders
   a. Fatigue is common in persons with arthritis and other rheumatological diseases
   b. Nighttime pain can interfere with effective consolidation of sleep
3. Traumatic brain injury
   a. Sleep abnormalities (including high incidence of nocturnal awakenings) occur most frequently in the first 6 months following traumatic brain injury (Askenasy & Rahmani, 1988)
   b. Reorganization of sleep tends to be normalized for the individual as rehabilitation progresses, with positive relationship between cognitive improvement and improvement in percentage of REM sleep (Culebras, 1992a)
4. Spinal cord injury
   a. Persons with high-level spinal cord lesions commonly report sleep disturbances and alterations in breathing due to increased diaphragmatic workload that results when they are in a supine or a prone position (Culebras, 1992a)
   b. Discomfort from nocturnal spasms can interfere with sleep and rest
   c. Sedating effects of antispasmodics can interfere with daytime activities and/or performance
5. Postpolio syndrome
   a. Characteristics
      1) Fatigue
      2) Appearance of weakness in muscles originally affected and previously unaffected
      3) Dysphagia
      4) Hypoventilation

5) Obstructive sleep apnea secondary to muscle weakness

b. Sleep studies should be done for postpolio clients with excessive daytime somnolence and/or respiratory complaints

c. Treatment strategies for respiratory-related sleep apnea in postpolio syndrome (Steljes, Kryser, Kirk, & Millar, 1990)
   1) Nasal CPAP to manage obstructive sleep apnea
   2) Nasal mask ventilation for hypoventilation syndrome and sleep apnea secondary to respiratory muscle weakness
   3) Long-term nasal mechanical ventilation for clients with postpolio fatigue who already use respiratory assistive devices (e.g., rocking beds) and have continuing respiratory problems
   4) Rest periods to generally relieve this condition, which peaks in late morning or early afternoon
   5) Use of energy conservation and work simplification techniques to achieve balance between rest and activity periods (Packer, Martins, Krefting, & Brouwer, 1991)

6. Multiple sclerosis (MS)
   a. Fatigue is a common complaint among MS clients
   b. Studies show that persons with MS have frequent sleep interruptions secondary to nocturnal myoclonus, spasticity, depression, and bladder disturbances (Clark et al., 1992)
7. Parkinson's disease and amyotrophic lateral sclerosis (ALS)
   a. Position changes in healthy persons might alter the sleep stage, but do not cause the extent of arousal seen with Parkinson's and ALS clients (Reimer, 1989)
   b. Parkinsonian tremors abate during sleep but might recur in association with body movements and arousals (Culebras, 1992a)
   c. High doses of levodopa have a stimulant effect; newer anti-Parkinsonian drugs might improve nocturnal sleep
8. Alzheimer's disease
   a. Sleep generally impaired in dementia disorders as result of neuroanatomic or functional brain abnormalities underlying these disorders (Vitiello, Bliwise, & Prinz, 1992)
   b. Reversal in sleep pattern, with nearly half of nighttime hours being spent awake and a large number of daytime hours spent asleep
   c. Daytime sleep often of poor quality, consisting of NREM Stage I and Stage II sleep (Vitiello & Prinz, 1989)
   d. Sundowning: Term used to describe exacerbation of delirium during evening or night, with improvement of delirium during day (Vitiello, Bliwise, & Prinz, 1992)
   e. Families and caregivers should be aware that as disease progresses, the patient's normal circadian sleep-wake rhythms will break down and nocturnal activity and daytime napping will increase
9. Myasthenia gravis
   a. Common sleep complaints
      1) Awakening at night
      2) Sensations of breathlessness
      3) Daytime somnolence
   b. Myasthenia gravis clients are prone to sleep apnea with potentially significant oxygen desaturation (Culebras, 1992a)
10. Other issues in sleep and chronic illness
   a. Studies indicate that quality of sleep in chronic illness deteriorates in presence of overlapping depression and/or affective disorders
   b. Rehabilitation professionals need to be aware of potential for masked depression as an etiological factor in both insomnia and daytime sleepiness (Hyyppa & Kronholm, 1989)

II. Nursing Assessment

A. Points to consider when taking a sleep history
   1. What is client's usual sleep pattern?
   2. What lifestyle changes or life events are occurring that interfere with sleep?
   3. What is the primary sleep problem?
      a. Difficulty with onset of sleep
      b. Frequent awakening
      c. Difficulty in getting back to sleep
      d. Waking earlier or later than desired
      e. Waking without feeling rested
      f. Feelings of sleepiness during the daytime
   4. How is sleep pattern disturbance affecting other areas of functioning?
   5. What specific activities or sleep-related hygiene measures does the client normally initiate to facilitate sleep and rest?
   6. What medications (prescription and/or over-the-counter) is client taking?
   7. Does client consume alcohol before bedtime and/or consume stimulants such as coffee?

B. Points to consider when observing sleep-wake behaviors
   1. What does bed partner or significant other report about client's sleep-wake behaviors?
   2. Does client snore at night, appear to be restless, or have periods when breathing stops?
   3. What overt or subtle clues regarding performance or behavior during the day suggest that the person might not be getting adequate sleep?
   4. Does client or significant other report excessive daytime somnolence or changes in daytime vigilance and alertness?

C. Points to consider when performing an environmental assessment
   1. What are noise and light levels in sleep environment?
   2. Are temperature and ventilation in sleeping environment conducive to sleep?
   3. Are there disturbances caused by roommates or other environmental factors that impair sleep?

III. Nursing Diagnosis

A. Sleep pattern disturbance

1. **Definition:** Disruption of sleep time causing discomfort or interference with desired lifestyle (NANDA, 1992)

2. **Major defining characteristics**

   a. Difficulty in falling asleep
   b. Complaints of not feeling rested
   c. Awakening earlier or later than desired
   d. Sleep interruptions
   e. Excessive daytime sleepiness
   f. Supporting cues
      1) Changes in behavior and/or performance
      2) Reports by families, significant others, or caregivers of changes in sleep quantity and/or quality
      3) Physical cues
         a) Listlessness
         b) Irritability
         c) Yawning

3. **Related factors/etiologies**

   a. Knowledge deficit
   b. Pain/discomfort
   c. Sleep interruptions
   d. Impaired mobility
   e. Depression, anxiety

4. **Interventions**

   a. Interventions for specific etiologies
      1) Knowledge deficit related to sleep hygiene
         a) Provide clients with strategies related to sleep hygiene—daily activities that promote high-quality restorative sleep and optimal daytime functioning (Bootzin & Perlis, 1992)
         b) Encourage use of specific sleep hygiene strategies
            (1) Avoiding daytime naps
            (2) Avoiding spending long periods of time in bed awake
            (3) Keeping regular sleep-wake schedules
            (4) Avoiding products known to interfere with sleep onset and/or maintenance
               (a) Caffeine
               (b) Nicotine
               (c) Alcohol
            (5) Avoiding exercise close to bedtime
            (6) Maintaining appropriate sleep environment
               (a) Clean bedding
               (b) Dark room
               (c) Cool temperature
               (d) Appropriate ventilation
               (e) Noise control
            (7) Avoiding going to bed hungry or soon after a large meal
            (8) Avoiding participating in activities that are emotionally upsetting or excessively stimulating close to bedtime
         c) Identify client's pattern of medication use (prescription and/or over-the-counter drugs) and teach client about medications that can impair sleep
         d) Help client accurately describe perception of sleep problems by suggesting use of a sleep diary
      2) Sleep disturbance related to pain and/or discomfort
         a) Administer pain medication on a schedule that will ensure maximum effect during onset of sleep
         b) Use positioning, back rubs, and nonnarcotic analgesics to relieve minor discomfort
      3) Sleep disturbance related to interrupted sleep
         a) Organize procedures to plan for fewest disturbances during the night
         b) Have client void before retiring and limit fluids in the early evening
         c) Minimize noise and other environmental distractions; noise control is one aspect of care in hospitals and long-term care facilities in which it is especially appropriate for nurses to intervene (Walgenbach, 1990)
         d) If interrupted sleep pattern is due to pathophysiological alterations in circadian rhythms (as in Alzheimer's disease and traumatic brain injury), advise family and caregivers to minimize client's daytime napping and to increase his or her daytime activity
         e) If depression or anxiety is interfering with onset of sleep, allow client some time to air feelings and express concerns before bedtime
      4) Sleep pattern disturbance related to impaired mobility
         a) When awakening a person with spasticity for turning or repositioning, move slowly and rouse him or her verbally before touching
         b) Plan strategies to accomplish position changes with minimal time and effort
         c) Use creative strategies to accomplish turning and repositioning, such as using satin sheets to decrease friction (Reimer, 1989)
         d) For persons with stroke, plan last turn of the night to be to affected side to normalize tone for morning activities (Gee & Passarella, 1985)

   b. Additional treatment strategies (Bootzin & Perlis, 1992)
      1) Stimulus control techniques to improve sleep efficiency
         a) Having client lie down to sleep only

when drowsy
b) Having client use bed only for sleep and sexual activities
c) Having client get out of bed if unable to fall asleep
d) Regulating sleeping and waking hours to be the same each day
e) Imposing sleep restriction to limit time spent sleeping
2) Chronotherapy
a) Used for circadian rhythm disorders in which client's sleep-wake pattern is out of phase with desired sleep pattern (e.g., jet lag)
b) Bedtime is progressively delayed by daily increments of 3 hours until onset of sleep matches desirable pattern
3) Bright light therapy
a) Therapy based on premise that exposure to bright light can shift sleep phases
b) Has been shown to benefit persons experiencing jet lag and seasonal affective disorder, and can have potential for management of circadian rhythm disturbances in persons with Alzheimer's disease
4) Relaxation training, meditation, and biofeedback
5) Referral to sleep disorder center may be indicated if chronic insomnia or excessive daytime somnolence is accompanied by any of the following factors (Moran & Stoudermire, 1992)
a) Failure to respond to customary sleep hygiene and therapy with hypnotic medications
b) Unacceptable side effects from controlled and supervised use of hypnotic medications
c) Potential and/or unconfirmed sleep apnea
d) Desire for consultation when sleep pattern disturbance has multiple etiologies or is resistant to traditional therapy

c. Pharmacologic approaches to treatment of insomnia
1) Indications for use of hypnotics in treatment of insomnia
a) Recommended therapeutic use (Vogel, 1992)
(1) Limited to low dose for intermittent insomnia in elderly clients
(2) Also limited to low dose for transient situational insomnia in young and middle-aged adults
b) Hypnotic drugs contraindicated for long periods or for treatment of chronic insomnia
c) Clients should be taught to view intermittent therapy with hypnotics as part of overall program whose goal is to restore and maintain normal sleep without medications (Walsh & Fillingim, 1990)
d) Hypnotic drugs are contraindicated for persons whose sleep problems are due to potential or actual sleep apnea
2) Benzodiazepine hypnotics are most frequently used agents for management of insomnia (Culebras, 1992b)
a) Benzodiazepine hypnotics are classified as short-acting, intermediate-acting, and long-acting, based on their pharmacokinetics
Editor's note: The list of products below is not intended to be comprehensive, nor does it constitute an endorsement by the editors or publishers. The products named serve only as examples.
(1) Short-acting benzodiazepines include midazolam (Versed®) and triazolam (Halcion®)
(2) Intermediate-acting agents include estazolam (Prosom®), quazepam (Doral™), temazepam (Restoril®), and lorazepam (Ativan® and others)
(3) Long-acting benzodiazepines include flurazepam (Dalmane®) and diazepam (Valium®)
b) Side effects of benzodiazepines
(1) Residual sedation: Sedation lasting into next waking period
(2) Anterograde amnesia: Lack of recall of events after medication was taken
(3) Rebound insomnia: Problems with sleep after medication is discontinued
c) Adverse effects might be seen in elderly clients, people with hepatic problems, and clients with psychiatric disorders
d) Considerations about dosage and length of action
(1) All side effects of benzodiazepines intensify with dosage; therefore, lowest effective dose should be used
(2) Long-acting agents, such as flurazepam, may last into next waking period and should be used only when daytime alertness is not required
(3) Intermediate-acting agents are useful for clients who have no problems related to sleep onset but need assistance with sleep maintenance
(4) Short-acting agents are most effective for problems with sleep onset and for problems with staying asleep during the majority of the sleep cycle (Walsh & Fillingim, 1990)
e) Adjustments with elderly clients
(1) Physiological alterations associated with aging affect drug absorption, distribution, and elimination

(2) Research indicates that triazolam (Halcion) dosage in elderly clients should be reduced by half (Roehrs & Roth, 1989)
(3) Use of smaller doses, short-acting agents, and drugs with simple metabolic pathways lessen risk of residual effects in elderly clients (Roehrs & Roth, 1989)

3) Effects of other medications on sleep
a) Average elderly client takes five to nine medications daily, many with potential to interfere with sleep (Monane, 1992)
b) Medications known to interfere with sleep
(1) Antihistamines
(2) Methylxanthines contained in coffee, tea, chocolate, soft drinks, and theophylline
(3) Over-the-counter medications such as headache remedies and diet aids
c) Over-the-counter sleep aids, which often contain antihistamines or scopolamine as active ingredients, can have undesirable effects
(1) Delirium due to drugs' anticholinergic effects in older patients
(2) Additive effects if client is taking other anticholinergic or sedating drugs
d) Use of diuretics should be monitored to minimize number of interruptions of sleep for voiding

5. Expected outcomes

a. Within the limits of his or her disability, client is able to establish a sleep pattern that produces high-quality restorative sleep and rest
b. Client and family verbalize ways to promote sleep and rest
c. Client and family report that client is able to return to sleep within a short period of time after planned awakening
d. Client is free of complications related to hypnotic therapy
e. Client's daytime performance is not negatively affected by lack of sleep or rest

References

Askenasy, J.J., & Rahmani, L. (1988). Neuropsycho-social rehabilitation of head injury. *American Journal of Physical Medicine, 66*, 315-327.

◆Beyerman, K. (1987). Etiologies of sleep pattern disturbance in hospitalized patients. In A. McLane (Ed.), *Classification of nursing diagnoses: Proceedings of the seventh conference of the North American Nursing Diagnosis Association* (pp. 381-394). St. Louis: The C.V. Mosby Company.

Biddle, C., & Oaster, T.R. (1990). The nature of sleep. *Journal of the American Association of Nurse Anesthetists, 58*(1), 193-198.

Bonnet, M.H., & Arand, D.L. (1989). Sleep loss in aging. *Clinics in Geriatric Medicine, 5*, 405-420.

Bootzin, R.R., & Perlis, M.L. (1992). Nonpharmacologic treatment of insomnia. *Journal of Clinical Psychiatry, 53*, 29-36.

Chenelly, S. (1989). Sleep and rest. In S. Dittmar (Ed.), *Rehabilitation nursing: Process and application* (pp. 227-240). St. Louis: The C.V. Mosby Company.

◆Clark, C.M., Fleming, J.A., Li, D., Oger, J., Klonoff, H., & Paty, D. (1992). Sleep disturbance, depression, and lesion site in patients with multiple sclerosis. *Archives of Neurology, 49*, 641-643.

Culebras, A. (1992a). Neuroanatomic and neurologic correlates of sleep disturbances. *Neurology, 42*(7), 19-27.

Culebras, A. (1992b). Update on sleep disorders and the sleep-wake cycle. *The Psychiatric Clinics of North America, 15*, 467-490.

Gee, Z., & Passarella, P. (1985). *Nursing care of the stroke patient: A therapeutic approach based on Bobath principles.* Pittsburgh: AREN Publications.

Haponik, E.F. (1992). Sleep disturbances of older persons: Physician's attitudes. *Sleep, 15*(2), 168-172.

◆Hyyppa, M.T., & Kronholm, E. (1989). Quality of sleep and chronic illness. *Journal of Clinical Epidemiology, 42*, 633-638.

Monane, M. (1992). Insomnia in the elderly. *Journal of Clinical Psychiatry, 53*(6), 23-27.

Moran, M.G., & Stoudermire, A. (1992). Sleep disorders in the medically ill patient. *Journal of Clinical Psychiatry, 53*(6), 29-35.

North American Nursing Diagnosis Association (NANDA). (1992). *NANDA nursing diagnoses: Definitions and classification 1992-1993.* St. Louis: Author.

◆Packer, T.L., Martins, I., Krefting, L., & Brouwer, B. (1991). Activity and post-polio fatigue. *Orthopedics, 14*, 1223-1226.

Pulling, C.A. (1991). The relationship between critical care nurses' knowledge about sleep and the initiation of sleep promoting nursing interventions. *Axon, 13*(2), 57-62.

Reimer, M. (1989). Sleep pattern disturbances related to neurological dysfunction. *Axon, 11*(3), 65-68.

Roehrs, T.A., & Roth, T. (1989). Drugs, sleep disorders and aging. *Clinics in Geriatric Medicine, 5*, 395-404.

Rosekind, M.R. (1992). The epidemiology and occurrence of insomnia. *Journal of Clinical Psychiatry, 53*(6), 4-6.

Schwartz, A.R., & Smith, P.L. (1989). Sleep apnea in the elderly. *Clinics in Geriatric Medicine, 5*, 315-330.

Steljes, D.G., Kryser, M.H., Kirk, B.W., & Millar, T.W. (1990). Sleep in postpolio syndrome. *Chest, 98*(1), 133-140.

Thorby, M.J. (1990). *International classification of sleep disorders: Diagnostic and coding manual.* Rochester, MN: American Sleep Disorders Association.

Vitiello, M.V., & Prinz, P.N. (1989). Alzheimer's disease: Sleep and wake patterns. *Clinics in Geriatric Medicine, 5*(2), 289-300.

Vitiello, M.V., Bliwise, D.L., & Prinz, P.N. (1992). Sleep in Alzheimer's disease and the sundown syndrome. *Neurology, 42*(7), 83-93.

Vogel, G. (1992). Clinical uses and advantages of low doses of benzodiazepam hypnotics. *Journal of Clinical Psychiatry, 53*(6), 19-22.

Walgenbach, J.C. (1990). Lullabye and not a good night? *Geriatric Nursing, 11*(6), 278-279.

Walsh, J.K., & Fillingim, J.M. (1990). Role of hypnotic drugs in general practice. *The American Journal of Medicine, 88*(3A), 34-38.

◆White, M.A., Williams, P.D., Alexander, D.J., Powell-Cope, G.M., & Conlon, M. (1990). Sleep onset latency and distress in hospitalized children. *Nursing Research, 39*(30), 134-139.

Suggested Readings

Ancoli-Israel, S. (1989). Epidemiology of sleep disorders. *Clinics in Geriatric Medicine, 5*, 347-362.

Aldrich, M.S. (1992). Narcolepsy. *Neurology, 42*(7), 34-43.

Becker, P.M., & Jamieson, A.O. (1992). Common sleep disorders in the elderly: Diagnosis and treatment. *Geriatrics, 47*(3), 45-48, 51-52.

Bliwise, D.L. (1989). Neuropsychological function in sleep. *Clinics in Geriatric Medicine, 5*, 381-394.

◆Buyesse, D., Browman, K., Monk, T., Reynolds, C., Fasiczka, A., & Kupfer, D. (1992). Napping and 24 hour sleep-wake patterns in healthy elderly and young adults. *Journal of the American Geriatric Society, 40*, 779-786.

Carpenito, L.J. (1989). *Nursing care plans and documentation.* Philadelphia: J.B. Lippincott Company.

Castor, D. (1991). Effect of sunlight on sleep patterns in the elderly. *Journal of the American Academy of Physician Assistants, 4*, 321-326.

Crosby, L.J. (1991). Factors which contribute to fatigue associated with rheumatoid arthritis. *Journal of Advanced Nursing, 16*, 974-981.

Culver, B.H. (1989). Pulmonary responses to sleep. *Respiratory Care, 34*, 510-515.

Davis-Sharts, J. (1989). The elder and critical care: Sleep and mobility issues. *Nursing Clinics of North America, 24*, 755-764.

◆De Konicnk, J., Lorrain, D., & Gagnon, P. (1992). Sleep positions and position shifts in five age groups: An ontogenic picture. *Sleep, 15*(2), 143-149.

Feijoo, M., & Bilbao, J. (1992). Seizures of sleep onset: Clinical and therapeutical aspects. *Clinical Pharmacology, 15*(1), 50-55.

◆Farney, R.J., Walker, J.M., Elmer, J.C., Viscomi, V.A., & Ord, R.J. (1992). Transtracheal oxygen, nasal CPAP, and nasal oxygen in five patients with obstructive sleep apnea. *Chest, 101*, 1228-1235.

Gates, D., & Norwessel, N. (1989). Night terrors: Strategies for family coping. *Journal of Pediatric Nursing, 4*(1), 48-53.

Gottlieb, G.L. (1990). Sleep disorders and their management. *The American Journal of Medicine, 88*, 295-335.

◆Greenblatt, D.J., Harmatz, J.S., Shapiro, L., Engelhardt, N., Gouthro, T.A., & Shader, R.I. (1991). Sensitivity to triazolam in the elderly. *New England Journal of Medicine, 324*, 1691-1698.

Greenblatt, D.J. (1992). Pharmacology of benzodiazepine hypnotics. *Journal of Clinical Psychiatry, 53*(6), 14-17.

Guilleminault, C., Stoohs, R., & Quera-Salva, M.A. (1992). Sleep-related obstructive and nonobstructive apnea and neurologic disorders. *Neurology, 42*(7), 53-60.

◆Hock, C.C., Buyesse, D.J., & Reynolds, C.F. (1989). Sleep and depression in late life. *Clinics in Geriatric Medicine, 5*, 259-272.

Hodgson, L.A. (1991). Why do we need sleep?: Relating theory to nursing practice. *Journal of Advanced Nursing, 16*, 1303-1310.

Horne, L.A. (1991). No more wakeful nights: Helping elderly people to sleep properly. *Professional Nurse, 6*, 383-385.

Jamieson, A.L., & Becker, P.M. (1992). Management of the 10 most common sleep disorders. *American Family Physician, 45*, 1262, 1268.

◆Johnson, J.E. (1991). A comparative study of the bedtime routines and sleep of older adults. *Journal of Community Health Nursing, 8*(3), 129-136.

◆Johnson, J.E. (1991). Progressive relaxation and the sleep of older non-institutionalized women. *Applied Nursing Research, 4*(4), 165-170.

◆Kedas, A., Lux, W., & Amodeo, S. (1989). A critical review of aging and sleep research. *Western Journal of Nursing Research, 11*(2), 196-206.

◆Kovacevic-Ristanovic, R., Cartwright, R., & Lloyd, S. (1991). Nonpharmacologic treatment of periodic leg movements in sleep. *Archives of Physical Medicine and Rehabilitation, 72*, 385-389.

Locsin, R.C. (1988). Sleeplessness among the elderly. *Rehabilitation Nursing, 13*, 340-341.

Metzgar, K.L., & Hiltunen, E.F. (1987). Diagnostic content validation of ten frequently reported nursing diagnoses. In A. McLane (Ed.), *Classification of nursing diagnoses: Proceedings of the seventh conference of the North American Nursing Diagnosis Association* (pp. 144-152). St. Louis: The C.V. Mosby Company.

National Institutes of Health Consensus Development Conference statement: The treatment of sleep disorders of older people. (1991). *Sleep, 14*(2), 169-175.

Monk, T.M. (1989). Circadian rhythm. *Clinics in Geriatric Medicine, 5*, 347-362.

O'Donnell, J. (1992). Obstructive sleep apnea syndrome. *Pediatric Nursing, 18*(2), 174-175.

◆Parsons, C., & Ver Beek, D. (1981). Sleep-awake patterns following cerebral concussion. *Nursing Research, 31*(5), 260-264.

Quine, L. (1991). Learning to sleep. *Nursing Times, 82*(48), 41-43.

◆Reimer, M. (1987). Sleep pattern disturbance: Nursing interventions perceived by patients and their nurses as facilitating nocturnal sleep in hospital. In A. McLane (Ed.), *Classification of nursing diagnoses: Proceedings of the seventh conference of the North American Nursing Diagnosis Association* (pp. 372-376). St. Louis: The C.V. Mosby Company.

Roth, T., & Roehrs, T.A. (1992). Issues in the use of benzodiazepine hypnotics. *Journal of Clinical Psychiatry, 53*(6), 14-17.

◆Rumble, R., & Morgan, K. (1992). Hypnotics, sleep, and mortality in elderly people. *Journal of the American Geriatric Society, 40*, 787-791.

Shaver, J.L., & Giblin, E.C. (1989). Sleep. *Annual Review of Nursing Research, 7*(4), 71-93.

◆Topf, M. (1992). Effects of personal control over hospital noise on sleep. *Research in Nursing and Health, 15*(1), 19-28.

Webb, W.B. (1989). Age-related changes in sleep. *Clinics in Geriatric Medicine, 5*, 275-288.

Wooten, V. (1992). Sleep disorders in geriatric patients. *Clinics in Geriatric Medicine, 8*, 427-439.

◆ indicates a research-based work

CHAPTER 16

Cognitive–Perceptual Pattern

Rehabilitation nurses encounter clients in all rehabilitation settings who are experiencing cognitive and perceptual alterations following injury or illness. The client's ability and capacity to learn new information is critical in the rehabilitation process, both for those recovering from cerebral insult and/or for those learning self-care and health maintenance. The client's ability to perceive and understand the environment and his or her own body functioning is an area requiring extensive nursing intervention. Educating the client and teaching about health maintenance are essential to success after the acute phase of rehabilitation in order to maintain health status. After trauma, injury, or illness, the client's sensory status may be impaired or the client may experience lifelong pain and perceptual cognitive impairment. Therefore, rehabilitation nurses must assess these areas and provide appropriate nursing interventions to promote adaptation at home, school, work, and in the community. Related nursing diagnoses included in this chapter are altered thought processes, knowledge deficit, uncompensated sensory deficit, sensory overload, sensory deprivation, unilateral neglect, and chronic pain.

Cognition

Rehabilitation nurses face increased challenges in assisting individuals with altered thought processes. Better on-site emergency care, advanced technology, and improved intensive-care services result in more patients surviving brain injury. Etiology, severity, health care, functional limitations, and the rehabilitation process all have an impact on whether these individuals will be able to return to their previous lifestyles.

Rehabilitation nurses may be involved in the continuum of care for clients with altered cognition, ranging from coma stimulation programs to inpatient rehabilitation and community reintegration. The rationale for managing deficits in thought processes includes "the supposition that specific deficits in cognitive functioning may be identified following various injuries to the brain; that the brain has both the ability to recover from such injuries and deficits, to a variable degree, and to acquire compensatory capabilities to replace deficits that are irrecoverable; and finally, that the extent to which such recovery occurs is significantly dependent on specific therapeutic remediation or training interventions" (Kottke & Lehmann, 1990, p. 1236). The ultimate expected outcome is coping effectively with the demands of daily living. While some individuals appear to make a full recovery, many never return to their preinjury status. Rehabilitation attempts to influence this process favorably, either to accelerate the restoration of function or to ensure that recovery or adjustment is more attainable than it would have been without treatment.

As thought is not a concrete entity, it is often conceptualized for the sake of assessment as a set of cognitive processes. These processes include orientation, memory, attention, judgment and intellectual functioning, problem solving, and motivation.

An alteration in cognition is a major issue in rehabilitation, because cognitive problems make it difficult to use the thinking skills that are needed in daily living.

I. Related Theory and Concepts (See Figure 16.1)

A. Importance of the nature of the insult or the disease
   1. Although the brain functions as a whole, lesions in specific areas of the hemispheres produce characteristic dysfunctions
   2. Location and nature of the insult or disease bear a direct relationship to physical or cognitive impairments that are incurred
      a. Stroke, gunshot wounds, multiple sclerosis, and brain tumors generally produce a localized injury; specific deficits result from injury to specific parts of the brain (DeLisa et al., 1988)
      b. Traumatic brain injury and anoxia usually create more widespread damage

B. Maturational considerations
   1. *Cognition in children*
      a. Cognitive deficits can have a profound effect on the life of a developing child; a child's knowledge base is not as well developed as that of an adult
      b. It is thought that a child under 5 years of age often can recover quite well after a focal injury (Sohlberg & Mateer, 1989)
      c. A child with a diffuse injury to the brain can have persistent cognitive impairments and behavioral problems, even more severe than those of an adult who has experienced a similar injury
      d. Alteration in thought processes in a child can become apparent immediately or years after injury
      e. As a child matures, he or she may experience failure and frustration due to not having attained appropriate cognitive development (Ylvisaker, 1989)
      f. Rehabilitation nurses need to understand a child's level of cognitive functioning, pattern of behaviors, and developmental level prior to developing a successful plan of care
   2. *Cognition in adults*
      a. Aspects unimpaired by aging

Figure 16.1. Lobes of the Brain and Specific Functions

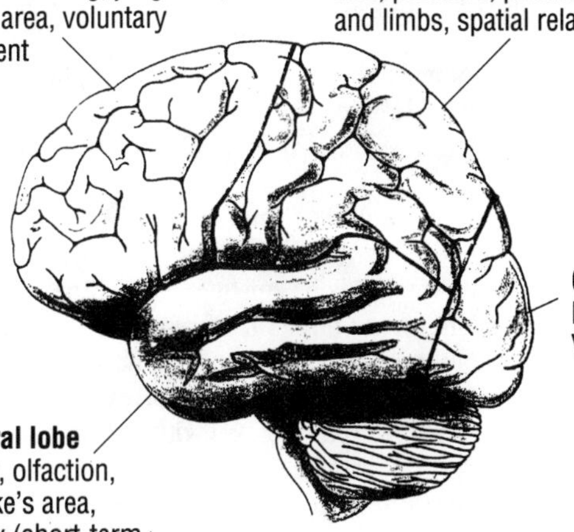

1) Many aspects of learning and memory remain relatively intact during normal aging
   a) Immediate memory of names and numbers
   b) Semantic memory of the context of a meaningful paragraph
   c) Remote memory's ability to retrieve information from long-term storage
   d) Retrieval of overlearned material
2) Some researchers believe that logical reasoning and abstract thinking do not decline as part of normal aging

b. Aspects impaired by aging
   1) Variety of cognitive skills are affected by aging and decline slowly throughout life
      a) Learning of new and complex information (DeBoskey, Hecht, & Calub, 1991)
      b) Learning of basic information that is not essential for daily living (DeBoskey et al., 1991)
      c) Short-term learning of information presented briefly (DeBoskey et al., 1991)
      d) Timed cognitive performance tasks
      e) Associative memory
      f) Logical reasoning
      g) Abstract thinking
   2) May be related to decrease in rate of elderly people's central information processing—that is, all thinking activities that require speed in processing of new information
   3) In general, the more complex the mental task, the greater the effects of aging appear to be (DeLisa et al., 1988)

c. Cognitive operations in elderly people
   1) "Elderly tend to rely more upon the automatic efforts to remember information as contrasted to active, intentional efforts often needed to assist encoding and later retrieval" (Maloney & Means, 1990, p. 26)
   2) Older persons have individual differences in their cognitive operations due to their varied life experiences and education; consequently, when an older person experiences an altered thought process, a rehabilitation nurse must keep in mind his or her preinjury cognitive baseline, life experiences, and other aging considerations

3. Prognosis for recovery: Regardless of age, individuals with altered thought processes can make a full recovery and return to their preinjury status

C. Cognitive skills most vulnerable to brain injury: Each individual with an injury to the brain has a unique pattern of deficits

1. *Orientation*
   a. Definition: Ability to know about oneself (name, age, date of birth, home), the time (current day, month, year), and facts about one's environment
   b. Individuals who experience disorientation lack very basic skills needed to participate in society (Rosenthal, Griffith, Bond, & Miller, 1990)
2. *Memory:* Crucial to all other aspects of cognition
   a. Types of memory
      1) Short-term memory involves recall of immediate or recent events
      2) Long-term memory involves storage and retrieval of information about oneself and the world
      3) Incidental memory is especially affected; involves spontaneous recall of information not intentionally memorized, such as where one puts his or her keys upon arriving home
   b. Memory functioning
      1) Information is coded and, when retrieved, seems to pass between long- and short-term storage
      2) Individuals with memory deficits cannot store and retrieve new information and, therefore, have difficulty learning new information
      3) Depending on location of the damage, memory problems can involve verbal/auditory information, visual information, or both
   c. Memory impairment after brain injury
      1) Posttraumatic amnesia (PTA): Inability to remember events and to learn new information since occurrence of brain injury
      2) Retrograde amnesia: Inability to remember events minutes to hours or longer prior to occurrence of brain injury
3. *Attention*
   a. Definition: Ability to respond to relevant information and to screen out unimportant information
   b. Is required for information to be coded and stored
   c. Enables a person to perform a task while conversation takes place in background

d. Characteristic behaviors of persons with attention and concentration deficits
   1) Distractibility by either internal or external events
   2) Going off on tangents when a single thought occurs to them
   3) Quick movement from one idea to another; that is, flight of ideas
   4) Failure to attend for any period of time

4. *Judgment and intellectual functioning*
   a. Definition: Involve remembering, planning, foresight, abstraction, ability to transfer information from one situation to another, and checking appropriateness of an action (Kreutzer & Wehman, 1991)
   b. Manifestations of problems in this area
      1) Individuals might misinterpret the actions and intentions of others
      2) Individuals might be unable to handle multiple pieces of information simultaneously
      3) Individuals might have inaccurate perception of their strengths and weaknesses
      4) Poor self-monitoring skills can lead to problems with safety and, ultimately, functional independence
5. *Problem solving*
   a. Definition: Involves high-level ability to consider important factors, recall them, organize them for analysis, and make the appropriate choice from more than one alternative
   b. Manifestations of problems in this area
      1) Individuals can have problems with planning and organizing their thoughts and behaviors
      2) There can be problems with formulating alternative solutions
      3) There can be problems with comprehending potential consequences of choices
6. *Motivation*
   a. Definition: Inner forces that regulate behavior in order to satisfy needs and achieve goals; multiple factors influence a person's motivation to participate in self-care and rehabilitation
   b. Barriers to motivation
      1) Memory impairment
      2) Inability to solve problems

D. Behaviors that often accompany alterations in thought

1. Confusion
   a. Definition: Results from an individual's inability to recall minute-to-minute, hour-to-hour, or day-to-day events
   b. Consequently, individual is unable to understand his or her current situation in light of what has happened or will occur in the future
2. Apathy, which has the following characteristics:
   a. Bland affect
   b. General lethargy
   c. Low motivation
   d. Absence of agitation
3. Lack of initiative
   a. Definition: Individuals are motivated to perform an activity, but cannot determine how to carry it out
   b. Might be evident when an individual does not experience self-starting and self-directed behavior
   c. Person might not be aware of this shortcoming
4. Denial of deficits
   a. Occurs because individuals lack insight into effects of their behavior on others
   b. Person might lack motivation for rehabilitation because he or she does not have internal feedback about his or her own capabilities and might blame others for frustrations
5. Impulsivity: Tendency to act without thinking
6. Depression: Sadness that may be evidenced by social withdrawal, crying, self-degrading comments, anxiety, and irritability
7. Perseveration
   a. Definition: Individual's reflexive repetition of certain behaviors (either verbalizations or actions)
   b. Perseveration often has a consistent theme, such as "I want to go home"
8. Confabulation
   a. Definition: Compensating for memory deficits and other deficits by inventing details to meet needs
   b. Although not done purposefully, often reflects person's inability to find other explanations for what is occurring to him or her and might serve a purpose, such as reducing anxiety
9. Emotional lability
   a. Definition: Inability to control emotions
   b. Generally evidenced in easily triggered bouts of crying or laughing even though the individual is not sad or happy
   c. Emotion can suddenly occur, perhaps appear to be exaggerated, and then disappear just as suddenly
10. Lack of inhibition, or disinhibition
    a. Definition: Inability to control verbalizations or behaviors in a socially appropriate way
    b. For individuals to function within the social and cultural norms of society, they must be aware of behavioral norms and the feelings and needs of others
11. Agitation
    a. Definition: Excesses of behavior
    b. Characteristics
       1) Restlessness
       2) Inability to focus or maintain attention
       3) Irritability
       4) Potential for combativeness (can escalate to this level)

E. Plan for management

1. Take into account that, combined with the cognitive impairments described above, cumulative effect of these emotional and behavioral changes often causes problems with personal and social relationships that can lead to increasing isolation for

individuals and their families

2. As primary goal of rehabilitation is a return to family and community, realize that simple containment or toleration of inappropriate behaviors is not enough because the community will not tolerate such behavior
3. Consider essential management goals
   a. Elimination of socially unacceptable behavior
   b. Restoration of self-regulated and socially acceptable responses to environmental demands
   c. Acknowledgment of an individual's limitations with assumption that, with structure and guidance, person can gain control over behavior
   d. Teaching family members about an individual's cognitive impairment and resulting behavior changes so that they can deal with the behaviors appropriately

F. Related theories

1. Piaget's theory of cognitive development (Cox et al., 1989)
   a. Defines normal pediatric cognitive operations
   b. States that intellectual behavior is composed of function and structure
      1) Describes function in terms of organization and adaptation
         a) Organization: Process that provides meaningful patterns and consistency to all activity
         b) Adaptation: Includes both assimilation and accommodation
            (1) Assimilation: Process by which individual integrates new perceptual data or events into existing patterns of behavior (previous experiences)
            (2) Accommodation: Process of changing the model that the individual has of the world by developing the mechanisms to adjust to reality
      2) Is composed of structural units (mental frameworks) at each developmental stage as the perceptual experiences of living offer meaning and organization (see pages 137-138 and Figure 16.2)
2. Right- versus left-brain function: Research continues in this area, and results are divergent
   a. Cerebral cortex hemispheres tend to specialize in different cognitive functions
      1) In most people, both halves of brain participate in thinking
         a) Processing information
         b) Approaching problems in different ways
      2) Left side of brain: Seat of logic
         a) Processes information in a logical, deductive, sequential manner
         b) Details and facts are important for logical thought
         c) Activities include language, planning, organizing, and a component of mathematics
      3) Right side of brain: Seat of intuition
         a) Processes information intuitively and conceptually
         b) Arrives at decisions based on subjective feelings
         c) Describes thoughts as images (visual)
   b. Individuals use both halves of brain, but one side becomes dominant in processing information and making choices
   c. Individuals can be taught to move thinking from one hemisphere to another and to develop each style of thinking
   d. Implications for rehabilitation nurses involve using different teaching and learning approaches based on individual's learning style and location of insult or disease

II. Nursing Assessment

A. Use data that predate disease or injury and alteration in thought processes
   1. Past medical history regarding thought processes
   2. Past cognitive and behavioral functioning
      a. Ask patient's family and friends to describe individual's preinjury behaviors and intellectual functioning
      b. Ask patient's family and friends about individual's preinjury recreational, social, and occupational activities
      c. Assess a child's level of preinjury development by talking with his or her parents and pediatrician
   3. History of medication use or alcohol and/or substance abuse
   4. History of activities of daily living
   5. History of sleep-wake pattern

B. Assess data immediately after an injury, the onset of disease, or alteration in thought
   1. Assess level of consciousness and/or cognition
      a. Glasgow Coma Scale: One of most commonly used scales in acute care (see Figure 8.1 on page 53)
      b. Rancho Los Amigos Levels of Cognitive Function Scale: Most commonly used scale in head injury rehabilitation (see Figure 8.4 on page 55)
   2. Identify gradual or sudden onset of symptoms and etiology of impairment
   3. Review medications and identify those that could alter thought processes
   4. Observe patient's posturing (Chipps, Clanin, & Campbell, 1992)
      a. Decerebrate
         1) Characteristics
            a) Rigid extension
            b) Arms fully extended
            c) Forearms pronated
            d) Wrists and fingers flexed
            e) Jaws clenched
            f) Neck extended
            g) Back may be arched
            h) Feet plantar flexed
         2) Manifestations can occur spontaneously, intermittently, or in response to a stimulus

b. Decorticate
1) Rigid flexion
2) Upper arms held tightly to the sides of body
3) Elbows, wrists, and fingers flexed
4) Feet plantar flexed
5) Legs extended and internally rotated
6) May be fine tremors or intense stiffness
5. Assess history of seizures
6. Note physical status and motor functioning
7. Assess verbal and nonverbal level of communication
8. Assess sensory and perceptual functions
a. Apply tactile stimulation to skin and monitor response
b. Note level of responsiveness
c. Note any alterations in visual or spatial perception

C. Use clinical data collected by nurses and other members of the rehabilitation team
1. Assess level of orientation, mental clarity, and memory
a. Use results of neuropsychological tests
1) Galveston Orientation and Amnesia Test (GOAT): Measures cognition, posttraumatic amnesia, and memory functioning (Rosenthal et al., 1990)
2) Wechsler Memory Scale-Revised (WMS-R): Measures verbal, nonverbal, and memory functioning (Rosenthal et al., 1990)
3) Mini-Mental State Examination (MMSE): Measures orientation, attention, short-term memory, ability to register new information, and recall (Chipps et al., 1992)
b. Use results of developmental screening tests commonly used for children
1) Denver II Developmental Screening Test (DDST)
2) Pediatric Evaluation of Disability Inventory (PEDI)
3) Bayley Scales of Infant Development
c. Assess general orientation to person, place, and time
d. Use common bedside assessment for memory
1) Test recall for immediate memory (0 to 60 seconds in past)
2) Test short-term memory (1 minute to 1 hour in past)
3) Test long-term memory (more than 1 hour in past)
e. Assess for deficits in attention span or concentration
2. Monitor judgment, intellectual functioning, and thought content
a. Examine ability to follow a sequence of commands
b. Assess ability to solve problems
1) Follow simple assignments and instructions
2) Solve problems and choose alternatives
c. Assess ability to use self-monitoring skills and to remain safe
d. Monitor for phobias, perseveration of thought, or delusions
3. Assess for changes in behavior

D. Observe motivation and cooperation with rehabilitation program

E. Assess community and social support systems

➤ III. Nursing Diagnosis: Altered Thought Processes

A. **Definition:** Discrepancy between manifested cognitive operations and expected cognitive operations for chronological age (Gordon, 1993)

B. Major defining characteristics

1. Disorientation or confusion
2. Impaired short-term or long-term memory
3. Decreased attention and concentration
4. Impaired judgment, intellectual functioning, and comprehension
5. Decreased problem-solving and decision-making ability
6. Decreased motivation, apathy, or lethargy
7. Agitated, combative, or hostile behavior
8. Inability to coordinate lifestyle

C. Related factors/etiologies

1. Neurological disease and/or injury
2. Brain tumor
3. Sensory deprivation
4. Drug intoxication
5. Infection
6. Cardiovascular and/or respiratory alterations
7. Pain and/or discomfort
8. Sleep disturbance
9. Medications

D. Interventions

1. Interventions for *cognitive skills*
a. Emphasize orientation
1) Reorient frequently
2) Maintain consistent daily routine
3) Structure the environment
b. Assist in developing memory skills
1) Assign consistent caregivers
2) Use memory aids and cues (e.g., calendars, clocks, photographs of family and friends)
3) Provide written daily activity schedule
4) Use memory devices (e.g., a daily logbook, activity board, maps, schedules, lists)
5) Provide repetition
6) Use verbal and visual cues
7) Encourage formation of mental pictures that integrate thoughts into a visual scene
8) Teach mnemonic strategies
c. Increase attention span
1) Keep messages short, simple, and basic
2) Monitor sensory stimulation
3) Remove all distractions
4) Provide safety precautions and constant supervision for agitated and/or combative individuals
5) Use physical and chemical restraints as last resort

6) Pace interactions and allow disengagement from one task or stimulus before proceeding to another

d. Develop judgment and intellectual functioning
   1) Associate new information with something familiar to patient
   2) Retrain patient from inappropriate social behaviors, for example, by videotaping an outburst and showing it to the individual while providing feedback
   3) Use games that typically are nonthreatening and selected appropriately
   4) Use computer-assisted interventions
   5) Reinforce self-monitoring
   6) Provide counseling for substance abuse or refer to appropriate source
   7) Provide age-appropriate programs and interventions based on patient's developmental level

e. Teach problem-solving skills
   1) Provide an explanation before beginning any activity
   2) Allow choices or alternatives to give patient control
   3) Encourage verbal rehearsal prior to implementation of tasks
   4) If patient is confabulating, provide nonthreatening feedback on the inaccuracy of the thought and then redirect individual's attention to another task
   5) Inform individual when he or she is demonstrating inappropriate behavior and provide him or her with an alternative behavior
   6) Role play to practice social skills
   7) Develop a problem-solving training program to give individuals practice in responding to common problem situations

f. Promote motivation
   1) Provide encouragement and praise
   2) In cases of apathy, involve individual in setting goals and setting contracts
   3) Reinforce positive behavior
   4) Refer to appropriate support or educational groups and resources

2. Interventions for *behavior modifications*
   a. Develop a behavior modification program
      1) Identify target behaviors; be concise in description of inappropriate behavior
      2) Identify causes and consequences of the behavior
      3) Record and rate occurrence of the behavior
      4) Identify alternative desired behaviors
      5) Identify potentially effective and readily controlled reinforcers
      6) Determine a schedule of reinforcement
      7) Implement and make changes in program based on outcomes
   b. Employ techniques of behavior modification
      1) Environmental management
         a) Provides a reinforcing learning environment
         b) Attempts to decrease the cause of the behavior
         c) Rewards patient for refraining from the behavior
         d) Calls for temporary cessation of positive reinforcement if the behavior occurs
         e) Identifies alternative behaviors
         f) Rewards patient for using alternative, socially acceptable behavior
      2) Physical management
         a) Is designed to contain dangerous behaviors or to suspend positive reinforcement
         b) Is employed only when necessary
         c) Uses staff with expertise in techniques to move the individual to a quiet, safe environment mechanically, smoothly, calmly, and without social contact
         d) Applies physical restraints or means to immobilize individual while maintaining safe environment (e.g., commonly used devices such as a locking bed belt, or protected bed environment)
      3) Pharmacological management
         a) Is used only after other available approaches have been considered
         b) Identifies different effects of medications given for behavioral management on each individual, depending on nature and amount of damage to brain
         c) Identifies unwanted effects of sedation, interference with cognitive processes, interference with speed and control of motor activity, production of movement disorders, and precipitation of epilepsy (Rosenthal et al., 1990)

E. Expected outcomes

1. Client improves memory for orientation and information
2. Client demonstrates developmentally appropriate cognitive and problem-solving skills
3. Client compensates for memory loss through use of aids and/or cues
4. Client demonstrates ability to self-monitor and self-correct inappropriate behavior
5. Client initiates and completes activities when appropriate structure is provided
6. Client avoids use of alcohol and drugs that contribute to altered mental ability
7. Client returns to preinjury environment, social interactions, and activities
8. Client uses resources and support groups

Learning

The learning process for rehabilitation clients begins at the moment of onset of the disability or chronic disease. Individuals and their families begin to acquire an understanding of the etiology of the neurological insult, disease, or trauma and its real or potential impact on their lives. The process continues as they learn how to carry out self-care tasks or to instruct others in performing these activities. As progress continues, the process focuses on health maintenance. Knowledge must be acquired and skills must be learned to help the individual remain at the highest level of wellness. At this point, the focus of the learning process is on the acquisition of knowledge and its application in the transition to the home and/or the community.

There are four basic reasons that a rehabilitation client might have a knowledge deficit (Thompson, McFarland, Hirsch, Tucker, & Bowers, 1989):

1. An individual might have undergone a change in health (e.g., a disability secondary to neurological disease or trauma), might be undergoing newly prescribed treatments or diagnostic tests, might be taking new medications, or might be entering a new developmental phase (e.g., adolescence, parenthood, aging). A knowledge deficit can exist because the individual has not experienced these conditions before.
2. Some individuals might not have access to information or know where to find it; others might not understand the information provided due to language or cultural differences.
3. There might be temporary or permanent deficits in the ability to learn due to cognitive limitations or the client's developmental age. These may be secondary to brain damage from trauma, cerebrovascular accident, or neurological disease such as multiple sclerosis. There also might be limitations in learning due to fatigue or because of the individual's immature developmental stage.
4. Another reason for a knowledge deficit is the lack of motivation to learn, often accompanied by anxiety or lack of adherence to a healthcare regimen.

I. Related Theory and Concepts

A. Applicability of learning theory to common rehabilitation disorders
  1. Rehabilitation clients and their families need information and education to deal with limitations and changes in lifestyle imposed by disease and disability that have an impact on the physical, social, emotional, economic, and vocational status of individuals and their families
  2. Rehabilitation nurses' role in recovery
    a. Rehabilitation nurses facilitate the recovery process by helping individuals to learn to be as independent and self-sufficient in self-care activities as possible
    b. Because learning can occur at all points on the healthcare continuum, all members of the interdisciplinary rehabilitation team must be knowledgeable and skillful in the rehabilitation teaching/learning process

B. Learning in adults and children: Knowles' theory
  1. Andragogy (education of adults) differs from pedagogy (education of children) (Knowles, 1984)
  2. Learning process for adults is distinguished from children's learning process by three major characteristics that are important for rehabilitation nurses to consider in teaching and learning activities
    a. Self-concept
      1) Unlike children, who are dependent and seek direction from teachers, adults make more of their own decisions about what they will do and learn
      2) Adults generally have been independent in life and resent being forced into dependent status in teaching and learning situations
      3) Teachers can best facilitate learning by encouraging learning and providing educational resources rather than directing learning opportunities
    b. Life experiences
      1) Children do not have an experiential base upon which to build as they learn, but because adults have more experience in living, they are able to relate new information to these experiences, allowing for more broadly based learning
      2) Rehabilitation nurses, as teachers, must point out the learner's past experiences that are similar to new experiences so that new concepts, information, and skills can be built upon past knowledge
      3) Individuals serve as resources for others by sharing experiences and insights; this also is the theory behind the teaching strategy of small-group discussion
    c. Learning readiness
      1) Children's readiness to learn is based on biological development and social pressure, whereas adults' readiness to learn is considered to be situational and rooted in developmental tasks required by adult social roles; this concept refers to taking advantage of that "teachable moment"
      2) Teachers of adults should be aware of where an individual is in life and developmental tasks for each life stage (listed below); these tasks can affect readiness to learn, and strategies to overcome obstacles must be planned
        a) Early adulthood
          (1) Selecting a mate
          (2) Rearing children
          (3) Beginning an occupation
        b) Middle age
          (1) Carrying out civic and social responsibilities
          (2) Adjusting to physiological changes of middle age
          (3) Adjusting to aging parents
        c) Later maturity
          (1) Adjusting to retirement
          (2) Adjusting to physical changes of aging
      3) Learning in children
        a) Children's learning centers on subjects and topics, whereas adult education is focused more on problems
        b) Nice-to-know content is not important until a child has skills and knowledge necessary to manage identified prob-

lems; when individuals are presented with a problem and potential solutions, they are more likely to apply the learning because it has relevance (O'Connor, 1986)

C. Piaget's description of stages of intellectual development (Cox et al., 1981; Hunt & Sullivan, 1974) (see Figure 16.2)
   1. Describes stages of direction and course of mental development
   2. Stages of development can be used as indicators of readiness for educational programs
   3. One stage must be attained before transition to the next stage can occur; development attained in earlier stages is integrated into that of advanced stages
   4. Each stage describes way of thinking that determines how child will experience (or fail to experience) and respond to activities in environment
   5. Intelligence: Process of adaptation and organization
      a. Adaptation: Equilibration, or balance between assimilation and accommodation, that occurs as a child interacts with his or her environment
         1) Assimilation: Incorporation of environment into present patterns of behavior
         2) Accommodation: Change in the intellectual structure a person makes in adjusting to demands of environment
      b. Organization: Integration of the adaptive actions of the child interacting with the environment
   6. Stages in learning development
      a. Sensorimotor stage (birth to 2 years)
         1) At birth, infant's reaction to environment is driven by inborn reflex
         2) Infants lack object permanence (e.g., if a toy is hidden, an infant does not search for it)
         3) An infant acquires knowledge through his or her own actions
         4) As concept of object permanence develops, an infant learns symbolic representation and, thus, the basic concepts of space, time, causality, and intentionality
         5) During this period of development, infant must be protected from hazards in environment, and caregiver must assume responsibility for educational and treatment program
      b. Preoperational stage and its phases (2 years to 7 years)
         1) Preconceptual thought (2 years to 4 years)
            a) Through symbolic play and language, objective world can be symbolized by thought processes that can be retained
            b) Children are unable to distinguish between the general and the particular (e.g., child who spots snails while walking through the woods does not know if he sees a succession of different snails or whether the same snail keeps reappearing)
            c) Children learn through trial and error, exploration, and repetition

Figure 16.2. Piaget's Stages of Development

Intellectual Stage	Age of Development *
Sensorimotor stage	Birth to 2 years
Preoperational stage	2 to 7 years
• Preconceptual thought	2 to 4 years
• Intuitive thought	4 to 7 years
Concrete operational thought	7 to 11 years
Formal operational thought	11 to 15 years

*Ages are approximate

Source Consulted

Cox et al. (1989). *Clinical applications of nursing diagnosis: Adult health, child health, women's health, mental health, home health* (pp. 15-17). Baltimore: Williams and Wilkins.

         2) Intuitive thought (4 years to 7 years)
            a) This stage marks transition from preconceptual thought into more advanced stage of concrete operations
            b) Simultaneous reasoning and logic do not occur (e.g., a child fills two identical small glasses with beads, one by one, until both are filled; first glass is emptied into a taller and thinner glass that has a larger capacity so it is not filled; child thinks there are more beads in the first glass, even though he sees that no beads were removed or added; child centers on one aspect of the glass, either height or width—but because he cannot hold the ideas simultaneously, he is unable to solve the problem; once the experimenter repeatedly empties the beads into even taller and thinner glasses, the child eventually will reply that there are fewer beads in the taller glass because it is narrow; the child sees the problem first from one point of view [height] and then from another [width])
            c) Important areas of concern at this developmental stage
               (1) Discipline
               (2) Accident prevention
               (3) Development of self-care proficiency related to eating, dressing, bathing, and dental hygiene
         3) Concrete operational thought (7 years to 11 years)
            a) Emergence of this stage is often sudden in child's development
            b) Intuitive thought is less rigid, but child is still unable to use secondary concepts
            c) Reasoning is tied to child's concrete experience (e.g., in the earlier example with the beads, the child, after a previous experience with beads, can see that the quantity of beads in both glasses is the same because if they are poured back

into the original glass, the two would be the same height again—or the quantity is the same now as it was before)

d) Thought is action-oriented

e) A child can take responsibility for personal hygiene and can be taught self-care skills, such as taking medications on a regular schedule; the emphasis should be on health education of the child in several areas

(1) Safety

(2) Nutrition

(3) Substance abuse

(4) Health information about puberty

4) Formal operational thought (11 years to 15 years)

a) This stage marks beginning of ability to solve problems beyond concrete experience

b) Adolescent thinker moves beyond the present and forms wide-ranging theories

c) Adolescent in this stage thinks about the world not only as it is, but also as it could be

d) Adolescent uses abstract logic and mathematics in problem solving

e) With guidance, adolescent can be responsible for total self-care

(1) In health education, emphasis should be on healthful living (e.g., topics such as sex education, skin care, nutrition, substance abuse, career choices, relationships)

(2) Risk-taking behavior is common at this developmental level

7. With increasing developmental age, a child has different intrinsic structures that enable him or her to process information in new and more complex ways as he or she gets older

D. Different levels of learning different skills and techniques (Baird, Schneier, & Laird, 1983)

1. Motor responses, memorization, and simple conditioning (e.g., learning transfer skills, describing importance of good skin care, pressure-relief techniques)
2. Adaptation involves gaining knowledge or adjusting to a simple environment (e.g., learning techniques of floor-to-wheelchair transfers)
3. Complex level involves integrating concepts—transferring knowledge from one situation to another (e.g., being able to carry self-care skills learned in rehabilitation hospital into home environment on therapeutic leave or a pass)
4. Advanced complex level deals with values (e.g., a person with TBI secondary to substance abuse or a motor vehicle accident becoming a speaker in a trauma prevention program)

E. Learner motivation (Pike, 1989)

1. Learning tends to be effective to the extent that an individual is properly motivated; motivation is a stimulus for acting or doing
2. Basic principles of creating motivation in others

a. Generate a need

b. Help client develop a sense of personal responsibility (one cannot motivate another individual; one can only provide an environment in which an individual can motivate himself or herself)

c. Create and maintain interest (use variety in teaching when trying to motivate the individual)

d. Structure experiences to help client apply the content to life

e. Give recognition, encouragement, and approval

f. Foster wholesome competition

g. Display enthusiasm about teaching-learning process

h. Establish long-range objectives (help individuals realize how they can benefit from learning)

i. See value of client's motives (find out what is really important to the individual)

j. Give individuals a choice; allow them some control and a variety of learning opportunities

F. Individual learning style

1. Definition: The way an individual receives and processes information in learning situations
2. Models incorporate individual development, learning theory, and personality types
3. Styles of learning

a. Visual learners learn best by seeing or reading

b. Auditory learners learn best by listening to instructions

c. Tactile or psychomotor learners learn best by doing

G. Learning domains

1. Learning behaviors fall into three domains: cognitive, psychomotor, and affective (Harold & Johnson, 1989)

a. Cognitive domain

1) Tasks: Those that reflect individual's intellectual abilities and problem-solving abilities

2) Teaching methods

a) Lecture

b) Demonstration

c) Audiovisual presentation

b. Psychomotor domain

1) Tasks: Those that are accomplished through physical or motor methods and that involve the ability to envision how a skill is performed

2) Teaching methods

a) Demonstrations

b) Return demonstrations

c. Affective domain

1) Abilities: Expressions of feelings, attitudes, emotions, and values

2) Makes a big impact upon readiness to learn

3) Teaching methods

a) Discussion

b) Listing alternatives and consequences

c) Clarifying values

2. Categorizing what an individual needs to learn in the appropriate domain helps to identify and evaluate the behaviors that the nurse wants the patient to achieve

II. Nursing Assessment

A. Premorbid data
1. Intellectual capacity and level of formal education
2. Language and cultural barriers to learning
3. Socioeconomic status
4. Environmental barriers to learning
5. Learning style
6. Presence of disease or disability

B. Current status
1. Knowledge about disease or disability
2. Knowledge of treatment regimen and self-care needs
3. Activity tolerance
4. Sensory deficits
5. Psychological response to current health or functional status (e.g., denial, anxiety, depression)
6. Identification of potential caregivers
7. Readiness to learn
8. Motivation to learn
9. Self-confidence and/or self-esteem
10. Stressors in individual's and/or caregiver's life
11. Ability to retrieve information taught
12. Ability to demonstrate skills previously taught
13. Ability to provide own care or direct care

➤ III. Nursing Diagnosis: Knowledge Deficit

A. Definition: Inability to state or explain information or demonstrate a required skill related to disease or disability management or activities required for daily living

B. Major defining characteristics

1. Verbal and/or nonverbal communication that indicates less-than-adequate recall of information or an inadequate understanding, misinterpretation, or misconception
2. Questions about health and self-care
3. Demonstration or verbalization of psychological alteration (anxiety, depression, apathy) as a result of misinformation or lack of information
4. Inaccurate follow-through after previous instruction
5. Inadequate performance of a test or demonstration of a skill
6. Inability to manage health maintenance program

C. Related factors/etiologies

1. No previous experience with disability or disease
2. Inadequate understanding or misinterpretation of information
3. Decreased motor skills due to disease and/or injury
4. Impaired cognitive and/or intellectual limitation
5. Lack of motivation to learn
6. Cultural and/or language differences
7. Denial regarding diagnosis and recommended health behaviors
8. Lack of belief in efficacy of treatment
9. Lack of access to resources and information in community

D. Interventions (Thompson et al., 1989)

1. Develop individualized behavioral goals and/or objectives for instructional experiences with individual and/or family; address their learning goals first
2. Encourage individual and family to be actively involved in making decisions about care
3. Integrate cultural and/or religious differences in teaching plan
4. Tailor information to conform to individual's and/or family's intellectual level
5. Provide opportunities for individual and family to practice self-care and health activities
6. Be creative with teaching approaches, especially with individuals who have neurological and/or perceptual learning deficits
7. Stimulate a variety of senses during teaching-learning process through use of written materials, audiovisuals, and hands-on practice
8. Provide written materials so that individuals and/or families can review new knowledge
9. Progress from simple to complex material
10. Provide atmosphere conducive to learning
11. Encourage demonstration, practice, and return demonstration if a skill needs to be learned
12. Check frequently throughout teaching-learning process to evaluate if individual and/or family understands what is being taught
13. Provide rewards for positive health behaviors and teach individual and family to reward themselves
14. Repeat information to reinforce learning
15. Facilitate participation in available health education, home care classes, and support groups

E. Expected outcomes

1. Client verbalizes or demonstrates knowledge about health behaviors and/or diagnosis, self-care activities, health actions, the need for assistance, and use of appropriate community resources in his or her own health maintenance program
2. Client verbalizes an increase in related knowledge
3. Client participates in decision making about treatment plan
4. Client verbalizes complications secondary to disability or disease and understands stressors related to health condition

Sensation and Perception

This section describes disturbances in the sensory and perceptual processes. Sensory and perceptual processes support the reception, interpretation, and integration of stimuli from external and internal environments. The processes are interrelated and are essential for survival. Through sensory perception, an individual receives information, comprehends the environment, and responds by reflexes, decisions, and behaviors.

Dysfunction related to sensory perception is significant for rehabilitation nurses due to its frequent occurence in clients with neurological injuries. Failure to assess sensory and perceptual problems accurately could result in a hypothesis that the client is emotionally disturbed or confused. Problems with sensory perception are frequently correctable (Cubelli, Nichelli, Bonito, De Tanti, & Inzaghi, 1991; Gray, 1990; Robertson, Gray, Pentland, & Waite, 1990).

Sensory and perceptual processes are significant for the pediatric client, because they provide a basis for perception, learning, and organizing behavior. The client who is still developing neurologically, in contrast to the mature adult client, might demonstrate developmental lags due to sensory and perceptual deficits in one area because he or she had not attained the prerequisite behaviors and learning during earlier developmental processes. The mature adult often can compensate because of stored data from the past, whereas the pediatric client might exhibit generalized irritability and/or delays in development.

With geriatric clients, the rehabilitation nurse is involved with individuals who may have multiple sensory and perceptual deficits. The elderly frequently experience problems with vision, hearing, pain perception, tactile sensitivity, and vibratory perception. Sensory and perceptual alterations experienced by older individuals must be recognized to prevent a mislabeling of the individual as disoriented or uncooperative. The rehabilitation nurse should also consider the impact of sensory and perceptual deficits in assessing the home environment; for example, impairment of the olfactory sense may make it unwise for an elderly individual to have a gas stove in the home, because he or she might not detect gas leaks.

Clients with sensory and perceptual deficits can often learn to meet their self-care needs through education and compensatory training. Nursing therapy that promotes a consistent plan of care, as well as cues and support, should contribute to successful rehabilitation.

I. Related Theory and Concepts

A. Sensory and perceptual process
1. Sensory
   a. Sensory processes are physiological in nature and relate to the reception and transmission of stimuli
      1) Visual
      2) Auditory
      3) Olfactory
      4) Tactile
      5) Kinesthetic
      6) Gustatory
   b. Sensory receptors for visual, auditory, olfactory, tactile, kinesthetic, and gustatory stimuli transmit information to the parietal lobe of the brain for interpretation (Schmitz, 1988)
2. Perceptual
   a. Perceptual component: Internal process of selection, integration, and interpretation of incoming stimuli
   b. Perceptual processes are psychological in character and involve interpreting the information through sensory receptors
   c. Reflexes, behavior, and decisions are based on the individual's interpretation of the sensory information
3. Perception of sensory information is affected by various factors
   a. Psychological factors (e.g., age, developmental level, values, beliefs, anxiety)
   b. Physiological factors (e.g., fatigue, pain, drugs, biological imbalances)
   c. Social and cultural factors (e.g., learning, habits, social status)

B. Transmission of sensory and perceptual input
1. Depends on central and peripheral nervous systems and a normally functioning neuroendocrine system
   a. Sensory data are analyzed and processed through perception
   b. Peripheral nerves and ganglia transmit impulses to the spinal cord; from the spinal cord, they are transmitted to the brain, specifically to thalamus and to parietal lobe of cerebrum
   c. Nondominant parietal lobe is site of integration of sensory input
   d. Cerebral arteries (anterior, middle, and posterior) supply parietal lobe
2. Provides for optimal level and variety of stimuli needed to support a waking state (McFarland & McFarlane, 1989)
   a. Individuals are driven to maintain an optimal amount of sensory stimulation (sensoristasis)
   b. Need for sensory stimulation varies according to age, environment, and culture
3. Provides for sensory integration and development of capacity to perceive, learn, and organize behavior (Pratt & Allen, 1989)
   a. Adaptation to our environment is a basic need to function effectively
   b. Perception of sensory stimuli is modified through thinking and learning
   c. Human response to sensory stimuli is modified by thinking and learning

II. Nursing Assessment

A. Determine if there were any previous problems with sensation or perception
1. Past behavior and responses to all stimuli
2. Successful past interventions for alterations
3. Use of adaptive and/or assistive equipment, for example, hearing aids, glasses
4. Related pathophysiological conditions

B. Determine current sensory and perceptual responses and behaviors
1. Visual acuity
2. Hearing ability
3. Smelling sensation
4. Touch sensation
5. Position sense
6. Taste (sour, salty, sweet, bitter)

C. Other considerations
1. Current medications that might affect sensation and/or perception
2. Current developmental level

3. Ability to perform activities necessary for daily living with particular emphasis on safety

III. Nursing Diagnoses

➤ A. Uncompensated sensory deficit

1. **Definition:** Uncompensated loss of acuity, or absence, of vision, hearing, touch, smell, or kinesthesia (Gordon, 1993)

2. **Major defining characteristics**

   a. Faulty interpretation of sensory stimuli
   b. Inability to see
   c. Inability to hear
   d. Inability to discriminate tactile sensation and perception
   e. Inability to identify odors
   f. Inability to identify movement of body or body part

3. **Related factors/etiologies**

   a. Altered sensory reception, transmission, or integration
   b. Environmental complexity and/or monotony
   c. Drugs
   d. Psychological stress

4. **Interventions** (McConnell, 1988)

   a. Visual
      1) Use appropriate adaptive equipment (e.g., glasses or contact lenses)
      2) Alter the environment
         a) Ensure that lighting is adequate
            (1) Prevent glare; use over-the-shoulder lighting, when possible
            (2) Prevent extremes in lighting intensity
            (3) Provide night-lights, when appropriate
         b) Use color contrasts to aid in visual discrimination and provide cues
         c) Provide reading material adapted to the degree of visual impairment
            (1) Large-print or braille books and papers
            (2) Clocks, calendars, and telephones with braille numerals or large numerals
      3) For clients with *homonymous hemianopsia*
         a) Teach client to visually scan; can use colored ruler or paper and left margin to assist in scanning
         b) Supply special glasses, if they are needed
         c) Approach client from unaffected side
         d) Place food so client can see all items
         e) Progressively involve both affected and unaffected sides in all activities

   b. Auditory
      1) Use appropriate adaptive equipment (e.g., a hearing aid or handheld assistive device)
      2) Alter environment
         a) Augment the environment through use of accentuated visual cues (e.g., flashing lights for doorbell and telephone)
         b) Reduce common background noises (e.g., those created by a radio, a television, or an air conditioner)
         c) Substitute written information, if necessary, or use written information to augment verbal information given

   c. Olfactory
      1) Provide variations in scents throughout home
      2) Provide stimulation by encouraging activities associated with scents (e.g., gardening, flower arranging)

   d. Tactile
      1) Provide variations in textures and temperatures throughout environment
      2) Provide stimulation by providing touch that is appropriate and comfortable for the client
      3) Teach safety measures to compensate for lack of touch sensation (e.g., advising caution with hot or cold items; teaching the client to use intact senses to compensate for lack of touch sensation)

   e. Kinesthetic
      1) Identify an exercise program that is appropriate for client's level of energy and endurance (e.g., rocking, walking, range-of-motion exercises)
      2) Provide safety checks, for example, assess heart rate and blood pressure during exercise

   f. Gustatory
      1) Provide foods of varying tastes and smells (prior to or between medications)
      2) Discuss with client his or her memories associated with different tastes
      3) Prepare and/or serve foods of various colors; arrange food attractively

5. **Expected outcomes**

   a. Client exhibits evidence of accurate sensory reception
   b. Client experiences no injuries related to impaired sensory perception
   c. Client practices and/or demonstrates compensatory strategies for alteration in sensation and/or perception

➤ B. Sensory overload

1. **Definition:** Environmental stimuli greater than habitual level of input and/or monotonous environmental stimuli (Gordon, 1993)

2. **Major defining characteristics**

   a. Disorientation to a person, place, or time
   b. Altered ability to resolve problems
   c. Irritability, agitation, anxiety
   d. Disturbed sleep patterns

3. **Related factors/etiologies**

   a. Complex environment (e.g., critical-care setting)

b. Continuous environmental stimuli (e.g., light, sound)

4. **Interventions**

a. Decrease and monitor stimulation due to noise, light, and touch
b. Provide at least 2 to 4 hours of uninterrupted sleep daily
c. Orient patient to person, place, and time
d. Limit number of visitors
e. Avoid multiple auditory stimuli (e.g., radio, TV, and conversations at the same time)
f. Keep a few familiar objects in a basically uncluttered room

5. **Expected outcomes**

a. Client reports satisfaction with amount of environmental stimuli and rest achieved
b. Client is oriented to person, place, and time

➤ **C. Sensory deprivation**

1. **Definition:** Reduced environmental and social stimuli relative to habitual (or basic orienting) level (Gordon, 1993)

2. **Major defining characteristics**

a. Intermittent episodes of disorientation and confusion
b. Limited environmental sensory stimuli
c. Hallucinations
d. Apathy

3. **Related factors/etiologies**

a. Isolation
b. Physical and/or environmental restrictions (e.g., immobility, traction)
c. Uncompensated sensory deficit (e.g., auditory, visual)
d. Dysphasia or impaired expression and reception of speech

4. **Interventions**

a. Orient patient to person, place, and time
b. Provide environmental stimuli in a structured pattern (e.g., turn on radio, television, favorite music, or family tapes for short periods of time)
c. Assist with resocialization and promote movement from bed and room
d. Consult therapeutic recreational specialist
e. Provide a consistent time for listening and communicating with client
f. Enhance stimulation of the intact senses
g. Refer client to support groups
h. Place calendar and clock near patient; provide newspaper

5. **Expected outcomes**

a. Client reports satisfaction with amount of environmental stimuli and rest achieved
b. Client is oriented to person, place, and time

➤ **D. Unilateral neglect**

1. **Definition:** The state in which an individual is perceptually unaware of and inattentive to one side of the body (NANDA, 1992)

2. **Major defining characteristics**

a. Failure to attend to affected side
b. Neglect of affected side with respect to sensory stimuli, positioning, and safety precautions
c. Visual bias toward unaffected side
d. Neglect of affected side during self-care

3. **Related factors/etiologies**

a. Hemianopsia
b. One-sided blindness
c. Neurological damage or illness related to stroke, tumor, or brain trauma

4. **Interventions**

a. Keep environment clean and uncluttered
b. Reorient client frequently
c. Implement protocol for safety precautions (e.g., safety vest, siderails)
d. Keep call light and telephone on unaffected side
e. During the early postinjury phase, approach client from unaffected side
f. Following acute phase, approach client from affected side to promote attention to affected side
g. Keep items of interest—including cards, pictures, television, clock, and calendar—on affected side to promote attention to that side
h. Involve family and friends in the plan
i. Provide client with verbal cueing to check affected side
j. Assist client with dressing and have the client check his or her attire in front of a mirror for easier visual scanning
k. Integrate affected extremity through sensory stimulation (e.g., apply cologne, lotion, or perfume to affected arm)
l. Provide reminders to check affected side by keeping patient's watch or a favorite ring or bracelet on affected arm
m. Teach patient to scan

5. **Expected outcomes**

a. Client demonstrates ability to scan self and environment visually
b. Client describes potential and actual safety risks
c. Client compensates for the sensory and motor deficit

Chronic Pain

While chronic pain can begin with an acute pain episode, it persists long after the initial cause of pain has been resolved (Burkhardt, 1990). Chronic pain often is referred to as the syndrome that results when pain interferes with all aspects of an individual's functioning. The consequences of the chronic pain experience are usually destructive to the individual's physical, social, financial, and psychological well-being. The impact of the syndrome is felt by the individual's family, friends, and coworkers.

Chronic pain is of significance to rehabilitation nurses in all settings, in terms of the prevalence with which individuals experience the problem. Between 25% and 30% of the population is estimated to experience chronic pain (Bonica, 1990). At least half of those with chronic pain are partially or completely disabled. Compounding the problem of chronic pain is the tendency of family members, friends, and the medical community to misunderstand the syndrome. There have been attempts to identify individuals who are prone to develop chronic pain (Burkhardt, 1990). Depression and psychological stress are ubiquitous among chronic pain patients and must be recognized and understood by rehabilitation nurses.

Rehabilitation nurses work across the healthcare continuum with individuals experiencing chronic pain. Not infrequently, chronic pain results from a work-related injury. Rehabilitation nurses functioning in the role of case managers are responsible for coordinating and supervising the client's rehabilitation program. Hospitalization may be necessary to manage a patient's pain and substance withdrawal. Rehabilitation nurses manage the rehabilitation programs of individuals with chronic pain and provide instruction in the use of nonpharmacologic methods of pain reduction, including biofeedback and relaxation techniques.

Nursing therapy with clients experiencing chronic pain is holistic in nature and includes the family and others in the patient's support system. As relief from pain is not usually a realistic goal, the rehabilitation nurse focuses on increasing the patient's functional ability and community involvement along with decreasing the client's pain behavior.

I. Related Theory and Concepts

A. The pain response

1. Tissue damage results in release of endogenous chemicals such as prostaglandins, bradykinin, histamine, and serotonin
   a. Chemicals are neuroactive and vasoactive
   b. Chemicals excite nociceptors
2. Stimulation of nociceptors results in liberation of substance P from peripheral nerve endings
   a. A-delta and C-nociceptor afferents relay transmission of sensation to substantia gelatinosa of dorsal column of spinal cord
      1) A-delta afferents relay sensations of touch, pressure, and temperature
      2) C-nociceptor afferents relay painful sensations
   b. Transmission is relayed to the thalamus, where it is interpreted as painful and indicative of tissue injury
3. Descending fibers from the cerebrocortex moderate the pain response
   a. Descending fibers are influenced by psychosocial variables
      1) Culture
      2) Personality
      3) Past experiences
   b. Descending fibers modulate pain response at substantia gelatinosa in dorsal column of spinal cord
4. Substantia gelatinosa is considered gate for pain response (see Figure 16.3)
   a. Stimulated ascending or afferent fibers relay the pain response
   b. Gate can be closed, or pain perception reduced, in two ways
      1) Descending, or efferent, fibers can be motivated to moderate pain response in one of two ways
         a) Distraction

Figure 16.3. Gate Control Theory of Pain

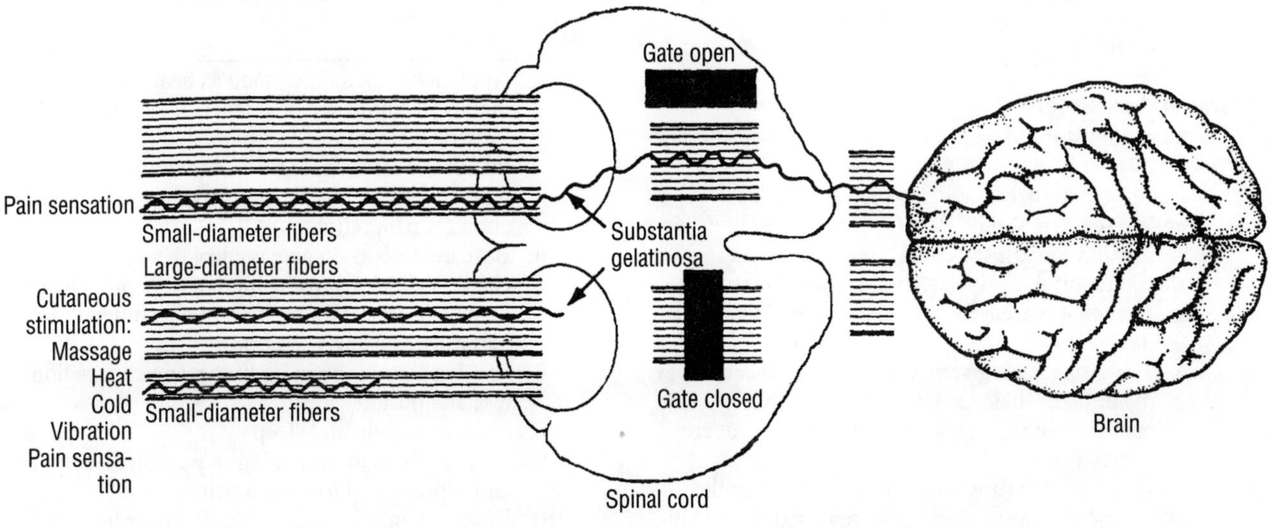

Reprinted with permission of W.B. Saunders Company and D.D. Ignatavicius from Ignatavicius, D.D., & Bayne, M.V. (1991). *Medical-surgical nursing: A nursing process approach* (p. 109). Philadelphia: W.B. Saunders Company. (Modified by permission from Potter, P.A., & Perry, A.G. [1989]. *Fundamentals of nursing: Concepts, process, and practice.* St. Louis: The C.V. Mosby Company.)

b) Hypnosis
2) Ascending, or afferent, A-delta fibers can be caused to block or limit the transmission by C-nociceptors by the presence of various stimuli
a) Touch, massage, and pressure
b) Ice, heat, and temperature change

B. The chronic pain cycle
1. Instinctive response to an acute injury is immobilization and a guarding of the site
2. Immobilization of body part has far-reaching consequences
a. Scar tissue forms around injured part
b. Synovial fluid production is reduced
1) Joint movement becomes stiff and painful, and range becomes limited
2) Movement leads to joint inflammation and tendonitis
c. Immobility results in decreased function and weakness
d. Cycle is reinforced by compensatory mechanisms
1) Alteration in gait, favoring injured part
2) Back pain, due to altered gait
3. Because of pain and immobilization, all aspects of life are affected
a. Employment becomes difficult because days are missed due to illness or loss of functional ability
b. Family and community involvement become limited because of pain secondary to activity
c. Reduced activity can lead to weight gain and further loss of endurance
d. Finances are expended as a search for a cause turns into a search for relief and, finally, to a search for healthcare professionals who will believe in the pain the patient is experiencing
e. Depression ensues because as the individual has little reason to look forward to the days to come, except the anticipation of more pain and disability

II. Nursing Assessment

A. Take a pain history: Assess pain experience as reported by client
1. Using standardized pain test, such as the visual analog scale or McGill Pain Questionnaire (Melzack, 1983), assess the client's pain; the client should report the pain perception when it is strongest, when it is weakest, and at the time of the interview
a. The visual analog scale consists of a 10-centimeter line, labeled at left endpoint with "no pain" and at right endpoint with "pain as severe as possible"
1) Client is instructed to mark the point on the line that best reflects pain being experienced
2) Line is measured from left endpoint to patient's mark to determine the quantity of pain patient perceives
b. McGill Pain Questionnaire (Melzack, 1983) is an example of a standardized and comprehensive pain inventory
1) Pain is conceptualized in the McGill Pain Questionnaire as having sensory, affective, and evaluative properties
2) Approximately 20 minutes are required to complete McGill Pain Questionnaire
2. Assess patterns of client's pain experience
a. Client should maintain a pain diary, indicating quantity (e.g., more or less with activity, position, resting) and quality (e.g., intensity) of pain he or she experiences over a period of several days
b. Does client do anything to alleviate pain?
c. What exacerbates or abates pain?

B. Complete a lifestyle history
1. Assess client's functional status and activity level
a. What is a typical day like?
b. How often does client exercise?
c. Does the pain have an impact on client's lifestyle?
2. Assess client's sleeping patterns
3. Assess client's use of addictive substances (e.g., alcohol, drugs)
4. Assess client's employment situation
5. Assess client's family and support system

➤ III. Nursing Diagnosis: Chronic Pain

A. Definition: State in which individual experiences pain that continues for more than 6 months (NANDA, 1992)

B. Major defining characteristic: Verbal reports of pain for 6 months or longer

C. Related factors/etiologies

1. Work-related injury (Gyldenvand & Tunick, 1988)
2. Traumatic injury (Gyldenvand & Tunick, 1988)
3. Chronic physical and/or psychosocial disability

D. Interventions

1. Apply local modalities such as heat and cold and therapeutic massage, and teach client the technique
2. Provide education in use of analgesic medications
3. Instruct or refer client for instruction in the use of biofeedback techniques, self-hypnosis, and relaxation for pain relief
4. Base treatments on gate control theory
5. Caution client against using fad or unproven cures
6. Teach client work-simplification techniques and necessity of using rest periods
7. Provide instruction in body mechanics, positioning, and posture
8. Monitor weight and sleep
9. Instruct client to keep a log of pain level, activities, and actions used to reduce pain
10. Refer patient to a comprehensive interdisciplinary pain management program based on a rehabilitation approach that includes counseling, physical reconditioning, behavior modification, and reduction in medications

E. Expected outcomes

1. Client verbalizes reduction in the pain experienced and in his or her own focus on pain
2. Client increases activity level
3. Client reduces or eliminates use of analgesics

References: Cognition

Chipps, E., Clanin, N., & Campbell, V. (1992). *Neurologic disorders.* St. Louis: Mosby-Year Book, Inc.

Cox, H., Hinz, M., Lubno, M., Newfield, S., Ridenour, N., & Sridaromont, K. (1989). *Clinical applications of nursing diagnosis: Adult health, child health, women's health, mental health, home health.* Baltimore: Williams and Wilkins.

DeBoskey, D., Hecht, J., & Calub, C. (1991). *Educating families of the head injured: A guide to medical, cognitive, and social issues.* Gaithersburg, MD: Aspen Publishers, Inc.

DeLisa, J., Currie, D., Gans, B., Gatens, P., Leonard, J., & McPhee, M. (1988). *Rehabilitation medicine: Principles and practice.* Philadelphia: J.B. Lippincott Company.

Gordon, M. (1993). *Manual of nursing diagnosis: 1993-1994.* St. Louis: Mosby-Year Book, Inc.

Kottke, F., & Lehmann, J. (1990). *Krusen's handbook of physical medicine and rehabilitation.* Philadelphia: W.B. Saunders Company.

Kreutzer, J., & Wehman, P. (1991). *Cognitive rehabilitation for persons with traumatic brain injury: A functional approach.* Baltimore: Paul H. Brookes Publishing Company.

Maloney, F.P., & Means, K.M. (1990). *Physical medicine and rehabilitation.* Philadelphia: Hanley and Belfus, Inc.

Rosenthal, M., Griffith, E., Bond, M., & Miller, J.D. (1990). *Rehabilitation of the adult and child with traumatic brain injury.* Philadelphia: F.A. Davis Company.

Sohlberg, M., & Mateer, C. (1989). *Introduction to cognitive rehabilitation: Theory and practice.* New York: The Guilford Press.

Ylvisaker, M. (1989, Fall). Key issues in pediatric/youth head injury. *Headlines*, pp. 2-11.

Suggested Readings: Cognition

Brewer, E., McPherson, M., Magrob, T.R., & Hutchins, U.L. (1989). Family-centered community based coordinated care for children with special health care needs. *Pediatrics, 83*, 1055-1061.

Deatrick, J., Knafl, K., & Walsh, M. (1988). The process of parenting a child with a disability: Normalization through accommodations. *Journal of Advanced Nursing, 13*, 15-21.

Frawley, P. (1990). Neurological observations. *Nursing Times, 86*(35), 29-34.

Gallagher, J., & Vietz, P. (1986). *Families of handicapped persons.* Baltimore: Paul H. Brookes Publishing Company.

Greenspan, S., & Greenspan, N. (1985). *First feelings: Milestones in the development of your baby and child from birth to age 4.* New York: Viking Penguin Books, Inc.

◆Herbel, K., Schermerhorn, L., & Howard, J. (1990). Management of agitated head-injured patients: A survey of current techniques. *Rehabilitation Nursing, 15*, 66-72.

◆Krajicek, M., & Tomlinson, A. (Eds.) (1983). *Detection of developmental problems in children.* Baltimore: University Park Press.

◆Kutz, N., Hefner, D., & Reuben, R. (1990). Measuring clinical change in cognitive rehabilitation of patients with brain damage: Two cases, traumatic brain injury and cerebral vascular accident. *Occupational Therapy Health Care, 7*(1), 23-43.

◆Mysiw, J., Corrigan, J., Carpenter, D., & Chock, S. (1990). Prospective assessment of post traumatic amnesia: A comparison of the GOAT and the OGMS. *Journal of Head Trauma Rehabilitation, 5*(1), 65-72.

◆Mysiw, W. J., Beegan, J.G., & Gatens, P.F. (1989). Progressive cognitive assessment of stroke patients before inpatient rehabilitation: The relationship of the neurobehavioral cognitive status examination to functional improvement. *American Journal of Physical Medicine and Rehabilitation, 68*(4), 168-171.

◆Prigatano, G.P., & Altman, I.M. (1990). Impaired awareness of behavioral limitations after traumatic brain injury. *Archives of Physical Medicine and Rehabilitation, 71*, 1058-1064.

◆Ryden, M., Bossenmaier, M., & McLachlan, C. (1991). Aggressive behavior in cognitively impaired nursing home residents. *Research in Nursing and Health, 14*(2), 87-95.

◆Sahgal, V., & Heinemann, A. (1989). Recovery of function during inpatient rehabilitation for moderate traumatic brain injury. *Scandinavian Journal of Rehabilitation Medicine, 21*, 71-79.

◆Sector, W. (1991). Cognitive impairment and disruptive behaviors among community-based elderly persons: Implications for targeting long-term care. *The Gerontologist, 31*(1), 51-59.

References: Learning

Baird, L.S., Schneier, C.E., & Laird, D. (Eds.). (1983). *The training and development sourcebook.* Amherst, MA: Human Resource Development Press.

Cox, H., Hinz, M., Lubno, M., Newfield, S., Ridenour, N., & Sridaromont, K. (1989). *Clinical applications of nursing diagnosis: Adult health, child health, women's health, mental health, home health.* Baltimore: Williams and Wilkins.

Harold, C.E., & Johnson, P. (Eds.). (1989). *How to teach patients.* Springhouse, PA: Springhouse Corporation.

Hunt, D.E., & Sullivan, E.V. (1974). *Between psychology and education.* Hinsdale, IL: The Dryden Press.

Knowles, M. (1984). *The adult learner: A neglected species.* Houston: Gulf Publishing Company.

O'Connor, A.B. (1986). *Nursing staff development and continuing education.* Boston: Little, Brown and Company.

Pike, R.W. (1989). *Creative training techniques handbook.* Minneapolis: Lakewood Books.

Thompson, J.M., McFarland, G.K., Hirsch, J.E., Tucker, S.M., & Bowers, A.C. (1989). *Mosby's manual of clinical nursing* (2nd ed.). St. Louis: The C.V. Mosby Company.

Suggested Readings: Learning

◆Boyd, S., Cleary, B., Coomer, M., Cooper, P., Cosner, D., Cummins, N., Decell, K., Kemper, B., Kirby, V., Sims, S., VanDen-Dries, D., & Wingate, L. (1991). Professional nursing roles: The reintegration of patient teaching. *Journal of Nursing Staff Development, 7*(2), 88-90.

◆Bucher, L. (1991). Evaluating the affective domain: Consider a Likert scale. *Journal of Nursing Staff Development, 7*(5), 234-238.

Haggard, A. (1989). *Handbook of patient education.* Rockville, MD: Aspen Publishers, Inc.

◆Naylor, M., & Shaid, E. (1991). Content analysis of pre- and post-discharge topics taught to hospitalized elderly by gerontological clinical nurse specialists. *Clinical Nurse Specialist, 5*(2), 111-116.

◆Schlueter, P., & White, C. (1991). Providers' and consumers' perceptions of quality health care. *Journal of Nursing Staff Development, 7*(1), 5-10.

◆Turner, S. (1991). Nursing process, nursing diagnoses and care plans in a clinical setting. *Journal of Nursing Staff Development, 7*(5), 239-243.

References: Sensation and Perception

Cubelli, R., Nichelli, P., Bonito, V., De Tanti, A., & Inzaghi, M. (1991). Different patterns of dissociation in unilateral spatial neglect. *Brain and Cognition, 15*, 139-159.

Gordon, M. (1993). *Manual of nursing diagnosis: 1993-1994.* St. Louis: Mosby-Year Book, Inc.

Gray, G. (1990). The remediation of attentional disorders following brain injury of acute onset. In R. Wood & I. Fussey (Eds.), *Cognitive rehabilitation in perspective* (pp. 29-47). New York: Taylor and Francis.

McConnell, E. (1988). Nursing diagnoses related to physiological alterations. In M. Matteson & E. McConnell (Eds.), *Gerontological nursing: Concepts and practice* (pp. 331-428). Philadelphia: W.B. Saunders Company.

McFarland, G., & McFarlane, E. (1989). *Nursing diagnosis and intervention: Planning for patient care.* St. Louis: The C.V. Mosby Company.

North American Nursing Diagnosis Associatio (NANDA). (1992). *NANDA nursing diagnoses: Definitions and classification 1992-1993.* St. Louis: Author.

Pratt, P., & Allen, A. (1989). *Occupational therapy for children* (2nd ed.). St. Louis: The C.V. Mosby Company.

◆Robertson, I., Gray, J., Pentland, B., & Waite, L. (1990). Microcomputer-based rehabilitation for unilateral left visual neglect: A randomized controlled trial. *Archives of Physical Medicine and Rehabilitation, 71*, 663-668.

Schmitz, T. (1988). Sensory assessment. In S. O'Sullivan & T. Schmitz, *Physical rehabilitation: Assessment and treatment* (2nd ed.) (pp. 79-92). Philadelphia: F.A. Davis Company.

Suggested Readings: Sensation and Perception

Ayres, A.J. (1985). *Sensory integration and the child.* Los Angeles: Western Psychological Services.

Danek, M. (1990). Issues and strategies in the rehabilitation of hearing impaired persons. In M. Eisenberg & R. Grzesiak (Eds.), *Advances in clinical rehabilitation* (Vol. 3) (pp. 148-166). New York: Springer Publishing Company.

Esposito, M., Tracey, C., & McCourt, A. (1988). Nursing diagnosis: Potential for disuse syndrome. In R.M. Carroll-Johnson (Ed.), *Classification of nursing diagnoses: Proceedings of the Eighth Conference of the North American Nursing Diagnosis Association* (pp. 464-468). Philadelphia: J.B. Lippincott Company.

Glass, L. (1990). Hearing impairment in geriatrics. In B. Kemp, K. Brummel-Smith, & J. Ramsdell (Eds.), *Geriatric rehabilitation* (pp. 235-252). Boston: Little, Brown and Company.

Kim, M., McFarland, G., & McLane, A. (1991). *Pocket guide to nursing diagnosis.* St Louis: The C.V. Mosby Company.

Lyke, E.M. (1992). *Assessing for nursing diagnosis: A human needs approach.* Philadelphia: J.B. Lippincott Company.

Mehr, E., & Shindell, S. (1990). Advances in low vision and blind rehabilitation. In M. Eisenberg & R. Grzesiak (Eds.), *Advances in clinical rehabilitation* (Vol. 3) (pp. 121-147). New York: Springer Publishing Company.

Segalowitz, S. (1983). *Two sides of the brain: Brain lateralization explored.* Englewood Cliffs, NJ: Prentice-Hall, Inc.

Vernon, M., & Duncan, E. (1990). Advances in rehabilitation of deaf-blind persons. In M. Eisenberg & R. Grzesiak (Eds.), *Advances in clinical rehabilitation* (Vol. 3) (pp. 167-186). New York: Springer Publishing Company.

◆Warren, M. (1990). Identification of visual scanning deficits in adults after cerebrovascular accident. *The American Journal of Occupational Therapy, 44*, 391-399.

Weinreb, R., Freeman, W., & Selezinka, W. (1990). Vision impairment in geriatrics. In B. Kemp, K. Brummel-Smith, & J. Ramsdell (Eds.), *Geriatric rehabilitation* (pp. 223-234). Boston: Little, Brown and Company.

Wood, R. (1990). Toward a model of cognitive rehabilitation. In R. Wood & I. Fussey (Eds.), *Cognitive rehabilitation in perspective* (pp. 3-26). New York: Taylor and Francis.

Wood, R. (1987). Neuropsychological assessment in brain injury rehabilitation. In M. Eisenberg & R. Grzesiak (Eds.), *Advances in clinical rehabilitation* (Vol. 1) (pp. 47-76). New York: Springer Publishing Company.

References: Chronic Pain

Bonica, J. (1990). *The management of pain* (2nd ed.). Philadelphia: Lea & Febiger.

Burkhardt, C. (1990). Chronic pain. *Symptom Management, 25*, 863-870.

Gyldenvand, T., & Tunick, P. (1988). Validation of the nursing diagnosis alteration in comfort: Chronic pain. In R.M. Carroll-Johnson (Ed.), *Classification of nursing diagnoses: Proceedings of the Eighth Conference of the North American Nursing Diagnosis Association* (pp. 284-290). Philadelphia: J.B. Lippincott Company.

Ignatavicius, D.D., & Bayne, M.V. (1991). *Medical-surgical nursing: A nursing process approach.* Philadelphia: W.B. Saunders Company.

Melzack, R. (1983). *Pain measurement and assessment.* New York: Raven Press.

North American Nursing Diagnosis Association (NANDA). (1992). *NANDA nursing diagnosis: Definitions and classification 1992-1993.* St. Louis: Author.

Suggested Readings: Chronic Pain

Anderson, L., & Rehm, L. (1984). The relationship between strategies of coping and perception of pain in three chronic pain groups. *Journal of Clinical Psychology, 40*, 1170-1177.

Carpenito, L. (1991). *Handbook of nursing diagnosis* (4th ed.). Philadelphia: J.B. Lippincott Company.

◆Dolce, J., Crocker, M., & Doleys, D. (1986). Prediction of outcome among chronic pain patients. *Behavioral Research Therapy, 24*, 313-319.

Field, E. (1991). Chronic pain in older persons. *Topics in Geriatric Rehabilitation, 6*(4), 17-24.

Forman, W., & Stratton, M. (1991). Current approaches to chronic pain in older patients. *Geriatrics, 46*(7), 47-52.

Gordon, M. (1991). *Manual of nursing diagnosis: 1991-1992.* St. Louis: The C.V. Mosby Company.

◆Linton, S. (1986). Behavioral remediation of chronic pain: A status report. *Pain, 24*, 125-141.

Lyke, E.M. (1992). *Assessing for nursing diagnosis: A human needs approach.* Philadelphia: J.B. Lippincott Company.

McFarland, G., & McFarlane, E. (1989). *Nursing diagnosis and intervention: Planning for patient care.* St. Louis: The C.V. Mosby Company.

Riley, J., Ahern, D., & Follick, M. (1988). Chronic pain and functional impairment: Assessing beliefs about their relationship. *Archives of Physical Medicine and Rehabilitation, 60*, 579-582.

Smith, I., Airey, S., & Salmond, S. (1990). Part II: Nontechnologic strategies for coping with chronic low back pain. *Orthopedic Nursing, 9*(4), 21-32.

Sparks, S., & Taylor, C. (1991). *Nursing diagnosis reference manual: An indispensable guide to better patient care.* Springhouse, PA: Springhouse Corporation.

◆Turk, D., & Rudy, T. (1990). Neglected factors in chronic pain treatment outcome studies—referral patterns, failure to enter treatment, and attrition. *Pain, 43*, 7-25.

Whipple, B. (1990). Part I: Neurophysiology of pain. *Orthopedic Nursing, 9*(4), 21-32.

◆ indicates a research-based work

CHAPTER 17

Self-Perception–Self-Concept Pattern

The self-perception–self-concept pattern involves the disabled individual's feelings of self-worth, perceptions about his or her body, and feelings about control over personal destiny. These processes are dynamic and are influenced not only by a person's current health situation, but also by past experiences, social relationships, and the previous view of himself or herself. Developmental stages beginning from early childhood through adolescence and late adulthood also will influence self-concept. Evaluating the client's self-perception–self-concept is necessary for rehabilitation nurses to understand the whole person as well as the impact of the disability.

The self-perception–self-concept pattern is important to rehabilitation nurses for several reasons. First, rehabilitation clients usually have experienced a change in body function as a result of an injury or illness. These changes in body function can result in the loss of familiar roles as well as feelings of dependence, helplessness, and anxiety—and, thus, pose a threat to a person's self-concept or self-esteem. Changes in body function, such as those experienced as a result of cervical spinal cord injuries, burns, or amputation, might be obvious; in other cases, such as strokes and minor head injury, the changes in functioning might be more subtle. Regardless of the degree and visibility of the impairment, a person's self-perception and self-concept might be challenged.

Another consideration is the influence of self-perception–self-concept on learning. Disturbances in self-esteem and self-concept and/or feelings of anxiety and powerlessness can make learning difficult. Rehabilitation clients are expected to participate actively in learning self-care tasks and health management behaviors. Understanding these concepts will enhance the rehabilitation nurses' abilities to assess their clients' needs and choose appropriate interventions to address disturbances in self-perception–self-concept.

Finally, successful rehabilitation requires the integration of the new view of the self. Clients must acknowledge and understand the bodily changes brought about by their illness or injury in order to achieve optimal levels of independence. The rehabilitation nurse plays a fundamental role in assisting clients toward successful reintegration of this new view of themselves into their self-perception–self-concept as well as into family and community life. Nursing diagnoses included in this chapter are anxiety, powerlessness, self-esteem disturbance, and body image disturbance.

I. Related Theory and Concepts

A. Anxiety: A feeling state from a source that is nonspecific or unknown; anxiety is self-protective and occurs when self-esteem is threatened

1. Levels of anxiety (the first three levels are most common in rehabilitation clients) (Peplau, 1963)
   a. Mild
   b. Moderate
   c. Severe
   d. Panic
2. Results of anxiety
   a. Physiological responses, including increased autonomic activation
   b. Behavioral responses, including altered ability for psychomotor skills
   c. Affective responses, including varying emotional reactions
   d. Cognitive responses, for example, altered cognitive functioning
3. Theories about the origins of anxiety
   a. Behaviorists view anxiety as resulting from frustration that occurs when a person is unable to reach a desired goal; inability to reach one goal might prevent the person from achieving other goals and result in feelings of failure and anxiety
   b. Experimental psychologists view anxiety as a drive that is learned because of an inherent desire to avoid pain, which is attached to a particular stimulus that may become generalized to other similar stimuli; thus, anxiety becomes self-protective to avoid the pain experience
   c. Some speculate that anxiety arises through conflict
      1) Conflict occurs when two opposing forces clash and the person must choose between them
      2) Four kinds of conflict have been identified
         a) Approach-approach: Occurs when a person has to choose between two equally desirable options
         b) Approach-avoidance: Arises when a person wants to both pursue and avoid the same goal
         c) Avoidance-avoidance: Arises when a person must choose between two equally undesirable goals
         d) Double approach-avoidance: Occurs when a person can see both positive and negative aspects of both alternatives
4. Anxiety occurs across developmental levels and throughout life span, with some persons more

prone to experiencing anxiety than others

a. Due to the increasing stresses associated with aging, particular attention has been given to anxiety in the elderly
   1) Many situations that might not produce stress in one person can be very stressful for the aging individual
   2) Potential sources of anxiety in the elderly
      a) Multiple losses
      b) Fewer resources
      c) Environmental changes
b. Rehabilitation clients with cognitive impairment might be at risk for anxiety due to distortions in cognitive processing that can cause a situation to be perceived as more stressful than it actually is

B. Power and powerlessness

1. Power
   a. Defined as the potential or actual ability to influence thinking, attitudes, behaviors, and/or emotions of oneself or another person
   b. Feeling of power creates potential for human beings to experience affirmation and assertion of the self
2. Powerlessness
   a. Defined as feeling that a person's own actions will not significantly affect the outcome of a situation
   b. Feeling of powerlessness and its behavioral consequences are one dimension of feeling alienated due to a loss of control of events and decision making (Seeman, 1959)
   c. Feelings of powerlessness can lead to apathy and helplessness
   d. Powerlessness in the context of Rotter's (1954) social learning theory
      1) Social learning theory suggests that the degree to which a person expects certain circumstances to occur is related to the extent to which the person feels he or she has control of the situation
      2) A person's locus of control can be external or internal
         a) A person who views events as being controlled by forces such as luck, fate, or chance is said to have an external locus of control
         b) A person who believes that events can be controlled by his or her own actions is said to have internal locus of control
      3) Relationships have been suggested between locus of control and learning, willingness to adopt positive health behaviors, and seeking and using information for personal decision making
      4) Extent to which a person with a disability believes he or she has control over a situation can affect problem-solving and decision-making skills and willingness or ability to learn health-management behaviors
      5) A person must distinguish between things that can or cannot be controlled in order to lessen feelings of helplessness or powerlessness

C. Self-perception

1. Can be positive or negative depending on factors such as age, life situation, and roles
2. Formed by related concepts of self-concept and self-esteem
   a. Self-concept: How a person sees himself or herself; cognitive component of self-perception
   b. Self-esteem: How a person evaluates or judges personal values; affective component of self-perception; develops across life span and is influenced by four critical elements
      1) Relationships with significant others
         a) Significant others are individuals who take on special importance for the development of self-esteem during a particular life phase
         b) Relationships with significant others that are affirming and supportive will enhance self-esteem
      2) Social role expectations
         a) General societal requirements for persons of a particular group (that is, age, sex, ethnicity, socioeconomic status)
         b) Critical in formation of self-esteem; a person's compliance or noncompliance with role expectations affects how that person judges his or her own self-worth
      3) Psychosocial developmental crises: Erikson's psychosocial stage theory of ego development proposes eight stages with implications for development of self-esteem (Erikson, 1964)
      4) Communications and coping style: Patterns of coping that effectively resolve stress with minimum of emotional residue will help individual adapt to change
3. Persons who can accurately appraise their strengths and weaknesses and who hold a positive view of self will have the skills to incorporate new behaviors and modify their lifestyle to successfully accommodate changes brought about by a disability

D. Body image

1. Defined as conscious and unconscious mental picture that a person has of shape, size, and mass of his or her body and its parts
2. Is one aspect of self-concept; influences a person's self-esteem, self-confidence, and personal identity
3. Dimensions of body image
   a. Physical body image: A person's perception of body as an object in space
   b. Cognitive body image: Way a person thinks about and evaluates his or her body
   c. Affective body image: A person's emotional experience based on beliefs and feeling about body
   d. Physical, cognitive, and affective body images are learned from experiences in environment and are influenced by the perceptions and/or re-

actions of others, developmental conditions, and changes in body due to health and illness

4. Disturbance in body image
   a. Actual or perceived disruption in way a person perceives his or her body; can result from developmental influences, chronic illness, or trauma; when a person's physical self is altered, his or her fundamental view of self changes
   b. Disturbance in body image reflects a view that is not a realistic representation of reality; for example, a stroke patient may perceive that a body part does not belong to him or her
5. Changes in body image must be integrated as events occur across life span to allow perception of body image to remain consistent with reality
   a. Sudden changes, such as those resulting from trauma, are more difficult to integrate than gradual changes
   b. Covert or internal changes (e.g., subtle cognitive or sensory losses) are more difficult to manage than overt or external changes such as visible motor weakness and/or paralysis and amputations

II. Nursing Assessment

A. Anxiety
   1. Feelings of anxiety
   2. Effects of injury or illness on ability to meet a person's own needs
   3. Stresses experienced since onset of injury and/or illness
   4. Past methods of dealing with anxiety
   5. Presence of physiological indicators of anxiety (e.g., agitation, tachycardia, shortness of breath)

B. Powerlessness
   1. Feelings about injury and/or illness
   2. Effects of injury and/or illness on life
   3. Feelings of lack of control over own life
   4. Situations that client thinks can be controlled
   5. Situations that client thinks cannot be controlled
   6. Past methods of dealing with difficulties
   7. Successful coping strategies
   8. Present method of dealing with difficulties brought on by illness and/or injury

C. Self-esteem
   1. Client's perception of self since onset of illness/injury
   2. Client's perception of how illness and/or injury will affect previous roles and lifestyle
   3. Client's assessment of own strengths or capabilities

D. Body image
   1. Feelings about body since onset of illness and/or injury
   2. Client's assessment of own strengths or capabilities
   3. Client's assessment of own limitations
   4. Presence of family and/or friends to provide support
   5. Client's assessment of own self-care learning needs
   6. Client's perception of how others see him or her

III. Nursing Diagnoses

➤ A. Anxiety

1. **Definition:** Vague, uneasy feeling, source of which is often nonspecific or unknown to the individual (Gordon, 1993)

2. **Major defining characteristics**
   a. Dimensions
      1) Physiological
      2) Psychological/behavioral
      3) Cognitive
   b. Severity level
      1) Mild anxiety
         a) Slight sympathetic arousal with minimal increase in heart rate, respirations, and blood pressure
         b) Positive behaviors and feelings
         c) Awareness of relationship among factors in the situation
      2) Moderate anxiety
         a) Activation of sympathetic nervous system
            (1) Muscle tension
            (2) Diaphoresis
            (3) Dilated pupils
            (4) Peripheral vasoconstriction
            (5) Notable increase in heart rate, respirations, and blood pressure
         b) Feelings of apprehension and tension
         c) Restlessness and difficulty in sleeping
         d) Difficulty in concentrating
         e) Attention focused on the situation of concern with little attention to extraneous events
      3) Severe anxiety
         a) Generalized sympathetic response, including a significant rise in heart rate, respirations, and blood pressure; can include trembling, sweating, palpitations, flushing or pallor, dry mouth, paresthesias, hot and cold flashes, urinary frequency
         b) Feelings of inadequacy, distress, and helplessness
         c) Attention directed to scattered details with learning greatly impaired

3. **Related factors/etiologies** (may be perceived or actual)
   a. Person's inability to meet his or her own basic human needs for food, air, comfort, and security (e.g., because of paralysis and/or cognitive impairment)
   b. Threat to self-concept
   c. Situational crises
   d. Change in health status (e.g., new disability or deteriorating function)
   e. Change in the environment (e.g., transfer to a new unit, facility, or home; new caregiver)

f. Change in roles, relationships, family and/or community (e.g., loss of job, inability to parent or participate in social activities)

4. Interventions

a. Develop consistent, honest, trusting relationship with client
b. Approach client with calm, reassuring, and nondemanding manner
c. Promote relaxed environment with appropriate level of sensory stimulation
d. Encourage client to express his or her thoughts and feelings
e. Help client explore experiences that precipitate feelings of anxiety
f. Give feedback regarding behaviors
g. Teach problem-solving strategies
h. Help identify adaptive strategies
i. Encourage client to use positive coping behaviors
j. Provide appropriate levels of information to reduce anxiety
k. Encourage social activities, new interests, and hobbies
l. Refer client to appropriate community resources
m. Provide instruction in muscle-relaxation exercises
n. Encourage client to practice assertive communication skills
o. Promote use of music for relaxation
p. Encourage physical activities, as tolerated, to promote relaxation
q. Collaborate with interdisciplinary team to promote a consistent approach for managing symptoms

5. Expected outcomes

a. Client verbalizes decreased feelings of anxiety
b. Client identifies actual and/or perceived threats
c. Client implements adaptive coping strategies
d. Client experiences improved physiological and psychological comfort

➤ B. Powerlessness

1. **Definition:** Perceived lack of control over a situation and belief that actions will not significantly affect an outcome (Gordon, 1993)

2. Major defining characteristics

a. Expression of having no control or influence over situation (e.g., course of illness, recovery, self-care, life events)
b. Expression of feelings of despair, hopelessness, and helplessness
c. Unwillingness or impaired ability to participate in decision-making activities or self-care
d. Exhibition of acting-out behaviors (e.g., aggressiveness toward others, hostility, anger)
e. Expression of feelings of apathy, resignation, and passivity
f. Depression
g. Inability to seek information about care
h. Dependence on others

3. Related factors/etiologies

a. Nature and severity of illness or disability
b. Hospitalization or institutionalization
c. Loss of control over body function
d. Loss of control of mental functions
e. Diminished physical strength or reserves
f. Inability to communicate
g. Inability to perform role responsibilities
h. Social isolation: Decreased interpersonal interaction
i. Lack of knowledge about the disability or treatment
j. A previous lifestyle characterized by helplessness

4. Interventions

a. Create environment that promotes independent behavior and responsibility
b. Adapt environment to promote independence
c. Promote client's and family's participation in client's care
d. Encourage client to personalize his or her own space
e. Help client express his or her feelings about condition, concerns, and involvement in self-care
f. Avoid being overprotective; promote healthy risk-taking behaviors
g. Help client to develop decision-making skills by providing him or her with opportunities to make decisions and also by respecting and supporting those decisions
h. Help client to distinguish between events that can and cannot be controlled
i. Mutually set short- and long-term behavioral goals that are attainable
j. Help client identify strengths and coping strategies for health management
k. Provide information relevant to the person's disability
l. Encourage questions and provide time for discussion

5. Expected outcomes

a. Client identifies factors in his or her life that can be controlled
b. Client perceives and demonstrates increased control of situations and outcomes
c. Client asks appropriate questions; demonstrates increased understanding of care and treatment
d. Client participates effectively in decision making about his or her own care
e. Client demonstrates health-management behaviors

➤ C. Self-esteem disturbance

1. **Definition:** Negative self-evaluation and feelings about one's own capabilities that may be expressed directly or indirectly (Gordon, 1993)

2. Major defining characteristics

a. Negative self-assessment
b. Difficulty in accepting positive feedback
c. Minimization of strengths and abilities
d. Failure to care for self
e. Lack of eye contact
f. Slumped posture
g. Feelings of inadequacy, worthlessness, helplessness
h. Lack of follow-through
i. Setting of unreasonable standards for self
j. Preoccupation with failure

3. Related factors/etiologies

a. Physical illness and/or disability
b. Disfigurement due to surgery or trauma
c. Absence of at least one consistently available person for support, especially after trauma
d. Abusive relationships early in life
e. Repeated negative experiences with interpersonal relationships
f. Loss of significant roles

4. Interventions

a. Assist client with self-care
b. Promote client's involvement in self-care
c. Mutually negotiate short-term goals that allow for success
d. Acknowledge client's feelings
e. Provide consistent, respectful, and honest approach to promote trust
f. Provide encouragement and supportive environment
g. Inspire reality-based hope
h. Promote laughter and humor
i. Accept client as a worthwhile, unique person
j. Provide information related to health regimen
k. Engage client in decision-making process
l. Encourage client's participation in social activities, including use of day and weekend passes

5. Expected outcomes

a. Client initiates self-care health management activities
b. Client communicates feelings and needs in an assertive way
c. Client sets and achieves realistic goals
d. Client demonstrates self-valuing behaviors
e. Client verbalizes thoughts and feelings spontaneously
f. Client participates in social and therapeutic activities

➤ D. Body image disturbance

1. **Definition:** Negative feelings or perception about characteristics, functions, or limits of one's body or body parts (Gordon, 1993)

2. Major defining characteristics

a. Feelings of disgust or negative beliefs about one's body
b. Inability to look at and/or touch one's changed body
c. Hiding or overexposure of the affected body part
d. Feelings of helplessness, hopelessness, or powerlessness about one's body
e. Preoccupation with loss or change of body function
f. Fear of rejection by others
g. Refusal to acknowledge change
h. Lack of knowledge about potential capabilities

3. Related factors/etiologies

a. Loss of body part or function
b. Disfigurement from surgery or trauma
c. Cognitive disturbances that distort one's self-perception (e.g., neglect)
d. Progressive debilitating disease
e. Uncontrollable pain
f. Dependence on mechanical devices (e.g., ventilators, gastrostomy tubes)
g. Psychological or drug-induced disturbances
h. Inability to integrate disability-related changes into sociocultural environment

4. Interventions

a. Encourage client to express feelings about his or her body
b. Actively listen and provide support
c. Support client in grieving process
d. Accept client as he or she is
e. Compliment client on his or her appearance
f. Assist client with adaptive clothing to enhance appearance
g. Encourage client to look at and touch changed body area
h. Encourage family to treat client in normalizing manner
i. Educate client about his or her capabilities for self-care and participation in social activities
j. Facilitate goal setting so that client can assume self-care responsibilities
k. Promote appropriate levels of involvement in self-care

5. Expected outcomes

a. Client shares feelings about his or her self-concept
b. Client recognizes negative feelings about himself or herself and identifies affirmations to counteract them
c. Client expresses feelings of sadness, loss, or anger
d. Client performs self-care activities
e. Client uses appropriate adaptive equipment
f. Client dresses and grooms to enhance appearance
g. Client participates in social activities without hiding affected body part(s)

References

Erikson, E.H. (1964). *Childhood and society* (2nd ed.). New York: W.W. Norton.

Gordon, M. (1993). *Manual of nursing diagnosis 1993-1994.* St. Louis: Mosby-Year Book, Inc.

Peplau, H. (1963). A working definition of anxiety. In S. Burd & M. Marshall (Eds.), *Some clinical approaches to psychiatric nursing* (pp. 323-327). New York: MacMillan Publishing Company.

Rotter, J.B. (1954). *Social learning and clinical psychology.* Englewood Cliffs, NJ: Prentice-Hall, Inc.

Seeman, M. (1959). On the meaning of alienation. *American Sociological Review, 24*, 783-791.

Suggested Readings

Carpenito, L.J. (1992). *Nursing diagnosis: Application to clinical practice* (4th ed.). Philadelphia: J.B. Lippincott Company.

◆Green, B.C., Pratt, C.C., & Grigsby, T.E. (1984). Self-concept among persons with long-term spinal cord injury. *Archives of Physical Medicine and Rehabilitation, 65*, 751-754.

Koehler, M.L. (1989). Relationship between self-concept and successful rehabilitation. *Rehabilitation Nursing, 14*, 9-12.

McFarland, G.K., & Thomas, M.D. (1991). *Psychiatric mental health nursing: Application of the nursing process.* Philadelphia: J.B. Lippincott Company.

◆Muhllenkamp, A.F., & Sayles, J.A. (1986). Self-esteem, social support, and positive health practices. *Nursing Research, 35*, 334-338.

◆Mullins, D. (1993). Nursing diagnosis of powerlessness: Concept analysis and validation of the defining characteristics and related factors. In R.M. Carroll-Johnson (Ed.), *Classification of nursing diagnoses: Proceedings of the tenth NANDA conference* (in press). Philadelphia: J.B. Lippincott Company.

Mumma, C.M. (Ed.). (1987). *Rehabilitation nursing: Concepts and practice—A core curriculum* (2nd ed.). Evanston, IL: Rehabilitation Nursing Foundation.

Norris, J., & Kunes-Connell, M. (1985). Self-esteem disturbance. *Nursing Clinics of North America, 20*, 745-761.

Olson, B., Ustanko, L., & Warner, S. (1991). The patient in a halo brace: Striving for normalcy in body image and self-concept. *Orthopædic Nursing, 10*(1), 44-50.

Roberts, S.L., & White, B.S. (1990). Powerlessness and personal control model applied to the myocardial infarction patient. *Progress in Cardiovascular Nursing, 5*(3), 84-94.

◆Samonds, R.J., & Cammermeyer, J. (1989). Perceptions of body image in subjects with multiple sclerosis: A pilot study. *Journal of Neuroscience Nursing, 21*, 190-194.

Spielberger, C.D. (1972). *Anxiety: Current trends in theory and research.* New York: Academic Press.

Stanwyck, D.J. (1983, August). Self-esteem through the life span. *Family and Community Health*, pp. 11-28.

Taft, L.B. (1985). Self-esteem in later life: A nursing perspective. *Advances in Nursing Science, 8*(1), 77-84.

Vogel, C.H. (1982). Anxiety and depression among the elderly. *Journal of Gerontological Nursing, 8*(4), 213-216.

◆ indicates a research-based work

CHAPTER 18

Role–Relationship Pattern

The role–relationship pattern involves personal performance as expected by the individual and others. The expected behaviors are based on personal values and beliefs as well as cultural influences. The evaluation of role–relationship patterns focuses on family life, work or school, and social activities. This chapter includes related nursing diagnoses of alteration in family processes, disturbance in role performance, social isolation, impaired verbal communication, unresolved conflicts about independence and dependence, and the relocation stress syndrome.

I. Related Theory and Concepts

A. Family processes

1. Family roles
   a. Depend on age, physical health, and cognitive abilities of family members
   b. Have a long-term impact; can be independent, interdependent, or dependent
   c. Can comprise one or more of the following roles: spouse, partner, parent, child, sibling
2. Family tasks
   a. Physical maintenance
   b. Resource allocation
   c. Division of labor
   d. Reproduction and nurturance of children
   e. Socialization
      1) Parents transmitting culture to children
      2) Parents helping children mature to adulthood
      3) Adult children caring for aged parents
   f. Maintenance of order and behavior
      1) Family rules governing behavior of each family member
      2) Family rules governing the individual and expectations of others in family
      3) Family rules governing the individual and interactions with the outside world
   g. Meeting essential emotional needs such as belonging, affecting, and worth
3. Family systems theory (Satir, 1964)
   a. Family must have the ability to expand and reshape itself over the lifetime
   b. Family members move into the family system and eventually, with maturity, out of primary family system
   c. Families exert much effort both overtly and covertly to achieve and maintain a balance in relationships (often referred to as *homeostasis*)
   d. All family members are affected to some degree by an event involving any individual family member; disability can have a long-term effect on family processes
   e. Characteristics of open and closed family systems
      1) Open system
         a) Family adapts by having rules that permit it to change openly, directly, clearly, and appropriately and that allow for growth of individual family member and family as a whole
         b) Adapts to and copes with change by acknowledging it realistically
      2) Closed system: Family attempts to handle change by maintaining status quo and/or denying or distorting reality of change

B. Socialization: Human need for contact and interaction with others

1. Healthy socialization involves the following behaviors
   a. Making choices and decisions based on accurate perceptions of individual and others
   b. Behaving as a separate and unique individual
   c. Dealing with reality, not wishing for or expecting unreal situations
   d. Learning and exploring throughout life
   e. Coping and adapting through negotiation, giving, and receiving
2. Impairments in socialization
   a. Disability due to physical, cognitive, and/or communication defects can impair socialization
   b. Interactions involving friendships, recreational, and community activities can be affected
3. Reasons for social isolation among those who have disabilities
   a. Lack of self-esteem
   b. Feelings of inferiority
   c. Fatigue
   d. Depression
   e. Failure to cope with and adapt to life changes
   f. Environmental barriers or socioeconomic factors that do not permit socialization or social activities
4. Effects of social isolation
   a. Personal growth is stifled
   b. Physical health can be negatively affected

C. Communication

1. Sharing of ideas, needs, purposes, feelings, and intentions
2. Communication abilities influence and affect fam-

ily relationships, success at work or school, social success, and enjoyment of recreation
3. Client's ability to communicate effectively is valued highly by family, friends, and others
4. Levels of communication
   a. Denotative: Literal content
   b. Metacommunicative: Literal content in combination with attitudes, feelings, intentions, facial expressions, and posture
5. Important components of communication
   a. Verbal
      1) Includes communication that consists of statements, clarification, qualification, and feedback of one's needs, thoughts, and ideas
      2) Can lead to growth, creativity, individuality, and productivity
   b. Nonverbal
      1) Occurs on behavioral and emotional levels
      2) Expresses one's self-esteem, emotional status, and cultural characteristics
      3) Can include incomplete or nonfunctional communication that leads to a stalemate, retarded growth, and pathology
   c. Symbol interpretation skills
      1) Includes an understanding of letters, numbers, signs, and shapes
      2) Involves essential rules (Markarian, 1989)
         a) Appropriately ordering sounds to form words
         b) Applying the correct meaning to words
         c) Appropriately ordering statements
         d) Applying appropriate word tense and number
   d. Language skills: Involves expression of information (speech and ability to write) and the reception of information (auditory comprehension and ability to read)

D. Conflict between independence and dependence

1. Healthy balance between independence and dependence is necessary
   a. Balance leads to increased self-esteem, which in turn leads to increased independence and confidence
   b. Increased self-esteem is characteristic of maturing adult
2. The balance between independence and dependence can be difficult to achieve, particularly with a disability as changes occur over the term of the disability
3. The balance can be influenced by the individual's family, friends, employers, educators, and others
4. Maladjustments: Have negative effects on both client and family
   a. Maladjusted dependence
      1) Involves a person with a disability not maintaining optimal level of self-care, family responsibilities, decision-making, and/or success with work, school, and/or play
      2) Creates the following problems
         a) Gives control of individual to others
         b) Reduces the individual's peace and contentment
         c) Creates resentment by the dependent person because of loss of self-control
         d) Creates resentment by dependent person as well as the one who has accepted responsibility
         e) Perpetuates a negative cycle of interpersonal dependency and control
   b. Maladjusted independence
      1) Involves a person with a disability who overestimates his or her cognitive and physical capabilities and energy level
      2) Safety of the disabled person can become a major issue

E. Relocation and stress

1. Relocation stress syndrome: Consequence of catastrophic injury or debilitating disease often augmented by a required transfer from one healthcare unit or living arrangement to another
2. Reasons for stress
   a. Sense of security, trust, and confidence that has been established in triad of client-family-nurse is disrupted by relocation
   b. Change opens client and family to another unknown, although relocation often is a signal of physical improvement
   c. If transfer is due to a worsening of the client's condition, stress and anxiety are magnified
3. Types of relocation in which stress is an important consideration
   a. Transfer from acute care to rehabilitation and from rehabilitation to community setting
   b. Transfer to and within long-term care facilities (Manion, 1991; Rantz & Egan, 1987)
   c. Transfer from critical care to step-down or acute care units (Barnhouse, 1987; Harkulich & Brugler, 1991)
   d. Community reentry
4. Planning for relocation
   a. Should attempt to minimize physiological and/or psychological disturbances triggered by moving
   b. Should include nursing interventions so as to ensure patient's progress toward independence and prevent setbacks in rehabilitation

II. Nursing Assessment

A. History: Questions to ask the client
1. What is your family's current structure?
2. Did your family have problems in the past that were difficult to handle?
3. Do members of your family or others depend on you?
4. How has your disability affected family life?
5. How has the injury and/or illness affected major life goals?
6. What support systems are available to you?
7. How has the injury and/or illness affected activities of daily living, work or school, social or recreational activities, and friendships?
8. Can you make your needs, feelings, desires, and

ideas known to others?
9. Which form of communication—verbal, written, or nonverbal—is best for you?
10. Do you understand the communication of others?
11. What impairs your ability to function at an optimal level?
12. Would you like to function at a higher level?
13. Do you feel others allow you to function optimally?
14. How do you feel about being transferred to this unit and/or facility?
15. Do you understand the goal and purpose of your transfer to the new environment?
16. Have you been informed of the resources available for your care in the new environment?

B. Observation
1. How does client interact with family members and/or friends?
2. Does the client communicate feeling a satisfying sense of belonging, caring, and interest in the family?
3. Can client communicate needs and desires?
4. Does client understand others' speech, voice intonation, gestures, facial and body language?
5. Can client attend, speak, write, hear, comprehend, and listen? (Compare current status with premorbid levels)
6. Has client resumed an appropriate role within his or her family?
7. Has client formulated realistic plans for the future?
8. Do family and friends include client in social activities?
9. Does client verbalize discomfort in social situations?
10. Does client have physical characteristics of social isolation (fatigue, insomnia, restlessness, vague aches, and/or anxieties)?
11. Does client exhibit behavioral responses of social isolation (overeating, alcoholism, drug abuse, and/or excessive sleeping)?
12. Are there environmental barriers that inhibit socialization?
13. Are there special physiological problems, such as incontinence, that might inhibit socialization?
14. Has client formulated realistic plans for work and/or school?
15. How have client and family been affected by the move to a new environment?
16. Did client and family feel involved in decision to move to a new environment?
17. Do client and family feel involved in decisions related to rehabilitation goals and program?
18. Have there been noticeable changes in appetite, sleep patterns, communication levels, mood, and/or motivational levels since the move?

III. Nursing Diagnoses

➤ A. Alteration in family processes

1. **Definition:** Inability of family system to meet needs of its members, carry out family functions, or maintain communications for mutual growth and maturation (Gordon, 1993)

2. **Major defining characteristics**

a. Family system is unable or unwilling to meet emotional, social, and physical needs of its members
b. Lack of shared goals within family
c. Changes in effective family patterns of behavior and coping
d. Changes in roles and responsibilities within family
e. Inability to cope with changes in family structure, roles, and responsibilities
f. Inability to accept and respect client as part of family with regard to injury, illness, or disability

3. **Related factors/etiologies**

a. Physical, cognitive, and communication deficits
b. Lack of prior family ability to cope with change
c. Depression
d. Social isolation
e. Denial
f. Rejection
g. Lack of or changes in financial support
h. Role conflicts within the family

4. **Interventions**

a. Provide support to client and family members regarding altered roles and responsibilities
b. Support communication between client and family members
c. Provide privacy for client and family within rehabilitation facility
d. If appropriate, give family members accurate information regarding client's status and abilities
e. Be an active listener; allow client and family members to express frustration, anger, hopelessness, and powerlessness
f. Include client and family members in short-term and long-term planning
g. Include family members in client's care
h. Arrange and support family conferences; refer to community family support groups
i. Consult with a rehabilitation psychologist and social worker
j. Recommend opportunities for social interaction within the community

5. **Expected outcomes**

a. Client and family establish adaptive coping for functions, roles, responsibilities
b. Client communicates effectively regarding goals and activities of family life
c. Client's family members participate in care of client and/or support client's independence

➤ B. Disturbance in role performance

1. **Definition:** Disruption in ability to perform one's usual social, vocational, educational, or family roles (Cox et al., 1989)

2. **Major defining characteristics**
   a. Change in perception of an individual's role held by himself or herself and/or others
   b. Change in physical abilities required for assuming former roles
   c. Change in usual responsibilities
   d. Denial of roles and responsibilities
   e. Lack of knowledge regarding current or future responsibilities
   f. Denial of abilities and/or disabilities
   g. Refusal to discuss abilities and/or limitations
   h. Feelings of worthlessness
   i. Increasing dependence
3. **Related factors/etiologies**
   a. Long-term disability or incapacitation
   b. Change in cognitive function
   c. Knowledge deficit
   d. Depression
   e. Fatigue
4. **Interventions**
   a. Provide opportunities for client and family to express thoughts and feelings regarding roles and responsibilities
   b. Provide opportunities for client and family to maintain personal roles and responsibilities
   c. Encourage client and family to participate in self-care activities
   d. Encourage client and family to be aware of current assets, knowledge, and strengths
   e. Encourage client and family to prioritize roles and responsibilities
   f. Define modified or new roles with the family and community
   g. Secure volunteer or noncompetitive role (job reflective of client's abilities)
5. **Expected outcomes**
   a. Client communicates the need for change regarding roles and responsibilities
   b. Client continues to function in prior roles as much as possible
   c. Client and family work together to revise and modify roles and responsibilities as indicated by current abilities

➤ C. **Social isolation**
1. **Definition:** Interpersonal interactions below a level desired or required for personal integrity (Gordon, 1993)
2. **Major defining characteristics**
   a. Behavior or statement indicating desire for increased human interaction
   b. Expression of feeling different from others
   c. Expression of loneliness or feeling of rejection
   d. Sad, dull affect
   e. Uncommunicative and withdrawn behavior; lack of eye contact
   f. Hostile, irritable behavior
   g. Insecurity in public
   h. Inability to concentrate and make decisions
   i. Feelings of uselessness
   j. Low level of contact with family, peers, and community
3. **Related factors/etiologies**
   a. Chronic illness or disability
   b. Depression
   c. Hopelessness
   d. Powerlessness
   e. Changes in roles and responsibilities
   f. Support system deficit
   g. Environmental barriers
4. **Interventions**
   a. Involve client and family in setting goals for making decisions about care
   b. Encourage client's independence in activities of daily living
   c. Encourage activities through recreational therapy
   d. Identify and involve client with successful role models
   e. Involve client with those who have shared interests
   f. Provide environment conducive to interpersonal interaction
   g. Inform client and family about vocational, educational, recreational, and social resources available in community for people with disabilities
   h. Invite client and family to support group activities
   i. Inform client and family about transportation resources for people with disabilities
   j. Encourage consultations with a chaplain, social worker, counselor, recreational therapist, or psychologist
5. **Expected outcomes**
   a. Client participates in activities that support vocational, educational, recreational, and social needs
   b. Client communicates feelings regarding resocialization
   c. Client communicates feelings regarding loneliness

➤ D. **Impaired verbal communication** (also see Chapter 6, pages 38-39)
1. **Definition:** Inability or reduced ability to use or understand language in human interactions (NANDA, 1992)
2. **Major defining characteristics**
   a. Difficulty with verbal expression
      1) Expressive aphasia (impaired verbal output, rhythm, and grammar)
      2) Apraxia (impaired fluency, word substitution, and inconsistent speech)
      3) Dysarthria (slowed, slurred speech)

b. Difficulty with writing
c. Difficulty with receiving verbal language
   1) Impaired hearing
   2) Inability to comprehend speech
   3) Fluent but inappropriate speech
d. Difficulty with reading

3. Related factors/etiologies

a. History of neurologic or neuromuscular injury or disease
b. Impaired level of communication skills prior to disability or disease
c. Age, developmental stage, and educational status
d. Cultural differences

4. Interventions

a. General interventions
   1) Encourage communication between client and family members
   2) Promote unhurried atmosphere
   3) Minimize distractions and avoid overstimulation
   4) Speak to client in a normal tone of voice and establish eye contact
   5) Speak in short, simple sentences
   6) Maintain interactions and conversations at an age-appropriate level
   7) Use or reinforce alternative methods of communication (communication boards, assistive communication systems)
   8) If inappropriate laughter or crying persists, remove client from the interaction
b. Interventions for *expressive (nonfluent) aphasia*
   1) Encourage verbal attempts and be patient, allow mistakes, and expect anger and frustration
   2) Praise client for any attempts at verbal communication and for small accomplishments
   3) If patient's frustration level is escalating, help by supplying the word you think client is attempting to say
   4) Teach family members to allow client to talk and to avoid habitually interrupting him or her
   5) Serve as a role model for good speech patterns
   6) Provide varied opportunities for patient to listen to verbal communication (e.g., on radio or TV)
   7) With patients exhibiting severe expressive aphasia
      a) Use gestures, pictures and demonstrations
      b) Establish yes/no reliability
c. Interventions for *receptive (fluent) aphasia*
   1) Provide feedback to client and acknowledge awareness of client's language problem
   2) Set limits concerning when and how much to verbalize
   3) Provide quiet, brief exchanges and social activities
   4) Speak in concrete terms
   5) Admit your inability to understand client
   6) Use touch and behavior to portray calmness and assurance
   7) Do not speak loudly
   8) Offer important information first, because client might understand only a few statements (Boss, 1991)

5. Expected outcomes

a. Client comprehends, speaks, and writes at the highest possible functional level
b. Client, family, and rehabilitation staff will establish a reliable and functional means of communicating
c. Client communicates effectively during educational, vocational, recreational, and social exchanges

➤ E. Unresolved independence–dependence conflict

1. Definition: Lack of resolution of need and desire to be dependent/independent with expectation (therapeutic, maturational, or social) to be dependent/independent (Gordon, 1993)

2. Major defining characteristics

a. Maladaptive dependence
   1) Lack of interest in activities of daily living that facilitate independence
   2) Difficulty making decisions
   3) Need for excessive reassurance
   4) Passivity and submissiveness
   5) Hesitation about trying new situations
   6) Perception of inability to cope with situations
   7) Powerlessness
b. Maladaptive independence
   1) Overconfidence or underconfidence regarding abilities
   2) Denial
   3) Impulsivity
   4) Avoidance of sharing decisions with family

3. Related factors/etiologies

a. Physical abilities and limitations
b. Cognitive abilities and limitations
c. Age and developmental stage
d. Work and educational status
e. Financial status
f. Available support systems

4. Interventions

a. Maladaptive dependence
   1) Support client's examination of his or her own assets and abilities
   2) Support client's evaluation of impact of his or her illness or injury on work, education, family, social, and recreational life
   3) Encourage client to assume activities associated with daily living
   4) Support client's ability to make decisions

5) Inform client of resources available that promote independence (e.g., options for transportation)
6) Encourage communication within family unit regarding independent, interdependent, and dependent roles
7) Encourage work and/or school activities

b. Maladaptive independence
1) Watch for situations that could cause injury
2) Increase client's and family's safety awareness
3) Monitor client's ability for self-care
4) Provide environmentally safe situations
5) Monitor physical, cognitive, and sensory deficits
6) Encourage the use of prosthetics or assistive devices
7) Provide appropriate level of supervision

5. Expected outcomes

a. Client assumes adaptive dependent, interdependent, and independent roles
b. Client performs optimal self-care activities
c. Client performs role at optimal level

➤ **F. Relocation stress syndrome**

1. Definition: Physiological and/or psychosocial disturbances as a result of transfer from one environment to another

2. Major defining characteristics

a. Change in environment or location
b. Anxiety
c. Apprehension
d. Increased confusion (especially in elderly populations)
e. Depression
f. Loneliness

3. Related factors/etiologies

a. Little or no preparation for impending move
b. Moderate to high degree of environmental change
c. Losses involved in decision to move
d. Feelings of powerlessness
e. Past, concurrent, and recent losses
f. Lack of adequate support system
g. History and types of previous transfers
h. Impaired psychosocial health status
i. Decreased physical health status
j. Limited capacity to comprehend the move

4. Interventions

a. Inform client and family about goals, programs, and resources of new environment
b. Encourage client and family to visit new unit or health facility prior to client's transfer
c. Communicate client's physical, psychological, social, and spiritual needs to new healthcare professionals
d. Encourage client's verbalization of feelings
e. Communicate with family regarding client's adjustment to relocation
f. When possible, encourage choice (e.g., space, room)

5. Expected outcomes

a. Client verbalizes positive statements concerning both acceptance of new environment and reasons for leaving previous environment
b. Client and family are motivated by goals of rehabilitation and reentry into community
c. Client expresses feelings of control and self-confidence
d. Client demonstrates stress management techniques
e. Client expresses trust in new care providers

References

Barnhouse, A. (1987). *The development of the nursing diagnosis of translocation syndrome with critical care patients.* Unpublished manuscript. Akron, OH: Akron City Hospital.

Boss, B. (1991). Managing communication disorders in stroke. *Nursing Clinics of North America, 26,* 985-996.

Cox, H.C., Hinz, M.D., Lubno, M.A., Newfield, S.A., Ridenour, N.A., & Sridaromont, K.L. (1989). *Clinical applications of nursing diagnosis.* Baltimore: Williams & Wilkins.

Gordon, M. (1993). *Manual of nursing diagnoses: 1993-1994.* St. Louis: Mosby-Year Book, Inc.

Harkulich, J., & Brugler, C. (1991). Nursing diagnosis: Relocation stress. In K. Gettrust (Ed.), *Interventions for nursing diagnosis: Guides for comprehensive care planning* (pp. 461-468). Albany, NY: Delmar Publishing.

Manion, P. (1991). *Translocation syndrome: Validation of a nursing diagnosis.* Unpublished master's thesis, Southern Illinois University at Edwardsville.

Markarian, F.M. (1989). Communication: Speech and language. In S. Dittmar (Ed.) *Rehabilitation nursing: Process and application* (287-310). St. Louis: The C.V. Mosby Company.

North American Nursing Diagnosis Association (NANDA). (1992). *NANDA nursing diagnosis: Definitions and classification 1992-1993.* St. Louis: Author.

Rantz, M., & Egan, K. (1987). Reducing death from translocation syndrome. *American Journal of Nursing, 87,* 1351-1352.

Satir, V. (1964). *Conjoint family therapy.* Palo Alto, CA: Science & Behavior Books.

Suggested Readings

Athreya, B.H. (1987). Impact of chronic illness on families. *Rheumatic Disease Clinics of North America, 13*(1), 123-131.

◆Back, J.R., Campagnolo, D.I., & Hoeman, S. (1991). Life satisfaction of individuals with Duchenne muscular dystrophy using long-term mechanical ventilatory support. *American Journal of Physical Medicine and Rehabilitation, 70*(3), 129-135.

Bronstein, K., Popovich, J., & Stewart-Amidei, C. (1991). *Promoting stroke recovery: A research-based approach for nurses.* St. Louis: Mosby-Year Book, Inc.

Brugler, C., Titus, M., & Nytaver, J. (1993). Relocation stress syndrome: A patient and staff approach. *Journal of Nursing Administration (JONA), 23*(1), 45-50.

◆Canan, C. (1987). Coping with feelings: Chronically ill children and their families. *Canadian Journal of Nursing Research, 19*(3), 9-21.

◆Casas, M.S. (1989). Experience in coping with stroke: A survey of caregivers. *Journal of Rehabilitation, 55*(4), 37-43.

Doenges, M.E., & Moorhouse, M.F. (1988). *Nursing diagnosis with interventions* (2nd ed.). Philadelphia: F.A. Davis Company.

◆Friedemann, M. (1991). An instrument to evaluate effectiveness in family functioning. *Western Journal of Nursing Research, 13*(2), 220-241.

Futcher, J.A. (1988). Chronic illness and family dynamics. *Pediatric Nursing, 14*, 381-385.

Gillies, D.A. (1988). Role supplementation to overcome intrafamily role insufficiency following physical disability. *Rehabilitation Nursing, 13*, 19-22.

Gleenon, T.P. (1990). Questions asked by patients and their support group during family conferences on inpatient rehabilitation units. *Archives of Physical Medicine and Rehabilitation, 71*, 699-702.

Gordon, M. (1987). *Nursing diagnosis: Process and application* (2nd ed.). New York: McGraw-Hill Book Company.

Groher, M.E. (1990). Speech and language assessment. In M. Rosenthal, E. Griffith, M.R. Bond, & J.D. Miller (Eds.), *Rehabilitation of the adult and child with traumatic brain injury* (2nd ed.) (pp. 294-309). Philadelphia: F.A. Davis Company.

◆Heller, K., Thompson, M.G., Vlachos-Weber, I., Steffen, A.M., & Trueba, P.E. (1991). Support interventions for older adults: Confidant relationships, perceived family support, and meaningful role activity. *American Journal of Community Psychology, 19*(1), 139-146.

◆Hendryx, P.M. (1989). Psychosocial changes perceived by closed-head injured adults and their families. *Archives of Physical Medicine and Rehabilitation, 70*, 526-530.

Johnson, J.R., & Higgins, L. (1987). Integration of family dynamics into the rehabilitation of the brain injured patient. *Rehabilitation Nursing, 12*, 320-324.

◆Killen, J.M. (1990). Role stabilization in families after spinal cord injury. *Rehabilitation Nursing, 15*, 19-21.

◆McBride, P.S. (1991). Comparative analysis of three instruments designed to measure self-care agency. *Nursing Research, 40*(1), 12-16.

McColl, M.A. (1988). Concepts and measurement of social support in the rehabilitation setting. *Canadian Journal of Rehabilitation, 3*(4), 42-50.

McCourt, A. (1991). Syndromes in nursing: A continuing concern. In R.M. Carroll-Johnson (Ed.), *Classification of nursing diagnosis: Proceedings of the ninth conference* (pp. 79-82). Philadelphia: J.P. Lippincott Company.

McLane, A.M. (Ed.). (1987). *Classification of nursing diagnoses: Proceedings of the seventh conference of the North American Nursing Diagnosis Association*. St. Louis: The C.V. Mosby Company.

Moch, S.D. (1988). Promoting health and role-reversal couples. *Journal of Community Health Nursing, 5*(3), 195-202.

◆Packard, N.J., Haberman, M.R., Woods, N.F., & Yates, B.C. (1991). Demands of illness among chronically ill women. *Western Journal of Nursing Research, 13*, 434-457.

Payne, M.B. (1988). Utilizing role theory to assist the family with sudden disability. *Rehabilitation Nursing, 13*, 191-194.

Phillips, A. (1987). Alternative systems of communication. *Geriatric Nursing Home Care, 7*(8), 25-27.

Remer, D., Buckwalter, K.C., & Maas, M. (1991). Translocation syndrome. In M. Maas, K.C. Buckwalter, & M. Hardy (Eds.), *Nursing diagnoses and interventions for the elderly* (pp. 493-504). Redwood City, CA: Addison-Wesley Nursing.

Rosenthal, M. (1988). Effective family intervention after traumatic brain injury: Theory and practice. *Journal of Head Trauma Rehabilitation, 3*(4), 42-50.

Smith, B.A. (1986). When is "confusion" translocation syndrome? *American Journal of Nursing, 86*, 1280-1281.

◆ indicates a research-based work

CHAPTER 19

Sexuality–Reproductive Pattern

Sexuality and reproduction are important issues for rehabilitation clients. Nursing issues lie primarily in the areas of education; fostering self-esteem; and ensuring safety concerning contraception, childbearing, and the correct use of aids for sexual expression and prevention of sexually transmitted diseases (STDs).

Due to the presence of neurological, orthopedic, and cardiovascular diseases and injuries, as well as their associated endocrine problems, the majority of rehabilitation clients have temporary or permanent sexual dysfunction. Sexual dysfunction can be as direct as erectile dysfunction, retrograde ejaculation, and lack of sensation and orgasm; it also can be indirectly related to social skills, positioning problems, pain, or behavioral abnormalities.

There are many aids and alternative methods that allow most clients a successful, fulfilling means of sexual function and reproduction. Rehabilitation nurses can promote a client's sexual satisfaction and expression, which in turn facilitates self-esteem, body image, actualization, and effective social relationships. Therefore, rehabilitation nurses should clarify their own personal values in the area of sexuality in order to provide an atmosphere of permission and acceptance. They should develop care plans and teaching strategies that allow clients to learn about the effects that the injury or illness can have on sexual function and reproduction, as well as about the methods and aids they can use to enhance sexual expression and conception.

I. Related Theory and Concepts

A. Sexual response is highly individualized and complex, involving both neurophysiological and psychological processes; Masters and Johnson (1966) divided the sexual response cycle into four phases, which are similar for males and females (see Table 19.1)

B. Neurophysiological responses

1. *Males*
   a. Erection involves tumescence and engorgement of the penis
   b. Erection occurs in three phases
      1) Initiation
      2) Filling
      3) Storage
   c. Two components of the erection process exist in males, reflex and psychogenic; in able-bodied males, stimulation to elicit both components is needed to maintain a firm erection adequate for intercourse
      1) Reflex erections (see Figure 19.1) are initiated by noncortical stimulation and occur through a reflex arc at the S2-4 spinal segments
         a) Caused by two types of stimulation
            (1) External tactile stimulation of genitals (e.g., friction from bed linen or clothing; catheter manipulation; manual, sexual, or oral stimulation)
            (2) Internal stimulation (e.g., from a full bladder)
         b) In upper motor neuron (UMN) spinal cord injury, which results in a severing of the connection between the genitals and the brain, the sacral reflex arc remains intact; reflex erection occurs independently of the brain and of psychological control, because there is still thoracolumbar (e.g., parasympathetic nervous system) function (see Figure 19.1)
      2) Psychogenic erections (see Figure 19.2) are initiated by cortical brain stimulation involving a combination of visual, auditory, olfactory, and other information that the individual perceives as erotic
      3) In lower motor neuron (LMN) spinal cord injury, the sacral reflex arc is not intact
         a) When brain becomes aware of erotic stimuli, efferent impulses travel from the brain to the spinal cord
         b) Impulses then leave spinal cord through sympathetic trunk of the craniosacral system—for example, sympathetic nervous system
         c) Impulses travel to pelvic area, producing an erection
   d. Emission of semen into posterior urethra is controlled by sympathetic nervous system
   e. Ejaculation is also controlled by sympathetic nervous system and is triggered by emission
      1) Antegrade ejaculation: Normal process that occurs when motor impulses travel through spinal segments S2-4 and go out to perineal, pelvic, and internal sphincter muscles, causing them to contract; thus, semen is released through urethra
      2) Retrograde ejaculation: Occurs when internal sphincter does not contract; therefore, semen exits into bladder; this is a complication especially for those with sphincter dyssynergia (see Chapter 13, page 101)

Table 19.1. The Sexual Response Cycle in Males and Females

Phase	Male Response	Female Response
Excitement (vasocongestion and muscle tension)	Nipples become erect Skin flushes Penis becomes erect Scrotum rises Testicles rise and increase in size Pulse rate and blood pressure rise	Nipples become erect Skin flushes Vaginal lubrication occurs Vaginal walls and labia thicken Vagina expands, cervix elevates, clitoris increases in size Pulse rate and blood pressure rise
Plateau (continuation of excitement phase)	Muscles are tense Skin flushes Respiratory rate increases Pulse rate increases Penis is at full erection Sperm travels in vas deferens to seminal vesicles and prostate Testicles swell and pull close to abdomen Cowper's gland secretion occurs	Muscles are tense Skin flushes Respiratory rate increases Pulse rate increases Labia are bright red Clitoris retracts, uterus elevates Vaginal barrel expands Bartholin's gland secretion occurs
Orgasm (involuntary muscle contractions release the accumulated vasocongestion and muscle tension)	Body muscles contract Respiratory and pulse rates increase Penis, anal sphincter, and prostate contract Ejaculation occurs	Body muscles contract Respiratory and pulse rates increase Rectal and urethral sphincters contract Clitoris retracts
Resolution (dissipation of vasocongestion and muscle tension)	Muscle tension subsides Perspiration occurs Respiratory and pulse rates slow to normal Blood pressure returns to normal Sex organs return to normal state Refractory period begins	Muscle tension subsides Perspiration occurs Respiratory and pulse rates slow to normal Blood pressure returns to normal Sex organs return to normal state Return to orgasm is possible Cervix drops into the seminal pool

Source Consulted
Masters, W.H., & Johnson, V.E. (1966). *Human sexual response.* Boston: Little, Brown & Company.

f. Orgasm (see Table 19.1)

g. Anorgasmia: Absence of orgasm; can occur after stroke, TBI, and musculoskeletal disorders, but commonly occurs after SCI (Rabin, 1980)
   1) Percentages of males and females with SCI experiencing orgasm is difficult to classify due to subjectivity associated with orgasm
   2) Physical sensations similar to orgasm—body tension, relaxation, and psychological sensations attributed to reflex orgasms—have been reported

h. Reproductive capability (see Table 19.2)
   1) Characteristics of semen
      a) Sixty percent of sperm must be normally shaped for fertility
      b) Fifty percent must be moving rapidly
      c) Sperm count should be at least 20 million per millileter
      d) Semen volume is necessary for fertility
         (1) Semen volume should be greater than 1.5 ml
         (2) Semen volume less than 1.5 ml can indicate retrograde ejaculation in those with upper motor neuron spinal cord injury or urinary sphincter dyssnergia
   2) Ability to transfer semen to a partner
      a) Erectile dysfunction or impotence frequently emerges in stroke, TBI, SCI, and cardiovascular disease, thus interfering with fertility
      b) Repeated infectious processes can impair fertility
         (1) Clumping of agglutinated sperm suggests inflammation or immunologic problems
         (2) Neurogenic bladder syndromes can cause retrograde ejaculation or repeated genitourinary or other systemic infections
   3) MacLeod and Gold (1951), in a classic study of males with SCI, reported that fertility decreased greatly; sperm count, morphology, and motility could be affected by testicular atrophy due to loss of temperature regulating mechanisms; and hyperthermia

Figure 19.1. Neurophysiology of a Reflex Erection with Complete Injuries at T10-L2 or Above

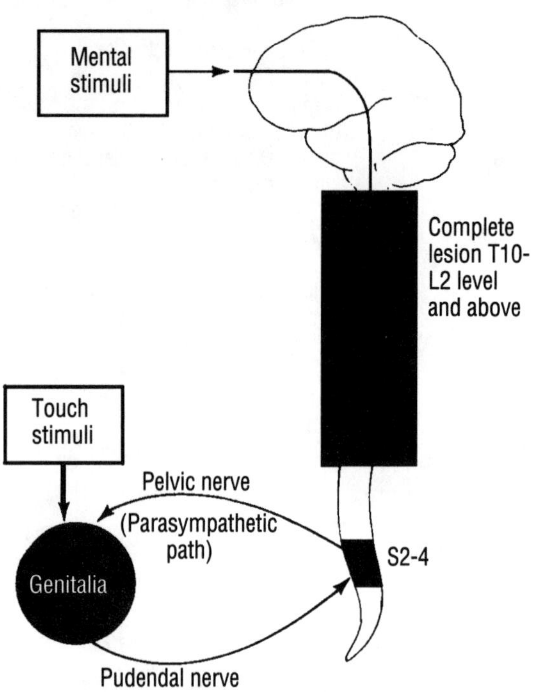

Reprinted with permission of Jones and Bartlett Publishers from Zejdlik, C.J. (1992). *Management of spinal cord injury* (2nd ed.) (p. 180). Boston: Jones and Bartlett Publishers. Copyright © 1991 Jones and Bartlett Publishers.

Figure 19.2. Neurophysiology of a Psychogenic Erection with Complete Injuries at S2-S4 and Below

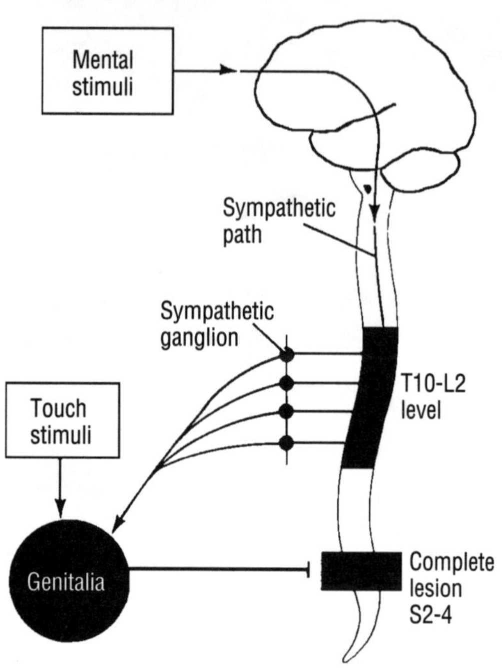

Reprinted with permission of Jones and Bartlett Publishers from Zejdlik, C.J. (1992). *Management of spinal cord injury* (2nd ed.) (p. 180). Boston: Jones and Bartlett Publishers. Copyright © 1991 Jones and Bartlett Publishers.

was common in the testicles and was associated with sterility in much the same way as a high fever

2. *Females*: Female sexual neurophysiology (see Table 19.1) has been investigated less often
   a. There is tumescence (swelling) and engorgement of the clitoris and labia minora
   b. Vaginal lubrication occurs
   c. Smooth muscle contractions in uterine wall occur during orgasm
   d. Sexual response cycle has not been studied extensively in disabled females; rather, it has been described in comparison to male functioning (Griffith & Trieschmann, 1975)
      1) Researchers have reported patterns of reflex and psychogenic vaginal lubrication (similar to that of reflex and psychogenic erections in males with UMN and LMN spinal cord injury) [Geiger, 1979; Berard, 1989)
      2) Orgasm (see Table 19.1)
      3) Reproductive capabilities are unchanged in females after stroke, arthritis, TBI, and SCI
         a) Menstrual cycle following most neurological traumas and disability is characteristically interrupted for 6 months, then resumes premorbid patterns
         b) Ovulatory cycles can be temporarily dysfunctional
         c) Pregnancy is viable because fertility is unaffected
         d) Uterine labor contractions are affected by SCI and other disabling conditions; the sensory component of labor is affected by complete SCI above T10; women do not feel labor pain, but they can deliver vaginally under close monitoring

II. Nursing Assessment

A. Take history of patient's sexual-reproductive pattern
   1. Choose private, unhurried time and environment
   2. Interview client and partner separately and then together
   3. Include questions that will provide a comprehensive assessment
      a. Masters and Johnson's (1970) extensive history format can be modified for use in a rehabilitation milieu; includes several useful components
         1) Inventory of personal values—moral and religious concerns pertaining to sexuality, reproductive patterns, parenting philosophy, and type of birth control practiced
         2) Determination of psychological and emotional status (examples of questions are

Table 19.2. Reproductive Capabilities After Disability

Diagnosis	Fertility	Pregnancy	Childbirth	Parenting
Arthritis (includes hip and knee disease)	Unchanged	Increased pressure on joints due to weight gain	Potential need for cesarean section depending on joint involvement	Increased energy needs and pressure on joints required in child care
Brain injury	*Males:* Possible premature ejaculation due to decreased attention span *Males and females:* Poor libido and behavioral changes and social inappropriateness may interfere with sexual relationships	Cognitive deficits possibly requiring assistance to ensure good prenatal care	Spasticity and sensory deficits may necessitate planned labor induction and/or a cesarean section	Cognitive, temper control, memory, safety awareness, ADL, or mobility deficits possibly requiring client to obtain assistance
Stroke	*Females:* Unchanged (see the listing for "Brain injury" above) *Males:* Possible vascular or psychogenic impotence (see also the listing for "Brain injury" above)	Plan around fully stabilized CVA, especially hemorrhagic CVA, if possible	(see the listing for "Brain injury" above)	(see the listing for "Brain injury" above)
Spinal cord injury	*Females:* Temporary disruption of the menstual cycle and ovulation *Males:* Erectile dysfunction, retrograde ejaculation, and poor sperm count and quality due to the loss of temperature-regulating mechanisms	Need for close medical supervision, possible increase in spasms due to the weight of the fetus, increased fatigue, circulation problems, edema, more difficulty with ADLs and transfers, and bladder infections or autonomic dysreflexia due to pressure of the fetus	Inability to feel contractions in injuries at or above T10, possibility of induction of a cesarean section and vaginal delivery, possibility of dysreflexia during delivery	Need for home and equipment modifications

given below)

a) Presence of depression: "How do you feel about the way your disability (disease) has affected your sexual function?"

b) Self-perception and body image: "Do you feel as sexually attractive since your stroke? If not, in what ways do you feel less attractive?"

c) Fears and concerns: "You've probably thought a lot about going home. What are your concerns about sexual functioning once you're at home?"

3) Gauge of client's level of psychosexual development

a) Knowledge of sexual functioning, reproduction, contraception, and effects of disability or disease on these processes

b) Social skills status, including concerns about dating, relationship issues, and communication with partners in light of changed body image

c) Comfort in discussing sexuality and reproduction

b. Assess medication and/or substance use and schedule; discuss types of medication that might interfere with sexual function or libido

1) Antihypertensives
2) Antidepressants
3) Antihistamines
4) Sedatives and tranquilizers
5) Narcotics
6) Diuretics
7) Antispasmodics

c. Assess premorbid and current sexual and/or reproductive patterns

1) Frequency of sexual activity, including sexual interest and libido
2) Techniques, practices, and erogenous zones
3) Partner availability, gender, and relationship history

4) Past changes or problems in sexual functioning and their type and onset
5) Receptivity to alternative methods of sexual expression and reproduction
6) Menstrual history and present state of menstrual cycle, any pre- or postmenopausal symptoms
7) Knowledge about contraceptives and history of personal use
8) Previous reproduction (number of pregnancies and outcome, number of children living in or out of household)
9) Previous fertility, childbearing, or parenting problems
10) Delineation of pain and types of movement or positions that cause pain, anxiety, shortness of breath, spasms, or syncope during sexual activity

B. Consider other assessment factors *(Note: Although the rehabilitation nurse does not order laboratory tests or perform extensive studies of sexual function, the nurse should be aware of their existence in order to plan educational programs, counseling, and referral.)*

1. Laboratory studies
   a. Testosterone test (for males): Can rule out organic causes of low libido or erectile dysfunction
   b. Glucose test: Can rule out diabetes-induced erectile dysfunction in men
2. Sensorimotor testing: Performed to determine sexual stimulation capabilities and, in females, the ability to feel labor contractions
   a. Tactile sensation in genital and/or perineal area
   b. Sacral 1, 2, 3 dermatome intactness of buttocks and legs; identification of hypersensitive dermatomes for potential erogenous zones that can be stimulated
   c. Motor function of lower extremities
3. Genitourinary (GU) examination and/or studies
   a. Urinary and rectal sphincter tone and strength
   b. Bulbocavernosus reflex (to assess the reflex arc between pelvic floor and spinal cord)
   c. Observation for penile lesions (in males) and genitorectal lesions (in males and females)
   d. Erectile studies (in males), including penile Doppler studies to assess for penile blood flow and lower extremity Doppler studies to assess for pulses and penile blood flow
4. Pharmacologic erection testing with agents such as Prostaglandin E_1, papaverine, or a combination of papaverine and phentolamine
   a. Good response suggests adequate penile vascular status
   b. Increased response is seen with neurogenic diseases or injuries
   c. Poor response occurs in males with incompetent penile systems
5. Penile cavernosogram and/or cavernosometry further explores the vascular system; used to further determine appropriate treatment alternatives
6. Nocturnal penile tumescence monitoring is used to confirm absence of rapid eye movement (REM) sleep erections, thus indicating organic erectile dysfunction; also used to rule out psychogenic erectile dysfunction and malingering

➤ III. Nursing Diagnosis: Altered Sexuality Patterns

A. Definition: State in which physical conditions or sexual behaviors cause an individual to express concern regarding his or her sexuality

B. Major defining characteristics

1. Reported difficulties in sexual behaviors or activities
2. Limitations in sexual behaviors or activities
3. Changes in sexual behaviors or activities

C. General related factors/etiologies

1. Knowledge deficit concerning alternative responses to health-related problems
2. Altered body structure or function
3. Impaired relationship with significant other
4. Availability of significant other for sexual relationship
5. Pain
6. Behavioral and/or cognitive abnormalities
7. Positioning problems
8. Mobility deficit
9. Depression
10. Altered elimination pattern

D. Additional disability-specific related factors

1. Stroke
   a. Sensory deficits
   b. Communication deficits
   c. Visual-perceptual deficits
   d. Personality changes
   e. Fear of further stroke
   f. Emotional lability
   g. Fatigue
   h. Decreased or increased libido
2. Arthritis
   a. Fatigue
   b. Mucosal dryness
   c. Inflammation
   d. Fear
3. TBI
   a. Impulsivity
   b. Sexual acting out
   c. Inappropriate social skills
   d. Personality changes
   e. Impaired libido
4. SCI
   a. Paralysis
   b. Loss of sensation
   c. Spasticity
   d. Autonomic dysreflexia
   e. Decreased self-esteem

E. Interventions

1. *General*
   a. Provide uninterrupted intimate time for client and partner

b. Provide information on expanded concept of sexuality that includes ways to achieve intimacy by means other than intercourse
   1) Touching
   2) Caressing
   3) Use of a vibrator
   4) Massage
   5) Mood music and/or lighting
   6) Oral and/or genital techniques
   7) Masturbation
   8) Penile implants
   9) Pharmacologic injections to achieve erections
   10) Vacuum erection devices
   11) Erotic fantasy
   12) Use of erotic audiovisuals
c. Offer educational materials about human sexuality and reproduction as well as information regarding effects of neurological injury and disease on sexual function, relationships, and reproduction
d. Discuss or refer to other healthcare professionals for alternatives to reproduction and infertility (e.g., donor insemination, in vitro fertilization, gamete intrafallopian transfer, electroejaculation, electrostimulation, surrogacy, adoption)
e. Explain effects of client's medications on sexual function; explore alteration of medications to help protect developing fetus and nursing newborn
f. Explore opportunities for social contact (e.g., clubs, hobbies, classes, tours) and role playing to assist with dating and initiation of communication and to help client deal with altered body image
g. Describe measures and/or devices for dealing with bladder control, such as emptying before and after sexual activity, restricting fluids for about 3 hours prior to sexual activity; provide counseling on social skills to deal with bladder accidents and need for thorough hygiene prior to and after sexual activity to prevent urinary tract infections
   1) Indwelling catheters (for males) should be bent over shaft of penis; a condom then can be placed over bent catheter (Nornhold, 1984)
   2) Indwelling drainage system with an antireflux valve should be used for males and females
   3) Indwelling catheters (for females) should be anchored or taped away from vagina onto thigh
   4) External condom catheters should be removed, the penis cleansed, and the catheter replaced after sexual activity
h. Stress importance of successful bowel program management and scheduling
i. Examine individualized birth control options that are acceptable and safe for patient
   1) Use of condoms, diaphragms, and contraceptive sponges requires dexterity or assistance; methods may not be practical for those with arthritis, brain injury, quadriplegia, or stroke
   2) Rhythm method requires adequate memory or another's assistance and may be difficult to maintain for those with brain injury or stroke
   3) Oral contraceptives are not indicated for females with SCI, circulatory problems, stroke, diabetes, or bed rest due to increased risk of thrombus formation (Garden, 1990)
   4) Intrauterine devices are contraindicated for females with spinal cord injury (SCI) because any migration into the uterine wall may go unnoticed due to loss of sensation
j. Discuss caregiving tasks preferred by partners that client finds distressing in terms of self-esteem and sexual identity; help identify alternate caregiving strategies to help maintain previous relationships and sexual roles (McCormick, Riffer, & Thompson, 1986; Sjogren, Damber, & Liliequist, 1983)
k. Refer client to appropriate healthcare providers, as necessary, for any of the aforementioned interventions

2. *Stroke*
   a. Instruct on positioning techniques for hemiplegia
      1) Suggest that patient lie supine or lie on the affected side supported with pillows, which leaves unaffected arm free to caress partner
      2) Use supine position if pain is present in affected shoulder
      3) Counsel partner to take active role and focus on caressing client's uninvolved side, regardless of positioning style (Conine & Evans, 1982; Garden, 1990)
   b. Emphasize that likelihood of sexual excitement's bringing on another stroke is unsupported by research in stabilized ischemic stroke; those with hemorrhagic stroke should consult their physician as to their readiness for the energy expenditure this activity requires (Burgener & Logan, 1989; Muckleroy, 1977)
   c. Consider methods of managing erectile dysfunction and penile vascular insufficiency
      1) Blood pressure medications
      2) Penile prosthesis
      3) Use of vacuum erection device
      4) Pharmacologic injections
3. *Arthritis (hip and knee disease)*
   a. Identify communication skills that couples can use to clarify what causes pleasure or discomfort during sexual activity to prevent misinterpretation
   b. Describe positions and use of pillows to maximize comfort and avoid weight on affected joints (Brandt & Potts, 1987)
   c. Give instructions on using therapeutic modali-

Table 19.3. Probable Sexual Dysfunctions Following Complete SCI

Sexual Reponses	Responses in Persons with Injury at T10-L1 and Above	Responses in Persons with Injury at L2 and Below
Genital sensations	Not possible because pathways between the genitals and the brain have been interrupted	Not possible, but vague internal feelings are possible; some visceral connections to the brain are still present
Erection created by touch or tactile stimulation	Still possible, if the sacral segments are still intact; reflex erections occur	Not usually possible; the reflex arc is lost
Erection created by mental stimulation	Not possible; fibers from the brain are interrupted	Possible; sympathetic pathways from the brain are open to bring signals to T10-L1
Ejaculation and/or orgasm	Not possible; the necessary genital-to-brain-to-genital contact is lost	Not possible; the necessary genital-to-brain-to-genital contact is lost
Erotic mental feelings	Possible when the intact areas are stimulated	Possible when the intact areas are stimulated

ties (e.g., warm baths, applying heat to joints, doing range-of-motion exercises, using water-soluble lubricants during massage) and analgesics prior to sexual activity; stress that these can be incorporated into foreplay (Brandt & Potts, 1987; Katz, 1989)

d. Instruct on ways to prevent dislocation of prostheses after hip open reduction and internal fixation (ORIF)
   1) Avoidance of vigorous thrusting until 6 to 8 weeks after surgery
   2) Avoidance of hip flexion to no more than 60 degrees
   3) Avoidance of hip abduction to no more than 30 degrees for involved hip; external rotation of no more than 45 to 60 degrees in unilateral hip disease
   4) Sometimes these restrictions are lifted 3 to 6 months after surgery (Fuchs & Salvati, 1989)
   5) Clients can position themselves on their unaffected side, facing toward or away from partner; the affected leg should be partially flexed at hip and/or knee and supported on a pillow; clients also can lie supine with their knees bent over side of bed (Fuchs & Salvati, 1989)
   6) Male clients can lie supine with their partners on top; in a position that allows rear entry; or a side-lying position with affected leg supported by pillow or partner's thigh (Brandt & Potts, 1987; Fuchs & Salvati, 1989); encourage partner to take an active role (Friedmann, 1977)

4. *Traumatic brain injury*
   a. Sexuality is influenced or related to several factors
      1) Sensorimotor impairments
      2) Impulsivity
      3) Sexual acting out
      4) Inappropriate social skills
      5) Poor memory
      6) Personality changes
      7) Communication impairments
      8) Libido impairments
   b. Enforce privacy and consistent daily routine
   c. Explain to client that self-exposure or masturbation is appropriate only in private
   d. Consistently and nonjudgmentally redirect inappropriate sexual behavior
      1) Describe inappropriate behavior
      2) Explain why behavior is inappropriate and what its effect on others is
      3) Explain and have client practice preferred behaviors
      4) Praise and/or reward client for appropriate sexual behavior
   e. Implement in-depth training in social skills and role playing about topics such as manners, eye contact, territorial space, social contacts, conversation, and dating
   f. Explain positioning options as described in the section on stroke interventions on page 165
5. *Spinal cord injury*
   a. Several factors can affect sexual function and/or relationships (see Table 19.3)
      1) Paralysis
      2) Sensation
      3) Spasticity
      4) Autonomic dysreflexia
   b. When treating client who has reflex or psychogenic reflex dysfunction that causes erections to be inadequate for intercourse, explain options such as a penile prosthesis, a vacuum erection device, and pharmacologic erection injections
   c. Explain causes of and options for dealing with anorgasmia
   d. Provide anticipatory counseling on communica-

tion skills, especially those concerning sexual activity with a new partner; discuss dating issues related to being in a wheelchair

e. Encourage exploration of methods to enhance sexual activity (e.g., using a firm surface to conserve motion or using a waterbed to enhance motion)
f. Explain electroejaculation and electrostimulation; explain how placing an electrical probe into rectum or using a vibratory device on corona of glans penis can be used to assist in conception (Smith, 1989; Szasz & Carpenter, 1989)

F. Expected outcomes

1. Client reports satisfying sexuality, sexual activity, and relationships
2. Client demonstrates adequate and safe use of birth control
3. Client achieves pregnancy as desired
4. Client verbalizes knowledge about prevention of sexually transmitted diseases

References

Berard, E.J.J. (1989). The sexuality of the spinal cord woman: Physiology and pathophysiology. A Review. In *Paraplegia, 27*(2), 99-112.

Brandt, K.D., & Potts, M.A. (1987). Arthritis in the elderly: Assessment and management of sexual problems. *Medical Aspects of Human Sexuality, 21*(3), 57-67.

◆Burgener, S., & Logan, G. (1989). Sexuality concerns of the poststroke patient. *Rehabilitation Nursing, 14*, 178-181, 195.

Conine, T.A., & Evans, J.H. (1982). Sexuality reactivation of chronically ill and disabled adults. *Journal of Allied Health, 11*(4), 261-270.

Friedmann, L.W. (1977). Sexual adjustment in patients with acute and chronic back pain. *Medical Aspects of Human Sexuality, 11*(11), 65-66.

Fuchs, M.D., & Salvati, E.A. (1989). Sexual counseling following total hip replacement. *Medical Aspects of Human Sexuality, 23*(4), 55-57.

Garden, F.H. (1990). Sex after stroke. *Medical Aspects of Human Sexuality, 24*(3), 27-30.

Geiger, R.C. (1979) Neurophysiology of sexual response in spinal cord injury. *Sexuality and Disability, II*(4), 257-266.

Griffith, E.R., & Trieschmann, R.B. (1975). Sexual functioning in women with spinal cord injury. *Archives of Physical Medicine and Rehabilitation, 56*, 18-21.

Katz, W.A. (1989). Arthritis in women: How does it affect sexuality? *Feminine Patient, 14*(11), 36.

MacLeod, J., & Gold, R.Z. (1951, September). The male factor in fertility and known fertility and in 1000 cases of infertile marriage. *Journal of Urology, 66*, 436-449.

Masters, W.H., & Johnson, V.E. (1966). *Human sexual response.* Boston: Little, Brown & Company.

Masters, W.H., & Johnson, V.E. (1970). *Human sexual inadequacy* (3rd ed.). Boston: Little, Brown & Company.

McCormick, G.P., Riffer, D.J., & Thompson, M.M. (1986). Coital positioning for stroke afflicted couples. *Rehabilitation Nursing, 11*(2), 17-19.

Muckleroy, R.N. (1977). Sex counseling after stroke. *Medical Aspects of Human Sexuality, 11*(12), 115-116.

Nornhold, P. (1984). Sex and the Foley catheter. *Nursing 84, 14*(5), 98-101.

Rabin, B.J. (1980). The *sensuous wheeler: Sexual adjustment for the spinal cord injured.* Long Beach, CA: Author.

◆Sjogren, K., Damber, J., & Liliequist, B. (1983). Sexuality after stroke with hemiplegia. *Scandinavian Journal of Rehabilitation Medicine, 15*(2), 55-61.

Smith, I. (1989). Shattering the myths: Sexuality in rehabilitation. *Rehabilitation Management, 3*(2), 28-34.

◆Szasz, G., & Carpenter, C. (1989). Clinical observations in vibratory stimulation of the penis of men with spinal cord injury. *Archives of Sexual Behavior, 18*, 461-474.

Zejdlik, C.J. (1992). *Management of spinal cord injury* (2nd ed.). Boston: Jones and Bartlett Publishers.

Suggested Readings

Barnett, K.M., & Desautels, R.E. (1989). Sexual dysfunction in diabetes. In L.P. Krall & R.S. Beaser (Eds.), *Joslen's diabetes mellitus* (pp. 686-697). Philadelphia: Lea and Febiger.

Brenner, H., & Sipski, M. (1991). Female sexual functioning following spinal cord injury. *Sexuality Update, 4*(1), 14-17.

Cole, T.M., & Cole, S.S. (1982). Rehabilitation of problems of sexuality in physical disability. In F.J. Kottke, G.K. Stillwell, & J.F. Lehmann (Eds.), *Krusen's handbook of physical medicine and rehabilitation* (pp. 889-905). Philadelphia: W.B. Saunders Company.

Gambert, S.R. (1990). Sex and type 2 diabetes. *Medical Aspects of Human Sexuality, 24*(5), 18-25.

Jain, H., Shamoian, C.A., & Mobarek, A. (1987). Sexual disorders in the elderly. *Medical Aspects of Human Sexuality, 21*(3), 15-16.

◆Sjogren, K. (1983). Sexuality after stroke. *Scandinavian Journal of Rehabilitation Medicine, 15*(2), 63-69.

Walbroel, G.S. (1990). Better sex for the older patient. *Medical Aspects of Human Sexuality, 24*(3), 15-16.

Wexler, N.R. (1985). Sexuality and the elderly. *Health Watch, 19*(11), 13, 31.

Williams, L. (1986). Strategies for sexual counseling. *Rehabilitation Nursing, 11*(5), 21-22.

Williams, L. (1989). Pharmacologic erection programs: A treatment option for erectile dysfunction. *Rehabilitation Nursing, 14*, 264-268.

◆ indicates a research-based work

CHAPTER 20

Coping–Stress Tolerance Pattern

Coping is a dynamic multidimensional process employed in response to internal, external, or system changes that alter or place stress on the individual and/or the ecological system. Stressors can arise from developmental (maturational) and situational events. Acute, traumatic, and chronic stressors can elicit differing coping behaviors. For example, an individual's responses, coping skills, and style; perceptions or definitions of the stressor; defenses (lines of resistance); and beliefs about control all influence the outcome. An individual can be coping with multiple combinations of stressors simultaneously. The nurse's assessment should incorporate temporal factors and the changing stages or steps common to coping processes.

Family and social support as well as individual strengths and needs are key indicators of outcome. They potentially promote wellness or, at other times, create incompatible styles that result in conflict or maladaptive coping. The nurse must have a repertoire of intervention strategies for working with individuals and families to improve coping skills. Coping behaviors are manifested through cognitive function, motor actions, affective responses, and psychological defense mechanisms.

Clients in rehabilitation experience varying degrees or levels of loss. These losses often result in an alteration of basic needs, cognition, or functional independence. Along with their families, they cope with irreversible chronic, progressive, or recurrent stressors. The clients' stressors require assisted care or adaptive devices and equipment to maintain optimal function, independence, quality of life, or survival. Effective coping skills establish patterns for managing environmental, economic, cultural, and psychosocial-emotional issues as well as for meeting physical needs. A client who is adapting to uncertainty, fear, concern about relationships, or loss of self may be vulnerable to acquiring dysfunctional coping patterns such as learned helplessness. Ineffective individual and family coping are included as the diagnostic categories in this chapter.

Rehabilitation nurses use theory-based assessments to plan therapeutic interventions and evaluate outcomes. They assist the client, family, community, and other rehabilitation team members with strategies for developing and maintaining effective long-term coping patterns. A client's coping is dynamic and ongoing 24 hours a day throughout the life span and changes with the client's status or perception of life events. Working within standards of practice, rehabilitation nurses set mutual goals with clients and their families. Rehabilitation nurses coordinate all levels of care and services, including nurse-to-nurse referrals with community agencies and transitions among levels or types of services such as those provided in schools, workplaces, or after-care settings.

I. Related Theory and Concepts

A. Stress

1. Classic theory identifying human responses to stress described a fight-or-flight reaction, detailing a set of universal physiological reactions generated when a person was confronted with stimuli evoking fear or anxiety (general adaptation syndrome) and physical adaptation to reattain homeostasis (Selye, 1956)
2. Researchers examined characteristics within coping styles that enabled individuals to experience differing outcomes as a result of similar stress-producing life events (Dohrenwend, 1973)

B. Family systems and social supports

1. Individuals and families have specific tasks assigned at progressive stages of development (Duvall, 1971)
2. Family dynamics, needs, and strengths change upon stressful encounters (Ackerman, 1958)
   a. Coping styles change
   b. A family's perception of disorganization following a stressful event can be charted by depth and extent of time, energy, and resources necessary to adapt its system to a tolerable, but not necessarily effective, outcome (Hill, 1949)
   c. Social support and networks are emerging as key factors in the individual's and the family's successful adjustment following crises
   d. Awareness of and concern about the often unrelenting burdens assumed by caregivers has targeted intervention by respite, advocacy, or discussion groups, or by supplemental services to support care
   e. Models used in rehabilitation assessment of family coping include the double ABCX model (McCubbin & Patterson, 1983), which guides interventions and addresses adaptation, adjustment, perception, and change
      1) A = stress and change
      2) B = family resources
      3) C = family perception
      4) X = family crisis and adaptation
   f. Preventive ecological approach addresses and improves outcome for individual, family, and

community; the family as a unit of service is a key factor enabling community living for many, especially children

C. Loss and change

1. Other early research findings document situational crisis responses among persons who are experiencing acute psychosocial-emotional events (Caplan, 1964) and among families who are acutely grieving lost members following disasters (Lindemann, 1944)
2. When an event surpasses an individual's capacity for coping and overwhelms his or her defensive lines of resistance (Neuman, 1982), or when chronic anxiety-producing situations multiply or recur, any attempts at coping become ineffective
3. Until recently, grieving and crisis resolutions were believed to occur within a limited time; however, ongoing studies reveal that coping may reflect recurrent or unresolved grieving or chronic sorrow for a perceived loss (Olshansky, 1962; Parad, 1965)
4. Loss due to impairment or disability places individual, family, and community at risk for ineffective coping (Vincent, 1985)
   a. Other factors influencing coping are related to amount or degree of stress individual or family is able or equipped to tolerate
   b. Whether the loss is situational or developmental, individual and family perceive a stressor, appraise it, and respond to eliminate or ameliorate anxiety at a tolerable level (Lazarus & Folkman, 1984)
   c. They call upon a repertoire of defense mechanisms to respond to anxiety-producing events; Roy refers to *innate or acquired mechanisms* (Roy, 1984)
   d. As a sequence of skills, selected defense mechanisms become incorporated into patterns, eventually forming a coping style; the patterns, or style, an individual or family chooses correlate with many factors

D. Decision-making and problem-solving patterns

1. Some coping styles are productive
   a. They lead to resolution, new behavioral responses for effective future problem solving, or ways of adapting to changes or completing a developmental task
   b. Problem-solving coping styles, rather than emotional styles, are related to effective decision making
2. Individuals with low self-esteem, altered body image, or external locus of control tend toward less effective decision making and emotional, rather than problem-solving, coping styles (Lazarus & Folkman, 1984)
3. Factors that influence response as defined by individual or family perception, culture, and meaning associated with an event
   a. Individual's personality and coping style prior to the stressor
   b. Individual's culture
   c. Individual's perception of the situation
   d. Previous successful experiences with problem solving
   e. Resources
   f. Hardiness (Pollock, 1989)
   g. Uncertainty (Mishel, 1990)
   h. Self-esteem
   i. Support systems
   j. Type or level and numbers of stressors
   k. Developmental stage

E. Systems responses

1. An ineffective coping style may alleviate an immediate anxiety while ultimately denying an opportunity for individual to develop successful problem-solving patterns and foster personal growth; however, as internal or external systems change, an individual or family may alter or modify coping styles to address new situations more effectively
2. Uncertainty about definition or outcome of an event prevents resolution and contributes its own stress
3. Effective coping behaviors arise in individuals who have a hardiness characteristic, who have an internal locus of control, and who are undaunted by change (Wallston & Wallston, 1982)
4. Dissatisfaction with or inadequacy of previous coping styles may become incentives for readiness to change; when in unresolved crisis, individual may regard any change as preferable to current anxiety, fatigue, and powerlessness

F. Change theory (see Chapter 23)

1. Planned change takes entire system into account, takes time, and provides for future building of problem-solving skills
2. Lewin (1958) suggested a theory for change
   a. Need for change occurs (unfreezing)
   b. Need is followed by working toward a new level (moving)
   c. Stabilization occurs (freezing)
3. Working toward change has a sequence
   a. Nursing diagnosis is made
   b. Alternatives are examined
   c. Action plans with goals are established
   d. Action plans are converted into change actions
4. Lack of adequate resources, multiple competing problems, or inability to detach from perceptions or environmental influences may interfere with or limit individual's motivation and capacity to implement changes
5. Nursing interventions to empower clients, families, and their communities improve outcomes for effective coping patterns

G. Learned helplessness

1. Psychological response to an adverse situation from which there appears to be no escape and which seems to have no solution
2. A belief that outcomes are uncontrollable; results in motivational, cognitive, and emotional deficits (Quinless & Nelson, 1988)

II. Nursing Assessment *(Author's note: Parents or significant caregivers should report for infants; the nurse should validate parents' reliability.)*

A. **History** is determined by asking questions about related factors

1. Perception of stressors; history of outcome with stressors
   a. What does this situation or event mean to you?
   b. Have you experienced similar events (or do you know others who have)?
   c. What are your major concerns apart from the immediate stressor?
   d. What do you think will happen as a result of this situation or event?
   e. Describe your feelings.
2. Past coping styles for managing stressful situations and outcome of using them
   a. Have you experienced losses in the past?
   b. How did you express stressful feelings or handle stress in the past?
   c. What do you think will be helpful to you?
3. Patterns of managing stress
   a. Has this situation or event produced changes in your lifestyle, health, occupation or education, functional independence, social system, quality of life, role in family, or values?
   b. What are your usual lifestyle coping patterns and behaviors?
   c. Do they include any of the following?
      1) Alcohol
      2) Drugs
      3) Food
      4) Sex
      5) Withdrawal or leaving
      6) Crying
      7) Acting out anger
      8) Medications
      9) Exercise
      10) Diversionary activities
      11) Other strategies
   d. Have these patterns and/or changes occurred since the situation or event?
   e. How does your family typically handle stress or loss?
4. Individual's perception of the loss, the extent of loss, and its severity
   a. What is most important to you at this time?
   b. How will this situation or event affect your life goals or your worth as an individual?
   c. Is this a chronic, episodic, or recurrent stressor?
   d. Before you experienced this situation or event, how did you perceive or describe another person who faced the disability or stressor you have?
   e. Why do you think this happened?
   f. Has this affected your ability to make decisions or the way you make decisions?
   g. Are you anxious or fearful?
   h. Are there other stressors in your life?
5. Type of crisis: Maturational, developmental, or situational
   a. What changes are occurring in your life now?
   b. Have you or your family recently added or lost a member (through marriage of a child, birth, death, divorce, or a long-distance move)?
   c. Are there unfulfilled needs or tasks in your life?
   d. What has produced or contributed to the current event?
   e. Who else in your family or support network is undergoing a crisis or stress?
6. Physical manifestations
   a. Will you be able to adhere to the medical regimen?
   b. Do you have pain, loss of ability, or questions about your condition?
7. Psychosocial and emotional manifestations
   a. What is your usual personality style?
   b. Since the situation or event, have you had difficulty with or changes in any of the following areas?
      1) Sleeping
      2) Eating
      3) Grooming
      4) Sexual activity
      5) Working
      6) Concentrating
      7) Communicating with others
      8) Practicing self-care skills
      9) Exhibiting emotions or thinking
   c. Are you concerned about how others will respond and who may reject you?
8. Knowledge about the condition or unmet needs
   a. What do you know about this situation or event?
   b. What do you think will happen as a result of this?
   c. How much or what kind of control do you have over what happens?
   d. Does anyone disagree with you about your responses to this situation? If so, who is it and what does he or she propose?
9. Assessment of internal and external resources, including education, income and employment, religion, supportive persons, pets, networks, living condition, assistive devices, other service agencies, interests or hobbies
10. Determination of the individual's personal goals
   a. What are your short-term and long-term rehabilitation goals?
   b. How much control do you think you will have in your planning and care?
   c. How do you think other people view you?
   d. What are your strengths and needs?
   e. Why do you think this event happened to you?
   f. How will this affect your future?

B. **Examination**

1. Monitor patient's vital signs and review body systems for symptoms of stress
   a. Cardiac: Racing pulse, palpitations, fainting
   b. Pulmonary: Shortness of breath, hyperventilation
   c. Gastro/urinary: Nausea, indigestion, burping,

diarrhea, constipation, irritable bowel, urinary frequency
d. Neuromuscular: Headache, pain, fatigue, neckache
e. General: Skin, posture, nervous habits
2. Inspect patient's physical appearance for signs of poor grooming, inadequate sleep, or crying
3. Inspect patient's altered body part or site of injury, impairment, or disability
4. Observe patient's affect, mood, or nonverbal cues such as crying, lack of eye contact or withdrawal response, anger or irritability, inappropriate type or level of activity, twitching or picking on body surfaces or clothing; in children, look for excessive sleeping, sucking on hands, or avoiding responding while seemingly engrossed in play
5. Elicit patient's current definition or denial of stressor; note his or her ability to describe it in present, to verbalize need for help, and to identify and/or describe situation accurately
6. Observe patient for self-destructive manifestations and signs of illness, injuries, or potential safety problems; measure weight gain or loss, possibility of eating disorder, excessive alcohol or drug use, or smoking
7. Evaluate sensory manifestations, concentration or memory loss, changes in speech pattern or communication, depression
8. Observe for signs of social or emotional deprivation
9. Assess patient's body image, excessive grieving, destructive or inappropriate mood swings or behavior, withdrawal, low self-esteem, or responses that represent worry, anxiety, or hopelessness, powerlessness, and/or helplessness
10. Assess family and social support; compare client's perspective on them with that of others and that of the nursing assessment; identify client's strengths, needs, and factors that affect his or her coping response

III. Nursing Diagnoses

➤ A. Ineffective individual coping

1. **Definition:** Temporary, recurrent, or permanent impairment of person's adaptive behaviors and problem-solving abilities in meeting life's demands and roles (Gordon, 1993)

2. **Major defining characteristics**

a. Inability to solve problems
b. Change in social interaction or participation
c. Change in communication patterns: Verbal manipulation, verbal hostility
d. Inability to meet own basic needs
e. Vulnerability to illness; high accident rate
f. Inability to meet age- and/or development-related role expectations or tasks
g. Destructive behavior toward self or others
h. Distorted belief and/or value system
i. Inappropriate behavior, activity, responses, and inability to delay gratification
   1) Chronic fatigue
   2) Depression
   3) Withdrawal
   4) Hyperactivity
   5) Denial of the problem
   6) Inability to ask for help
   7) Unresolved grieving
j. Substance abuse or addictive behavior
k. Poor self-esteem; external locus of control
l. Learned helplessness

3. **Related factors/etiologies**

a. Developmental and/or maturational crises
b. Situational crises
c. Individual vulnerability or resistance factors and/or defenses
d. Impaired cognition or neurological system
e. Long-term disability, resulting in many life changes
f. Altered sensory system and overload; chronic pain
g. Inadequate or complete lack of social and/or support systems
h. Altered locus of control; unrealistic perceptions
i. Low self-esteem; poor or distorted body image
j. Unresolved, chronic, or incomplete grieving
k. Childhood trauma or posttraumatic stress disorder
l. Unmet needs or development in a dysfunctional family situation
m. Inadequate basic health-wellness patterns (e.g., poor nutrition or inadequate sleep-rest patterns)
n. Cultural patterns, socioeconomic factors
o. Major change in life (e.g., moving to new location, employment problems, socioeconomic status)

4. **Interventions**

a. Maintain safe environment for the individual
b. Assess patient's coping skills; identify ineffective coping and degree of impairment
c. Promote and reinforce problem-solving and coping behaviors and techniques
d. Educate individual about the crisis or stressor and its related conditions and/or factors
e. Reinforce importance of decision making by including the individual in planning and goal setting
f. Restore or improve individual's self-esteem, maintain hope, and develop empowerment
g. Establish health prevention, maintenance, and a wellness and/or exercise program
h. Develop trust and rapport with client to guide open, honest communication
i. Resolve grieving and loss issues
j. Use interventions appropriate for client's developmental stage
k. Promote strengthening of family and social support systems
l. Evaluate assistive devices or equipment that could assist individual with independent living

or self-care activities

m. Employ therapeutic interventions such as relaxation techniques, reframing perceptions, participating in previously gratifying activities, or participating in structuring a schedule or regimen
n. Restore optimal level of independent self-care and decision making
o. Prevent further disability or complications
p. Assist client in finding access to resources, services, and activities for improving independence

5. Expected outcomes

a. Client gives evidence of improvement in coping skills and tolerance for stress
b. Client expresses increased psychological and physiological comfort
c. Client expresses feelings of greater control over stressors
d. Client gives evidence of improvement in problem-solving and decision-making skills

➤ B. Ineffective family coping

1. Definition: A significant other's behavior disables his or her own capacities and client's capacities to effectively address tasks essential to either person's adaptation to health challenge (Gordon, 1993)

2. Major defining characteristics

a. Neglect of client's basic needs (may be selective)
b. Denial or avoidance of assistance; neglect in obtaining care for illness or disability
c. Denial of client's health problem, severity of problem, or needs (prolonged denial may lead to abuse); abuse
d. Rejection, abandonment, or desertion of client
e. Detrimental or interfering family actions or decisions related to client's welfare and social or economic wellness
f. Disorganized, disintegrated, and dysfunctional family process and dynamics with disruption of structure, role functions, communication patterns, or interpersonal relationships
g. Demonstration of inadequate emotional problem-solving and decision-making abilities and poor verbalization skills
h. Maladaptive or negative family coping behaviors
   1) Blaming or fault finding
   2) Aggression
   3) Depression
   4) Abuse or neglect
   5) Hostility
   6) Stigmatizing
i. Lack of understanding or participation as well as a knowledge deficit about client's condition or prognosis
j. Overprotection and overconcern versus guilt, learned helplessness, powerlessness, or hopelessness
k. Impaired health maintenance behaviors (e.g., poor nutrition, inadequate sleep, decreased activity)
l. Inability to maintain and provide diversional or recreational activities or essential family services (e.g., child care, cleaning, shopping, family social activities)
m. Lack of social support networks or systems

3. Related factors/etiologies

a. Psychosomatic conditions (e.g., family members taking on symptoms of the client's illness), preoccupation with fear, anxiety, guilt, anticipatory grief, helplessness, and/or powerlessness
b. Family distress in values, beliefs, or spiritual strengths
c. Impaired understanding or knowledge deficit regarding client's perception of event, illness, or injury
d. Family crisis due to an inability to deal with family developmental tasks, multiple stressful changes; changes in membership status, resources, or lifestyle/events; or unresolved coping with previous events
e. Unresolved grieving, coping, or anxiety
f. Significant other who has chronic psychosocial and/or emotional symptoms such as guilt, despair, hostility, or anxiety
g. Impaired development
   1) Lack of sense of self as an individual
   2) Impaired independent living
   3) Breakdown in interpersonal relationships
h. Change in environment, social networks or supports, security, or socioeconomic status

4. Interventions

a. Help family members verbalize their perceptions of and knowledge about the stressor event
b. Encourage clarification and decision making within framework of problem-solving approaches to coping and resolution
c. Encourage family's active participation in therapeutic activities, planning, setting goals, and expected outcome
d. Educate family about event and client's condition, providing opportunities for improving capabilities and empowerment
e. Identify barriers to effective coping
f. Assist family in planning for scheduling and daily activities, managing resources, interacting with other agencies and services, meeting needs of other family members, and maintaining a lifestyle of wellness
g. Refer family to other resources or specialized services as appropriate
h. Reassess periodically, allowing for dynamic nature of change and a complex system
i. Use contracts, maintenance of daily or weekly records, and other techniques to help family meet goals

5. Expected outcomes

a. Family expresses realistic understanding, expectations, and support for individual members
b. Client and family develop realistic goals and means for achieving them through a problem-solving method
c. Client and family demonstrate positive family coping and decision-making mechanisms
d. Client's and family's strengths, needs, culture, spiritual values, and lifestyle are incorporated by client, family, and professional caregivers into the plan for the future
e. All family members, extended family, and social networks are addressed in plan
f. Family maintains daily activities, wellness, and work activities
g. Family members complete stage-related developmental tasks
h. Family is empowered and capable of getting access to resources, making transitions among services and agencies, and allocating resources
i. Family members are active participants in plan, are knowledgeable about event or condition, and encourage client's self-care and, therefore, maximum independence
j. Family members resolve their loss and grieving, thereby enabling members to continue with meaningful roles and have potential for growth
k. Family members recognize potential problems or changes and seek preventive assistance from professionals

References

Ackerman, N.W. (1958). *The psychodynamics of family life.* New York: Basic Books.

Caplan, G. (1964). *Principles of preventive psychiatry.* New York: Basic Books.

Dohrenwend, B.S. (1973). Life events as stressors: A methodological inquiry. *Journal of Health and Social Behavior, 14,* 167-175.

Duvall, E.M. (1971). *Family development* (4th ed.). Philadelphia: J.B. Lippincott Company.

Gordon, M. (1993). *Manual of nursing diagnoses: 1993-1994.* St. Louis: Mosby-Year Book, Inc.

Hill, R. (1949). *Families under stress.* New York: Harper & Row Publishers, Inc.

Lazarus, R., & Folkman, S. (1984). *Stress, appraisal, and coping.* New York: Springer Publishing Company.

Lewin, K. (1958). Group discussion and social change. In E. Maccaby (Ed.), *Readings in social psychology* (3rd ed.). New York: Holt, Rinehart, & Winston.

Lindemann, E. (1944). The symptomatology and management of acute grief. *American Journal of Psychiatry, 101,* 141-148.

◆McCubbin, H.I., & Patterson, J. (1983). The family stress process: The double ABCX model of adjustment and adaptation. In H. McCubbin, M. Sussman, & J. Patterson (Eds.), *Social stress and the family: Advances and developments in family stress theory and research* (pp. 7-37). New York: Haworth Press.

◆Mishel, M.H. (1990). Reconceptualization of the uncertainty in illness theory. *Image: Journal of Nursing Scholarship, 22,* 256-262.

Neuman, B. (1982). *The Neuman systems model: Application to nursing education and practice.* Norwalk, CT: Appleton-Century-Crofts.

Olshansky, S. (1962). Chronic sorrow: A response to having a mentally defective child. *Social Casework, 43,* 190-193.

Parad, H.J. (1965). *Crisis intervention: Selected readings.* New York: Family Service Association of America.

Pollock, S.E. (1989). The hardiness characteristic: A motivating factor in adaptation. *Advances in Nursing Science, 11*(2), 53-62.

Quinless, F.W., & Nelson, M.A. (1988). Development of a measure of learned helplessness. *Nursing Research, 37*(1), 11-15.

Roy, C. (1984). *Introduction to nursing: An adaptation model* (2nd ed.). Englewood Cliffs, NJ: Prentice-Hall.

Selye, H. (1956). *The stress of life.* New York: McGraw-Hill Publishing.

Vincent, K.G. (1985). The validation of a nursing diagnosis: A nurse consensus study. *Nursing Clinics of North America, 20,* 631-640.

Wallston, K.A., & Wallston, B.S. (1982). Who is responsible for your health? The construct of locus of control. In G.S. Sanders & J. Suls (Eds.), *Social psychology of health and illness* (pp. 65-95). Hillsdale, NJ: Lawrence Erlbaum and Associates.

Suggested Readings

◆Austin, J., Patterson, J., & Huberty, T. (1991). Development of the Coping Health Inventory. *Journal of Pediatric Nursing, 6*(3), 166-174.

◆Bach, J.R., Campagnolo, D.I., & Hoeman, S.P. (1991). Psychosocial aspects of long term mechanical, ventilatory support for patients with Duchenne muscular dystrophy. *American Journal of Physical Medicine and Rehabilitation, 70*(3), 129-135.

Bertino, L. (1989). Stress management with SCI patients. *Rehabilitation Nursing, 14,* 127-129.

◆Brillhart, B. (1986). Predictors of self-acceptance. *Rehabilitation Nursing, 11*(2), 8-12.

Brown, R. (1992). Psychosomatic problems in adolescents. *Adolescent Medicine: State of the Art Reviews, 3*(1), 87-96.

◆Buelow, J.M. (1991). A correlational study of disabilities, stressors, and coping methods in victims of multiple sclerosis. *Journal of Neuroscience Nursing, 23*(4), 247-252.

◆Call, J.G., & Davis, L.L. (1989). The effect of hardiness of coping strategies and adjustment to illness in chronically ill individuals. *Applied Nursing Research, 2*(4), 187-188.

◆Campbell, C.H. (1988). Needs of relatives and helpfulness of support groups in severe head injury. *Rehabilitation Nursing, 13,* 320-325.

◆Carmack, B.J. (1992). Balancing engagement/detachment in AIDS-related multiple losses. *Image: The Journal of Nursing Scholarship, 24*(1), 9-14.

Casas, M.S. (1989). Experience in coping with stroke: A survey of caregivers. *Journal of Rehabilitation, 55*(4), 37-43.

Cherry, D.B. (1989). Stress and coping in families with ill or disabled children: Application of a model to pediatric therapy. *Physical and Occupational Therapy in Pediatrics, 9*(2), 11-32.

Damrosch, S.P., & Perry, L.A. (1989). Self-reported adjustment, chronic sorrow, and coping of parents of children with Down's syndrome. *Nursing Research, 38*(1), 25-20.

DesRosier, M.B., Catanzaro, M., & Piller, J. (1992). Living with chronic illness: Social support and the well spouse perspective. *Rehabilitation Nursing, 17,* 87-91.

Dittmar, S. (1989). *Rehabilitation nursing.* St. Louis: The C.V. Mosby Company.

Dougherty, C.M. (Ed.). (1985). Nursing diagnosis. *Nursing Clinics of North America, 20,* 609-610.

Dubos, R. (1965). *Man adapting.* New Haven, CT: Yale University Press.

Ellis, J. (1991). How adolescents cope with cancer and its treatment. *Maternal Child Nursing, 16*(3), 157-160.

Engel, G. (1968). A life setting conducive to illness: The giving-up-complex. *Annals of Internal Medicine, 69*(20), 293-300.

Felton, B.J., Revenson, T.A., & Hinrichsen, G.A. (1984). Stress and coping in the explanation of psychological adjustment among chronically ill adults. *Social Science and Medicine, 18*, 889-898.

Frye, B.A. (1986). A model of wellness seeking behavior in traumatic spinal cord injury victims. *Rehabilitation Nursing, 11*(5), 6-14.

Gass, K.A., & Chang, A.S. (1989). Appraisals of bereavement, coping, resources, and psychosocial health dysfunction in widows and widowers. *Nursing Research, 38*(1), 31-36.

Gibbons, M.B. (1992). A child dies, a child survives: The impact of sibling loss. *Journal of Pediatric Health Care, 6*(2), 65-72.

Gillies, D.A. (1987). Family assessment and counseling by the rehabilitation nurse. *Rehabilitation Nursing, 12*, 65-69.

Graffi, S., & Minnes, P. (1989). Stress and coping in caregivers of persons with traumatic head injuries. *Journal of Applied Social Sciences, 13*, 295-315.

Grant, J.S., & Bean, C.A. (1988). Stress: An analysis and application to rehabilitation nursing. *Rehabilitation Nursing, 13*, 181-185.

Greene, J.W., Werner, M.J., & Walker, L.S. (1992). Stress and the modern adolescent. *Adolescent Medicine: State of the Art Reviews, 3*(1), 13-28.

◆Grey, M., Cameron, M.E., & Thurber, F.W. (1991). Coping and adaptation in children with diabetes. *Nursing Research, 40*(3), 144-149.

Hoeman, S.P. (1989). Cultural assessment in rehabilitation nursing practice. *Nursing Clinics of North America, 24*, 277-289.

Hoeman, S.P. (1990). *Rehabilitation/restorative care in the community*. St. Louis: The C.V. Mosby Company.

Keane, S., Chastain, B., & Rudisill, K. (1987). Caring: Nurse-patient perceptions. *Rehabilitation Nursing, 12*, 182-184.

◆Keefe, F.J., & Williams, D.A. (1990). A comparison of coping strategies in chronic pain patients in different age groups. *Journal of Gerontology, 45*(4), 161-165.

Kim, T-S. (1989). Hope as a mode of coping in amyotrophic lateral sclerosis. *Journal of Neuroscience Nursing, 21*, 342-347.

Kubler-Ross, E. (1969). *On death and dying*. New York: Macmillan Publishing Company.

◆Larsen, P.D. (1990). Psychosocial adjustment in multiple sclerosis. *Rehabilitation Nursing, 15*, 242-247.

Leidy, N.K., Ozbolt, J.G., & Swain, M.A. (1990). Psychophysiological processes of stress in chronic physical illness: A theoretical perspective. *Journal of Advanced Nursing, 15*, 478-486.

Lipsky, D.K. (1985). A parental perspective on stress and coping. *American Journal of Orthopsychiatry, 55*, 614-617.

Lubkin, I.M. (1990). *Chronic illness: Impact and interventions* (2nd ed.). Boston: Jones and Bartlett Publishers.

Mahon-Darby, J., Ketchik-Renshaw, B., Richmond, T., & Gates, E. (1988). Powerlessness in cervical spinal cord injury patients. *Dimensions of Critical Care Nursing, 7*, 346-355.

Maier, S. (1980). Learned helplessness and the schedule-shift hypothesis. *Journal of Research in Personality, 14*, 170-186.

Mandell, A.R., & Keller, S.M. (1986). Stress management in rehabilitation. *Archives of Physical Medicine and Rehabilitation, 67*, 375-379.

Maslow, A.H. (1968). *Toward a psychology of being*. New York: Van Nostrand Reinhold.

McCubbin, H.I., McCubbin, M.A., Patterson, J.M., Cauble, A.E., Wilson, L.R., & Warwick, W. (1983). CHIP—Coping Health Inventory for Parents: An assessment of parental coping patterns in the care of the chronically ill child. *Journal of Marriage and the Family, 45*, 359-370.

◆McCubbin, M.A. (1989). Family stress and family strengths: A comparison of single- and two-parent families with handicapped children. *Research in Nursing and Health, 12*(2), 101-110.

◆McNett, S.C. (1987). Social support, threat and coping responses, and effectiveness in the functionally disabled. *Nursing Research, 36*(2), 98-103.

Miller, J.F. (1983). *Coping with chronic illness: Overcoming powerlessness*. Philadelphia: F.A. Davis Company/Publishers.

◆Miller, P., Garrett, M.J., Stoltenberg, M., McMahon, M., & Ringel, K. (1990). Stressors and stress management 1 month after myocardial infarction. *Rehabilitation Nursing, 15*, 306-310, 318.

Moos, R.H. (Ed.). (1986). *Coping with life crises: An integrated approach*. New York: Plenum Press.

Norbeck, J.S. (1981). Social support: A model for clinical research and application. *Advances in Nursing Science, 3*, 43-59.

Nyhlin, K.T. (1990). Diabetic patients facing long-term complications: Coping with uncertainty. *Journal of Advanced Nursing, 15*, 1021-1029.

Piazza, D., & Foote, A. (1990). Roy's adaptation model: A guide for rehabilitation nursing practice. *Rehabilitation Nursing, 15*, 254-259.

Phillips, M., & Brostoff, M. (1989). Working collaboratively with parents of disabled children. *Pediatric Nursing, 15*(2), 180-185.

Power, P.W. (1985). Family coping behaviors in chronic illness: A rehabilitation perspective. *Rehabilitation Literature, 46*(3-4), 78-83.

◆Riffle, K.L. (1988). The relationship between perception of supportive behaviors of others and wives' ability to cope with initial myocardial infarctions in their husbands. *Rehabilitation Nursing, 13*, 310-315.

◆Sutton, T.D., & Murphy, S.P. (1989). Stressors and patterns of coping in renal transplant patients. *Nursing Research, 38*(1), 46-49.

Swanson, B., Cronin-Stubbs, D., & Sheldon, J.A. (1989). The impact of psychosocial factors on adapting to physical disability: A review of the research literature. *Rehabilitation Nursing, 14*, 64-68.

Tackett, P., Kerr, N., & Helmstadter, G. (1990). Stresses as perceived by children with physical disabilities and their mothers. *Journal of Rehabilitation, 56*(3), 30-34.

Van Clere, L. (1989). Parental coping in response to their child's spina bifida. *Journal of Pediatric Nursing, 4*, 172-176.

Wallander, J.L., & Varni, J.W. (1989). Social support and adjustment in chronically ill and handicapped children. *American Journal of Community Psychology, 17*(2), 185-201.

Wilson, H.S. (1989). Family caregiving for a relative with Alzheimer's dementia: Coping with negative choices. *Nursing Research, 38*(2), 94-98.

Wortman, C.B., & Silver, R.C. (1989). The myths of coping with loss. *Journal of Consulting and Clinical Psychology, 57*, 349-357.

Wright, B. (1983). *Physical disability: A psychosocial approach*. New York: Harper & Row Publishers, Inc.

◆ indicates a research-based work

CHAPTER 21

Value–Belief Pattern

This chapter addresses the concepts of values and beliefs and their impact on the rehabilitation client's sense of wholeness and sense of well-being. *Valuing* is the human response pattern involving the assigning of relative worth (Gordon, 1987), while *believing* is the human response pattern to developing faith, trust, or confidence in life as the rehabilitation client experiences it. Values and beliefs provide the basis for meaning in life. Viktor Frankl (cited in Bowers, 1987) wrote of the need to live meaningfully as a will or force in the individual. Distress of the human spirit occurs when this meaning is challenged or lost.

The advent of a disability creates a crisis in the life of a rehabilitation client that may test the client's and the family's values and beliefs. The rehabilitation nurse, as a result of his or her primary role in coordinating and overseeing the client's rehabilitation program, is in a position to identify distress of the human spirit and to develop a plan of care to assist the client in coping with and resolving it. If the client continues to demonstrate distress of the human spirit, the rehabilitation process will be affected; the client may withdraw, refuse to actively participate in the rehabilitation program, strike out at members of the rehabilitation team, and/or leave the rehabilitation program. The most effective intervention is the rehabilitation nurse's use of self, which can be a means of support and affirmation for the client. The rehabilitation nurse needs to be able to convey warmth, respect, and empathy. Spiritual well-being is achieved in the client who demonstrates a reality-based peace or who develops meaningful, purposeful behaviors. Only when the client is viewed holistically—as a composite of body, mind, and spirit—can the rehabilitation goals of optimal function and a sense of well-being be achieved.

I. Related Theory and Concepts

A. Disability results in disharmony among mind, body, and spirit

B. Spiritual dimension of an individual cannot be defined scientifically; although biologically not discernible, it is accepted in society as real (Piles, 1990)

C. Spirituality is a "quality that goes beyond religious affiliation, that strives for inspiration, reverence, and awe, even in those who do not believe in any God" according to Murray and Zentner (cited in Clifford & Gruca, 1987, p. 331)

D. Ruffing-Rahal stated that "spirituality involves a personal quest to find meaning and purpose in life and a relationship to the Mystery/God and the rest of the universe" (cited in Clifford & Gruca, 1987, p. 331)

E. Each person has a religious impulse, according to Maslow (cited in Hamner, 1990)

F. *Spirituality* refers to an activity of the human spirit that seeks or expresses a relationship with God or a higher power

G. The human spirit is nourished when spiritual needs are satisfied by experiencing transcendence, reaching out beyond oneself, and rising above painful circumstances; having a sense that life is meaningful and purposeful; finding opportunities to shape life creatively (Bowers, 1987)

H. Clients' and families' spiritual belief systems reflect the diversity of American culture

II. Nursing Assessment (Shelly & Fish, 1988; Stallwood, 1975)

A. Use religious values clarification scale

1. Questions to elicit client's beliefs about and involvement with God or a higher power and religious practice
   a. Are there any religious practices that are important to you?
   b. How is God or a higher power involved in your life?
   c. How would you describe God or a higher power?
2. Questions to determine extent to which client's religious practices serve as resource for faith and life
   a. Do you feel your faith is helpful to you? If so, how?
   b. How do prayer and other religious practices help you?
   c. Are religious books (e.g., Bible, *Koran*, *Book of Mormon*) helpful to you?
   d. Have any events or experiences changed your feelings about God or a higher power?
   e. Has your present disability made any difference in your faith?
3. Questions to assess whether client's resources for hope and strength are founded on reality
   a. In what ways is your faith important to you now?
   b. What helps you most when you feel alone or afraid?
   c. Is there anything you are hoping for right now?
   d. What is your source of strength right now?
4. Questions that give client an opportunity to accept spiritual help
   a. How can I help you in carrying out your faith?

b. Would you like me to pray for you or read the Bible or other religious books to you?
c. Would you like a visit from your pastor or the hospital chaplain?

B. Observe for presence of religious or spiritual articles (e.g., medals, texts, or clothing)
C. Observe for visits from a spiritual leader or adviser
D. Assess responses during interview on spiritual matters for presence of anxiety, depression, or anger
E. Listen and observe attentively while providing care

➤ III. Nursing Diagnosis: Spiritual Distress (Distress of the Human Spirit)

A. Definition: Distress of the human spirit is a disruption in the life principle that pervades a person's entire being and that integrates and transcends one's biologic and psychosocial nature (NANDA, 1992)

B. Major defining characteristics

1. Expression of concern about meaning of life and death and/or belief systems
2. Verbalization of inner conflict about beliefs and/or concerns about a relationship with a deity
3. Seeking of spiritual assistance
4. Inability to participate in usual religious practices
5. Questions about meaning of a person's own existence and/or suffering
6. Alteration in behavior or mood evidenced by anger, crying, withdrawal, preoccupation, anxiety, hostility, or apathy

C. Related factors/etiologies

1. Separation from religious and cultural ties
2. Challenged belief and value system
3. Sense of meaninglessness or purposelessness
4. Remoteness from God or a higher power
5. Moral or ethical nature of therapy
6. Intense suffering
7. Anger toward or blaming of God or a higher power
8. Pathophysiological factors such as loss of body part or function, debilitating disease, pain, or trauma (Thompson, McFarland, Hirsch, Tucker, & Bowers, 1986)

D. Interventions

1. Be aware of your own spirituality and what it means in your life and profession
2. Develop trust with your clients by listening and by being present and responsive to their needs
3. Assure clients that you or another nurse will be available to support them in times of suffering
4. Be available as an advocate for clients' needs
5. Refer to spiritual adviser that client chooses
6. Prepare clients for religious rituals of their choice and provide setting and/or opportunity for those to take place
7. Provide clients with environment conducive to prayer
8. Offer to obtain religious articles for clients
9. Offer to pray with clients
10. Offer to read scripture, meditations, or poetry
11. Help clients maintain a diet with religious restrictions when it is not detrimental to their health
12. Encourage spiritual rituals that are not detrimental to health
13. Make a tape recorder or notebook available for keeping a journal so that clients can focus on their thoughts and feelings
14. Help clients see that anger toward God or a higher power is a common reaction to a disability; help them recognize and discuss their feelings of anger
15. Use questions about past beliefs and spiritual experiences to help clients in putting their life events into a wider perspective (Carpenito, 1989)

E. Expected outcomes

1. Client uses spirituality to enhance adaptation to disability
2. Client demonstrates confidence in expressing spiritual concerns
3. Client clarifies values and beliefs
4. Client describes a spiritual belief system positively
5. Client demonstrates reality-based peace and develops meaningful, purposeful behavior

References

Bowers, C.C. (1987). Spiritual dimensions of the rehabilitation journey. *Rehabilitation Nursing, 12*, 90-91.

Carpenito, L.J. (1989). *Nursing diagnosis: Application to clinical practice* (3rd ed.). Philadelphia: J.B. Lippincott Company.

Clifford, M., & Gruca, J.A. (1987). Facilitating spiritual care in the rehabilitation setting. *Rehabilitation Nursing, 12*, 331-333.

Gordon, M. (1987). *Nursing diagnosis: Process and application.* New York: McGraw-Hill Book Company.

Hamner, M.L. (1990). Spiritual needs: A forgotten dimension of care? *Journal of Gerontological Nursing, 16*(12), 3-4.

North American Nursing Diagnosis Association (NANDA). (1992). *NANDA nursing diagnoses: Definitions and classification 1992-1993.* St. Louis: Author.

Piles, C.L. (1990). Providing spiritual care. *Nurse Educator, 15*(1), 36-41.

Shelly, J.A., & Fish, S. (1988). *Spiritual care: The nurse's role* (3rd ed.). Downers Grove, IL: Inter-Varsity Press.

Stallwood, J. (1975). Spiritual dimensions of nursing practice. In I. Beland & J. Psassos (Eds.), *Clinical nursing* (3rd ed.) (p. 1088). New York: MacMillan Publishing Company.

Thompson, J.M., McFarland, G.K., Hirsch, J.E., Tucker, S.M., & Bowers, A.C. (1986). *Clinical nursing.* St. Louis: The C.V. Mosby Company.

Suggested Readings

Benner-Carson, V. (1989). *Spiritual dimensions of nursing practice.* Philadelphia: W. B. Saunders Company.

Burnard, P. (1990). Learning to care for the spirit. *Nursing Standard, 4*(18), 38-39.

Doenges, M., & Moorhouse, M. (1988). *Nursing diagnosis with intervention* (2nd ed.). Philadelphia: F.A. Davis Company/Publishers.

Forbis, P.A. (1988, May/June). Meeting patients' spiritual needs. *Geriatric Nursing*, pp. 158-159.

Labun, E. (1988). Spiritual care: An element in nursing care planning. *Journal of Advanced Nursing, 13*, 314-320.

◆Mettolm, F.A. (1991). A nursing diagnosis validation study: Defining characteristics of spiritual distress. In R.M. Carroll-Johnson

(Ed.), *Classification of nursing diagnoses: Proceedings of the ninth conference of the North American Nursing Diagnosis Association* (pp. 112-119). Philadelphia: J.B. Lippincott Company.

Roche, S.J. (1989). Spirituality and the ALS patient. *Rehabilitation Nursing, 14*, 139-141.

Saylor, D.E. (1991). Pastoral care of the rehabilitation patient. *Rehabilitation Nursing, 16*, 138-140.

◆Sodestrom, K.E., & Martinson, I.M. (1987). Patient's spiritual coping strategies: A study of nurse and patient perspectives. *Oncology Nursing Forum, 14*(2), 41-46.

◆ indicates a research-based work

Section IV
The Rehabilitation Team

In rehabilitation, the combined efforts of various individuals are critical because rehabilitation involves a holistic and comprehensive approach to health care. These individuals include the patient, healthcare professionals, and family members. They compose what practitioners in rehabilitation commonly refer to as *the team*. Team activity is synergistic, producing more than what each professional in the group could accomplish individually and separately (Melvin, 1980). The responsibility for rehabilitation does not belong to any single healthcare discipline, but, rather, to all those involved. This section includes the following topics that contribute to the success of the rehabilitation process: the rehabilitation team, the phenomenon of change, accreditation, quality improvement, and program evaluation.

Reference

Melvin, J.L. (1980). Interdisciplinary and multidisciplinary activities and American Congress of Rehabilitation Medicine. *Archives of Physical Medicine and Rehabilitation, 61,* 379-380.

CHAPTER 22

The Rehabilitation Team: Composition, Models, Functions, and Issues

Of all the members of the rehabilitation team, the rehabilitation client is considered most significant, having unique and complex physical, psychosocial, and spiritual attributes contributing to his or her identity. Alterations in any of these areas affect the function of the total being (Dittmar, 1989). By establishing and striving toward the achievement of common goals, the team strives to maintain client individuality and promote client autonomy within the parameters of the disability or chronic illness.

Because the mission of rehabilitation is to treat the multiple needs of the whole person, coordinated efforts by many specialists are necessary to enable the client to reach maximum potential (Keith, 1991). The Joint Commission on Accreditation of Healthcare Organizations (JCAHO, 1993) identifies the physician, rehabilitation nurse, physical therapist, occupational therapist, speech-language pathologist, and social worker as core team members (see Table 22.1). In addition to this group, the Commission for Accreditation of Rehabilitation Facilities (CARF, 1993) includes the psychologist and therapeutic recreational therapist. Depending on the setting, client population, and individual client needs, other professional team members may include the following: audiologist, chaplain, driving evaluator/instructor, nutritionist, orthotic/prosthetic specialist, pharmacist, rehabilitation engineer, respiratory therapist, and vocational counselor.

The team approach for the delivery of care and services to persons with disabilities has been the foundation of rehabilitation. In light of the current healthcare crises in the United States, however, alternative treatment models may be indicated as government and third-party payers demand tighter cost controls and resource utilization (Keith, 1991). Today's challenge, then, is to demonstrate and support the effectiveness of team functioning in order to ensure and provide quality care to the individuals whom we serve.

I. Rehabilitation Team Models: Common Characteristics, Unique Benefits, and Limitations

A. Types of models: Various team models are used both in facilities and the community; the models can be described as interdisciplinary, transdisciplinary, or multidisciplinary; they are hierarchically related, with the transdisciplinary model being the most sophisticated and the multidisciplinary model being the least sophisticated

B. Facility-based models
   1. Interdisciplinary model
      a. Characteristics
         1) *Interdisciplinary* refers to activities performed by team members from different disciplines to reach a common goal
         2) The interdisciplinary model is required by both the Joint Commission on Accreditation of Healthcare Organizations (JCAHO) (1993) and the Commission on Accreditation of Rehabilitation Facilities (CARF) (1993)
         3) This model involves members who are engaged in problem solving beyond the confines of their own discipline (Diller, 1990)
         4) Team meetings are held regularly (weekly or biweekly) to share information and discuss progress toward goals
         5) Team meetings should be a high-priority activity for nursing; accurate assessment of a client's progress without the input of nurses who coordinate client activities is difficult (O'Toole, 1992)
      b. Benefits
         1) Interdisciplinary model provides the team with a holistic view of client needs
         2) A comprehensive, consistent, nonfragmented approach fosters optimal client outcome
         3) Effective interdisciplinary team has the ability to reduce healthcare costs and improve client outcomes (O'Toole, 1992)
      c. Limitations (Melvin, 1989)
         1) Model is more complex and time-consuming than multidisciplinary approach
         2) Can create controversy over who should be considered team leader

Table 22.1. Core Members of the Rehabilitation Team and Their Functions

Core Team Members	Major Functions
Rehabilitation nurse Assists patient in achieving maximum independence 24 hours per day, 7 days per week	• Performs activities that maintain and restore function and prevent complications and further loss • Provides direct care • Directs carryover of skills taught and practiced during therapies • Coordinates daily schedule and team activities • Provides a therapeutic environment • Provides patient and family education • Acts as a patient and family advocate
Physician Typically a physician who specializes in physical medicine and rehabilitation	• Establishes a medical diagnosis and prognosis and provides medical management • Interprets results of radiologic and laboratory findings and special testing results • Prescribes treatments, medications, and therapeutic aids • Guides the progress of the treatment plan
Physical therapist Assists patient in functional restoration of mobility	• Addresses range of motion, strength, reflexes, tone, posture, gait, orthotic or prosthetic fit and function, and sensorimotor performance • Uses treatment modalities of heat and cold, hydrotherapy, electrical stimulation, massage, joint mobilization, and exercise • Trains patient in locomotion activities using orthoses, prostheses, crutches, canes, walkers, and wheelchairs
Occupational therapist Helps patients to restore function for optimal participation in activities of daily living, including work, school, family, community, and leisure activities	• Assists with activities of daily living and independent living skills • Addresses joint function and protection, coordination, endurance, body mechanics, and positioning • Guides the use of adaptive equipment and prosthetic devices; designs, fabricates, and applies orthotic devices • Evaluates home management, prevocational activities, and social skills • Participates in adaptation of physical and social environment
Speech-language pathologist Assists with communication disorders and dysphagia related to stroke, head trauma, and other neurologic conditions or surgical procedures	• Treats disorders of verbal and written language, articulation, fluency, and interactive communication • Treats comprehension, memory, and cognitive deficits • Coordinates use of appropriate verbal and nonverbal augmentative communication system • Directs treatment plan for patients with dysphagia
Social worker Assists with personal issues affected by disability	• Assesses coping history and current psychosocial adaptation to disability • Assesses availability of immediate or extended family members and support networks; provides counseling and support • Addresses housing, living arrangements, education, and employment issues • Discusses healthcare costs and coverage, financial resources, and transportation issues • Facilitates discharge planning and acts as a liaison between the patient and the family and community resources
Psychologist Evaluates and treats psychological and neuropsychological impairments relating to disability	• Assesses cognitive and emotional status of client to facilitate psychological treatment and adaptation to disability; counsels client and significant others with respect to limitations of and expectations about disability
Therapeutic recreational therapist Assists client with individual or group activities to promote social skills and constructive use of leisure time	• Involves client in recreational and leisure activities appropriate for age, disability, and environment; group activities and resocialization are a major focus in both hospital and community settings

Sources Consulted

Commission on Accreditation of Rehabilitation Facilities. (1993). *Standards manual for facilities serving people with disabilities.* Tucson: Author.

Dittmar, S.S. (1989). *Rehabilitation nursing.* St. Louis: The C.V. Mosby Company.

Joint Commission on Accreditation of Healthcare Organizations. (1993). *Accreditation manual for hospitals.* Oakbrook Terrace, IL: Author.

Rothberg, J.S. (1992). Knowledge of discipline, roles, and functions of team members. In *American Congress of Rehabilitation Medicine guide to interdisciplinary practice in rehabilitation settings* (pp. 44-71). Skokie, IL: American Congress of Rehabilitation Medicine.

2. Transdisciplinary model (Diller, 1990)
   a. Characteristics
      1) *Transdisciplinary* refers to reinforcing and teaching across all disciplines
      2) Is similar to interdisciplinary model; however, one or two individual healthcare professions are responsible for implementing the treatment plan
      3) Members of individual disciplines are available for consultation
      4) A high degree of communication and interaction, staff development, and flexible thinking are involved (Hoeman, 1992)
   b. Benefits
      1) Client experiences less stimulation and stress working with a limited number of individuals; this model is particularly beneficial for patients with a cognitive disorder—such as a traumatic brain injury or a developmental disability—who have greater difficulty tolerating multiple and frequently changing healthcare providers
      2) Staff resources are conserved
   c. Limitations (Melvin, 1989)
      1) Primary healthcare provider may not demonstrate expertise in all areas of the treatment plan
      2) Relative cost savings and effectiveness have not yet been demonstrated
3. Multidisciplinary model (Howard, 1991)
   a. Characteristics: *Multidisciplinary* refers to the activities of individuals from various disciplines who are required to know only the skills of their own discipline
   b. Benefits
      1) Minimal coordination is required
      2) Less time is required for team meetings
   c. Limitations
      1) Patient and/or family participation in the rehabilitation process is not encouraged
      2) Collaborative goal setting and evaluation of interventions are limited
      3) Treatment is fragmented, services are duplicated, creativity is limited, and effectiveness of care is compromised

C. Community-based models
   1. "Rehabilitation in a community setting is becoming recognized as a logical and essential step in the complex health system commonly encountered by persons with chronic, developmental, or disabling conditions" (Hoeman, 1992, p. 32)
   2. Principles and concepts related to community-based rehabilitation include the following: collaborations (interdisciplinary, transdisciplinary, and interagency); holistic and comprehensive services; self-care, maximum function, and prevention; focus on family and cultural values; and client and/or family as unit of service in the community (Hoeman, 1992)
   3. Case management model (see Chapter 25)
      a. Case manager performs overall coordination, possible supervision, and determination and/or selection of patient services (Rothberg, 1992)
      b. Case managers traditionally have been used by insurance companies, industries, and governmental agencies to coordinate services and control benefit utilization and costs; this model is receiving considerable attention as a way to coordinate care, achieve expected patient outcomes, and control costs on inpatient units (Pierog, 1991)
   4. Team-managed care (Leath, 1991)
      a. Case management and multidisciplinary models are combined
      b. Case manager coordinates team's efforts
      c. Team determines priority of client's needs and provides services to meet those needs
   5. Community-oriented primary care model (Tollman, 1991)
      a. Community-oriented primary care is a formalized way to practice primary health care in the community; its philosophy is to provide accessible health care to the entire community
      b. Defined and accessible programs are set up to address needs of a community
      c. Curative and preventive interventions are provided
      d. Community is involved in health promotion
      e. Multidisciplinary model is recommended
   6. Religion-based community care model
      a. Churches and synagogues are often the first places to which people turn when problems arise (Olson, Reis, Murphy, & Gehm, 1988); religious institutions have a history of responding to the physical, emotional, and social needs of members as well as their spiritual needs (Denny, 1990)
      b. Some religion-based programs collaborate with healthcare institutions and use case managers or advanced practice nurses to coordinate client services

II. Core Functions of the Rehabilitation Team

A. Core functions of the rehabilitation team (CARF, 1993; JCAHO, 1993)
   1. Assessment of the patient's needs and functional ability
   2. Development and documentation of an interdisciplinary treatment plan based on client's and team's goals
   3. Implementation of the treatment plan in an interdisciplinary manner
   4. Evaluation of the treatment plan to the extent to which goals are achieved by the patient
   5. Planning for patient discharge

B. Performing assessments
   1. Making initial assessments of patient's biologic and psychosocial needs
   2. Assessing capacities and disabilities
   3. Continually monitoring results of interventions

C. Setting goals
   1. Purpose

a. Goals serve as a foundation for planning treatment strategies
b. Goals help caregivers evaluate the rehabilitation process in relation to client-centered outcomes
c. Goals help the team to promote carryover of newly learned skills from therapy sessions to nursing unit
d. Goals help the healthcare team provide high-quality care in conjunction with cost containment

2. Characteristics of well-defined goals (Fralish, 1991)
   a. Meaningful to client and family
   b. Clear and specific
   c. Realistic and attainable
   d. Measurable and verifiable and related to projected outcomes
   e. Congruent with available funding sources
3. Types of goals (Fralish, 1991)
   a. Short-term goals: Related directly to achievement of long-term goals (e.g., the client will lock wheelchair brakes before transferring from wheelchair to bed or commode)
   b. Long-term goals: Developed for each portion of client's rehabilitation program and related to achievement of outcome goals (e.g., the client will not sustain an injury related to falling)
   c. Outcome goals: Anticipated status of client at discharge and 3 months after discharge from rehabilitation unit; include the areas of living, working, and community (e.g., client incorporates safe practices while engaging in activities of daily living at home and in the community)

D. Planning and implementing interventions
   1. Planned interventions toward rehabilitation goal achievement are based on client's healthcare problems, their etiology, and established team goals
   2. Interventions among disciplines may be different even though goals are the same—for example, interventions for self-bathing deficit for nurse would be assisting and/or supervising with bathing, for physical therapist would be teaching transfer techniques, and for occupational therapist would be providing assistive devices for bathing, while the team's overall goal for the client would remain independence in bathing

E. Performing evaluations and monitoring outcomes
   1. All disciplines evaluate and review client's progress regularly; if progress is being made toward goal achievement, treatment plans are continued
   2. If goal is met, new goals are established for client
   3. If client is incapable of performing a task required to complete a goal, appropriate changes are made in treatment plan

F. Planning for discharge (Povse & Keenan, 1981)
   1. Discharge planning is part of goal setting early in rehabilitation process; discharge planning promotes continuity of care (JCAHO, 1993)
   2. Coordinated and timely discharge planning is critical to the success of controlling inpatient length of stay and healthcare costs
   3. Team responsibilities related to discharge planning
      a. One team member coordinates discharge plans
      b. Team members discuss client's discharge needs and communicate that information to person responsible for coordinating discharge
      c. Team members assess skills that client and family must have and provide information accordingly
      d. Team members give opportunities to the client, family, and significant others to provide client care and demonstrate that they have learned the information and techniques provided
      e. Team determines the need for equipment and supplies and provides a means for obtaining them
      f. Team makes referrals to appropriate, available, and accessible resources
      g. Team communicates client's status and anticipated needs to referral agencies both verbally and in writing to ensure continuity of care
      h. Team initiates disengagement process from client and family to promote their independence after discharge and facilitate their transition to discharge setting
   4. Benefits of discharge planning (Povse & Keenan, 1981)
      a. Optimal level of health for client is promoted
      b. Diseases and complications related to the disability are prevented or minimized
      c. Number of visits and readmissions to acute healthcare facility is decreased
      d. Services are available and appropriate to meet clients' needs
      e. Duplication of services is minimized
      f. Overall cost of care is reduced

III. Issues Associated with the Rehabilitation Team: Leadership, Collaboration, Communication, and Conflict Resolution

A. Leadership
   1. The manner in which the team is led is the single most important element in determining the quality of teamwork (Francis & Young, 1979)
   2. Campbell (1992) believes that team leadership is a set of behaviors and skills that can be taught and learned and that team leadership is not vested in one person, but is the responsibility of the entire team
   3. The effectiveness of the team is increased when leadership acts are based on competence, expertise, and information—not perceived status or authority—and when it is relatively balanced among all team members (Garner, 1988)
   4. The program manager
      a. CARF (1993) requires the designation of a program manager
      b. Primary functions
         1) Coordinating team activities
         2) Ensuring appropriate use of resources
         3) Facilitating timely discharge of clients

5. Leadership activities
   a. Team building (Farley and Stoner, 1989)
      1) Team building is the process of deliberately creating and unifying a group of people into an effective and efficiently functioning work unit so that specified goals are accomplished; the process should enable the group to become more adept at pursuing its objectives and in identifying and resolving its own work-related problems
      2) Effective teams are nurtured and developed through the efforts of team members who consciously work at the process of team development
   b. Team enhancement (Campbell, 1992) involves fostering and supporting creativity, risk taking, and controversy and avoiding stagnation

B. Collaboration: Occurs when team members communicate openly to work together successfully and harmoniously
   1. A collaborative team has a strong philosophy related to acknowledging the human dignity that resides in all team members (Roseman, 1985)
   2. Researchers have identified collaboration as a vital factor in patient outcomes (Baggs, 1989)
   3. Negotiations are used to seek creative, integrated solutions to problems
   4. Information is communicated clearly and decision-making responsibility is defined clearly and supported by group consensus
   5. Boundaries and roles are well-defined (Cohen, Rubin, & Gombash, 1992)

C. Communication
   1. Increased communication is an extremely important factor in the success of an interdisciplinary team (Moulder, Staal, & Grant, 1988)
   2. Results of ineffective communication (Garner, 1988)
      a. Team experiences frustration and stress
      b. Inappropriate actions may be taken due to incomplete information
      c. Patients and/or families receive conflicting messages and instructions from members of different disciplines who are supposedly working together
   3. An effective communicator has the following attributes: accepts differences in perspectives of others; functions independently; negotiates roles with other team members; forms new values, attitudes, and perceptions; tolerates constant review and challenge of ideas; takes risks; possesses personal identity and integrity; and accepts the team philosophy of care (Given & Simmons, 1977)
   4. Communication can be formal or informal
      a. Formal communication
         1) Team conferences are held to discuss progress toward goal achievement; conferences are required by accrediting agencies
         2) Periodically, family conferences are conducted to help promote open communication among the client, his or her significant others, and healthcare professionals
         3) Administrative meetings are used to evaluate team process, program goals, financial resources, and future directions
         4) Newsletters highlight program activities and current rehabilitation practices
         5) Computerized schedule sheets or scheduling boards communicate therapy and treatment schedules
         6) Administrative reports document team's contributions to patient outcomes
         7) Notices apprise team of official policy, procedures, and protocols
      b. Informal communication
         1) Impromptu confidential conversations in hallways, at lunch, and at bedside provide team with current information
         2) Informal communication networks often circulate information more quickly than formal communication channels

D. Conflict resolution
   1. Conflict between and among individuals is common and necessary for team development; conflict among team members may serve as a catalyst for needed change
   2. Unresolved conflict can undermine the effectiveness of a group whose mission is ensuring individual functioning at the highest level of independence (Frank & Elliot, 1992)
   3. Causes of conflict (Roseman, 1980)
      a. Status issues (e.g., controversy about team leadership, equality of members, and professional rivalries)
      b. Communication obstacles (e.g., use of professional jargon, poor listening habits, or time limitations)
      c. Practice issues (e.g., role ambiguity or overlap, questions of competence)
      d. Decision-making conflicts (e.g., value conflicts, authoritarian approach)
      e. Organizational issues (e.g., contradictory institutional priorities, time constraints)
      f. Feelings of burnout caused by large caseload or staffing shortages
      g. Ineffective conflict resolution (e.g., avoidance, competition, forceful confrontation)
   4. Stages of conflict (Marriner, 1980)
      a. Latent conflict: Conflict is anticipated based on certain conditions such as scarcity of resources and changes in environment
      b. Perceived conflict: Cognitive awareness that a stressful situation is present
      c. Felt conflict: Affective states (e.g., stress, tension, anxiety, anger, hostility) are present
      d. Manifest conflict: Overt behavior results from perceived or felt conflict and can be either constructive or destructive
      e. Conflict aftermath: Conflict is resolved or avoided
   5. Strategies for preventing conflict (Cornett-Cooke & Dias, 1984)

a. Identify roles
   1) Reach team consensus on roles of team members
   2) Identify role overlap
   3) Negotiate role boundaries
b. Identify team's purpose: Articulate and negotiate team's goals
c. Improve communication—for example, orient new members and encourage constructive criticism of team process
d. Provide support to new team members and those experiencing staffing shortages or treating complex and challenging clients
e. Facilitate the group process by identifying the role of the group, informal and formal leaders, and team responsibilities; foster team building and enhancement

6. Strategies for resolving conflict (Levenstein, 1984)
   a. Clarify the common purpose
   b. Keep discussion relevant
   c. Agree on terminology
   d. Concentrate on facts
   e. Look for potential trade-offs
   f. Listen to each other and avoid debating tactics
   g. Recognize the uniqueness of each individual
   h. Be logical
   i. Pursue multidimensional solutions

References

◆Baggs, I. (1989). Intensive care unit use and collaboration between nurses and physicians. *Heart and Lung, 18*, 332-338.

Campbell, L.J. (1992). Team maintenance and enhancement. In *American Congress of Rehabilitation Medicine guide to interdisciplinary practice in rehabilitation settings* (pp. 173-187). Skokie, IL: American Congress of Rehabilitation Medicine.

Cohen, H., Rubin, A.M., & Gombash, L. (1992). The team approach to treatment of the dizzy patient. *Archives of Physical Medicine and Rehabilitation, 73*, 703-708.

Commission on Accreditation of Rehabilitation Facilities (CARF). (1993). *Standards manual for facilities serving people with disabilities.* Tucson: Author.

Cornett-Cooke, P., & Dias, K.K. (1984). Team building: Getting it all together. *Nursing Management, 15*(5), 16-17.

Denny, M.S. (1990). Church-based geriatric care. *Nursing Administration Quarterly, 14*(2), 65-66.

Diller, L. (1990). Fostering the interdisciplinary team, fostering research in a society of transition. *Archives of Physical Medicine and Rehabilitation, 71*, 275-278.

Dittmar, S.S. (1989). *Rehabilitation nursing.* St. Louis: The C.V. Mosby Company.

Farley, M.J., & Stoner, M.H. (1989). The nurse executive and the interdisciplinary team. *Nursing Administration Quarterly, 13*(2), 24-30.

Fralish, K.B. (1991). Measures of progress and outcome. In P.M. Deutsch & K.B. Fralish (Eds.), *Innovations in head injury rehabilitation* (pp. 13A-1–13A-23). New York: Mathew Bender Company.

Francis, D., & Young, D. (1979). *Improving work groups: A practical manual for team building.* San Diego: University Press.

Frank, R.G., & Elliot, T.R. (1992). Conflict resolution and feedback. In *American Congress of Rehabilitation Medicine guide to interdisciplinary practice in rehabilitation settings* (pp. 143-157). Skokie, IL: American Congress of Rehabilitation Medicine.

Garner, H.G. (1988). *Helping others through teamwork.* Washington, DC: Child Welfare League of America.

Given, D., & Simmons, S. (1977). The interdisciplinary health care team. *Nursing Forum, 16*(2), 165-184.

Hoeman, S.P. (1992). Community-based rehabilitation. *Holistic Nursing Practice, 6*(2), 32-41.

Howard, M.E. (1991). Interdisciplinary team treatment in acute care. In P.M. Deutsch & K.B. Fralish (Eds.), *Innovations in head injury rehabilitation* (pp. 3-1–3-26). New York: Mathew Bender Company.

Joint Commission on Accreditation of Healthcare Organizations (JCAHO). (1993). *Rehabilitation services: Accreditation manual for hospitals.* Oakbrook Terrace, IL: Author.

Keith, R.A. (1991). The comprehensive treatment team in rehabilitation. *Archives of Physical Medicine and Rehabilitation, 72*, 269-274.

Leath, C. (1991). Team managed care for older adults: A clinical demonstration of a community model. *Journal of Gerontological Nursing, 17*(7), 25-28.

Levenstein, A. (1984). Negotiating vs. confrontation. *Nursing Management, 15*(1), 52-53.

Marriner, A. (1980). *Guide to nursing management.* St. Louis: The C.V. Mosby Company.

Melvin, J.L. (1989). Status report on interdisciplinary medical rehabilitation. *Archives of Physical Medicine and Rehabilitation, 70*, 273-276.

Moulder, T.A., Staal, A.M., & Grant, M. (1988). Making the interdisciplinary team approach work. *Rehabilitation Nursing, 13*, 338-339.

◆Olson, L.M., Reis, J., Murphy, L., & Gehm, J.H. (1988). The religious community as a partner in health care. *Journal of Community Health, 13*(4), 249-257.

O'Toole, M.T. (1992). The interdisciplinary team: Research and education. *Holistic Nursing Practice, 6*(2), 76-83.

Pierog, L.J. (1991). Case management: A product line. *Nursing Administration Quarterly, 15*(2), 16-20.

Povse, S.M., & Keenan, M.E. (1981). Discharge planning for the transition from a health care facility to the community. In N. Martin, N.B. Holt, & D. Hicks (Eds.), *Comprehensive rehabilitation nursing* (pp. 667-689). New York : McGraw-Hill Book Company.

Roseman, E. (1980). How to overcome intergroup conflict. *Medical Laboratory Observer, 12*(6), 41-44.

Roseman, E. (1985). Collaborative problem solving. *Medical Laboratory Observer, 17*(2), 59-62.

Rothberg, J.S. (1992). Knowledge of disciplines, roles and functions of team members. In *American Congress of Rehabilitation Medicine guide to interdisciplinary practice in rehabilitation settings* (pp. 44-71). Skokie, IL: American Congress of Rehabilitation Medicine.

Tollman, S. (1991). Community oriented primary care: Origins, evolution, applications. *Social Science and Medicine, 32*(6), 633-642.

Suggested Readings

American Nurses' Association and Association of Rehabilitation Nurses. (1986). *Standards of rehabilitation nursing practice.* Kansas City, MO: Author.

Condeluci, A. (1991). *Interdependence: The route to community.* Orlando, FL: Paul M. Deutsch Press, Inc.

Cronrath, P.R. (1991). Building teams through solving problems. *Nursing Management, 22*(10), 120q-120x.

Dean, B.Z., & Geiringer, S.R. (1990). Physiatric therapeutics: 6. The rehabilitation team/behavioral management. *Archives of Physical Medicine and Rehabilitation, 71*, S-275–S-277.

DeLisa, J.A., Martin, G.M., & Currie, D.M. (1988). Rehabilitation medicine: Past, present, and future. In J.A. DeLisa (Ed.), *Rehabilitation medicine: Principles and practice* (pp. 3-24). Philadelphia: J.B. Lippincott Company.

◆Fieger, S.M., & Schmitt, M.H. (1979). Collegiality in interdisciplinary health teams: Its measurement and its effects. *Social Science and Medicine, 13A*, 217-229.

Halstead, L.S. (1976). Team care in chronic illness: A critical review of the literature of the past 25 years. *Archives of Physical Medicine and Rehabilitation, 57*, 507-511.

◆Halstead, L.S., Rintala, D.H., Kanellos, M., Griffin, B., Higgins, L., Rheinecker, S., Whiteside, W., & Healy, J.E. (1986). The innovative rehabilitation team: An experiment in team building. *Archives of Physical Medicine and Rehabilitation, 67*, 357-361.

Lowe, J.I., & Herranen, M. (1981). Understanding teamwork: Another look at the concepts. *Social Work in Health Care, 7*(2), 1-11.

Margolis, H., Fiorelli, J.S., & Leonard, H.S. (1984). Resolving differences in the rehabilitation team. *Rehabilitation Nursing, 9*(3), 38-40.

Moulder, P.A., & Grant, M. (1988). Making the interdisciplinary team approach work. *Rehabilitation Nursing, 13*, 338-339.

Nichols, B. (1979). Dealing with conflict. *Journal of Continuing Education in Nursing, 10*(6), 24-27.

◆North, M., Meeusen, M., & Hollinsworth, P. (1991). Discharge planning: Increasing client and nurse satisfaction, *Rehabilitation Nursing, 16*, 327-329.

Peterson, C.R., Carnes, G.D., & Frank, R.G. (1981). Who's in charge here? The rehabilitation team: Anatomy, physiology, and pathology. *Science Digest, 3*, 3-8, 43-44.

Purtillo, R.B. (1988). Ethical issues in teamwork: The context of rehabilitation. *Archives of Physical Medicine and Rehabilitation, 69*, 318-322.

Rothberg, J. (1981). The rehabilitation team: Future directions. *Archives of Physical Medicine and Rehabilitation, 62*, 407-410.

◆Sands, R.G., Stafford, J., & McClellan, M. (1990). "I beg to defer": Conflict in the interdisciplinary team. *Social Work in Health Care, 14*(3), 55-72.

◆White, M.J., & Holloway, M. (1990). Patient concerns after discharge from rehabilitation. *Rehabilitation Nursing, 15*, 316-318.

◆ indicates a research-based work

CHAPTER 23

The Phenomenon of Change in Rehabilitation

The phenomenon of change as it relates to the human experience can be considered a central concern in nursing (DeFeo, 1990). This is especially true for rehabilitation nurses, who regularly interact with persons experiencing great change. Although the phenomenon of change is applicable to rehabilitation facilities and rehabilitation teams, the focus of this chapter is the individual patient, the central member of the rehabilitation team. Laughlin (1989) wrote, "Changed behavior of a disabled client is the ultimate goal of a change strategy" (p. 530). Understanding and promoting the change process are, therefore, integral parts of the role of the rehabilitation nurse.

I. Definition of Change: Alteration in the Status Quo in an Organism, Situation, or Process (Lippitt, 1973)

II. Types of Change
   A. Planned change: Systematic process directed toward producing improvement in function or output, or solving a problem (Bennis, Benne, Chin, & Corey, 1976); outcomes are predictable and deliberate
   B. Unplanned change or drift: Generally, is random with no effort made by the participants to prepare for onset of change process; outcomes are unpredictable and nondeliberate, but not necessarily negative

III. Principles Related to the Change Process (Bushnell, 1979)
   A. Person takes part in change to the extent that he or she participated in planning
   B. Person may respond to a gradual shaping of behavior; the consequent change is likely to be more effective and long-lasting than the response to rapid change strategies
   C. Person changes to the extent that the reward or benefit is greater than the pain or disruption of the status quo
   D. Person changes to the extent that he or she sees others as changing
   E. Person maintains the change behavior to the extent that it is rewarded, supported, and satisfying
   F. Person needs time to detach from old behavior patterns while exploring and acclimating self to new patterns
   G. Person who is highly anxious about or mourning a loss created by the change learns or applies little about desired changes

IV. Kurt Lewin's Classical Change Theory
   A. Historical perspective: Social scientist Kurt Lewin (1947) is credited as the classical theorist of change theory; much of his work was done in the 1940s
   B. Related concepts
      1. Lewin believed that behavior is a function of both personality and the environment and that interactions between the two are dynamic
      2. Lewin identified three stages of change: unfreezing, movement, and refreezing
         a. Unfreezing: Movement from a steady state to a state that is unsteady and amenable to change
            1) Discomfort with the present situation is induced or emerges
            2) Status quo is questioned
            3) Change relationship is established
         b. Movement: Movement to a higher level of behavior
            1) Problem is assessed and diagnosed
            2) Options and alternatives are identified
            3) Goals are established
            4) Action is taken
            5) Evaluation is made
         c. Refreezing: Integration and stabilization of new learning
            1) New responses are integrated into the lifestyle and relationships
            2) Change is complete
      3. Lewin formulated the concept of a force field related to change
         a. Definition: Forces that facilitate or impede the change process are constantly at work
         b. Types of forces
            1) Driving forces: Forces that facilitate the change process by moving the participant in the direction of a positive outcome
            2) Restraining forces: Forces that impede the change process
         c. Dynamics of the driving and restraining forces
            1) Identify both to capitalize on and benefit from the driving forces and to avoid and modify the restraining forces
            2) Change occurs when one outweighs the other; the status quo is maintained when forces are equal
   C. Application to rehabilitation (see Figure 23.1)

Figure 23.1. Clinical Application of Lewin's Change Theory

History

Terry is a 36-year-old male with an L4-5 incomplete spinal cord injury and subsequent areflexic neurogenic bowel. He has not achieved restoration of bowel regularity and continence.

Lewin's Stages of Change

Unfreezing: Terry experienced fecal incontinence with frequent oozing of liquid stool. He was not receptive to information about bowel care and repeatedly refused to participate in a daily bowel program. Therapies were often interrupted due to his incontinence and the foul-smelling odor (discomfort emerges with the present situation). He verbalized his embarrassment and frustration to his nurse (the status quo is questioned and a change relationship is established).

Movement: Through the therapeutic relationship established with Terry, the nurse was able to discuss issues related to fecal incontinence and bowel regularity (the problem is assessed and diagnosed). Alternate times for the bowel program were discussed (options and alternatives are identified). The following goals were mutually established: (a) patient education, (b) understanding of bowel care, (c) bowel regularity and continence, and (d) patient independence in bowel care (goals are established). The nurse provided education about bowel care, arranged a dietary consult, reviewed Terry's medications, and scheduled a daily bowel program (action is taken). The nurse took daily notes on the results of bowel care and Terry's response to interventions (an evaluation is made).

Refreezing: After a 3-week period, Terry demonstrated bowel regularity and continence with a bowel program every other day (qod) (new responses are integrated into lifestyle and relationships). Activities of daily living were no longer interrupted by incontinence, and Terry took responsibility for his own care (change is complete).

Lewin's Force Field

Driving forces: Fear of embarrassment, negative effects on the relationship with the significant other, soiled clothing

Restraining forces: Denial, uncomfortable feelings associated with discussion of bowel care, time and energy expended to learn bowel care

Source Consulted

Lewin, K. (1947). Frontiers in group dynamics: Concepts, methods, and reality in social science. *Human Relations, 5*(1), 5-42.

V. The Change Agent
   A. Definition: A person who deliberately promotes a change process (Mauksch & Miller, 1981)
   B. Characteristics (Lippitt & Lippitt, 1978)
      1. Flexibility, innovation, and creativity
      2. Self-motivation
      3. Sensitivity toward others
      4. Ability to deal successfully with ambiguity and adapt to unfamiliar situations
      5. Genuine desire to help others
      6. Integrity
      7. Optimism, self-confidence, and sincerity
      8. Charisma
   C. Functions of the change agent (Rogers, 1972)
      1. Develops a need for change
      2. Establishes a change relationship
      3. Diagnoses the problem
      4. Examines goals and alternative courses of action
      5. Translates intent into action
      6. Stabilizes change and attempts to prevent any discontinuance of the change behaviors
      7. Achieves closure

VI. Impediments to Change (Bailey, 1990)
   A. Resistance
      1. Behavior that will oppose, obstruct, or block movement in the change process
      2. Resistance is a common reaction to change and can be active or passive
   B. Other impediments
      1. The demoralizing effects of day-to-day management of chronic illness
      2. Deterioration of vigor, mobility, and comfort, which strains the pursuit of work, hobbies, and social activities
      3. Erosion of support systems
      4. Society's indifference to the needs of persons with disabilities

References

Bailey, B. (1990). Change agent. In I.M. Lubkin (Ed.), *Chronic illness: Impact and interventions* (pp. 262-278). Boston: Jones & Bartlett Publishers.

Bennis, W., Benne, K., Chin, R., & Corey, K. (1976). *The planning of change* (3rd ed.). New York: Holt, Rinehart, & Winston.

Bushnell, M. (1979). Institutions in transition. *Perspectives of Psychiatric Care, 17*(6), 260-265.

DeFeo, D.J. (1990). Change: A central concern of nursing. *Nursing Science Quarterly, 3*(2), 88-94.

Laughlin, J.A. (1989). Rehabilitation: Unlocking the gates to change. In S. Dittmar (Ed.), *Rehabilitation nursing: Process and application* (pp. 528-535). St. Louis: The C.V. Mosby Company.

Lewin, K. (1947). Frontiers in group dynamics: Concepts, methods, and reality in social science. *Human Relations, 5*(1), 5-42.

Lippitt, G.L. (1973). *Visualizing change: Model building and the change process.* La Jolla, CA: University Associates.

Lippitt, G., & Lippitt, R. (1978). *The consulting process in action.* San Diego: University Associates.

Mauksch, I.G., & Miller, M.H. (1981). *Implementing change in nursing.* St. Louis: The C.V. Mosby Company.

Rogers, E.M. (1972). Change agents, clients, and change. In G. Zaltman, P. Kotlteer, & I. Kaufman (Eds.), *Creating social change* (pp. 194-213). New York: Holt, Rinehart, & Winston.

Suggested Readings

Holt, F.M. (1990). The CNS embroiled in change. *Clinical Nurse Specialist, 4*(2), 97.

Kaplan, M.S. (1990). The nurse as change agent. *Pediatric Nursing, 16*, 603-605, 618.

Kievman, B., & Blacknun, S. (1989). Handling change: The family caregiver's perspective. *Caring, 8*(12), 4-5, 7-8.

Lancaster, J., & Lancaster, W. (1982). *The nurse as a change agent.* St. Louis: The C.V. Mosby Company.

McGovern, W.N., & Rodgers, J.A. (1986). Change theory. *American Journal of Nursing, 86*, 566-567.

Vanetzian, E. (1988). Force field analysis: A person-centered approach to behavioral change. *Rehabilitation Nursing, 13*(1), 23-25.

Walsh, K.C. (1989). Using planned change to implement a pressure sore program. *Journal of Neuroscience Nursing, 21*(4), 245-249.

CHAPTER 24

Accreditation, Quality Improvement, and Program Evaluation

The accreditation process has evolved into a means of ensuring that healthcare facilities are in compliance with established standards of practice. More recently, accrediting organizations such as the Joint Commission on Accreditation of Healthcare Organizations (JCAHO) and the Commission on Accreditation of Rehabilitation Facilities (CARF) have taken the lead in developing and applying new standards of care to healthcare institutions with an increased emphasis on quality improvement programs (CARF, 1993; JCAHO, 1992). Along with these advances, program evaluation has emerged with implications for improved treatment services and greater program efficiency. Accreditation, quality improvement, and program evaluation are essential for maintaining the accountability of the rehabilitation field and rehabilitation nursing to the larger society.

Accreditation: Joint Commission on Accreditation of Healthcare Organizations (JCAHO) and Commission on Accreditation of Rehabilitation Facilities (CARF)

I. Missions of JCAHO and CARF
   A. JCAHO: "To improve the quality of health care provided to the public; develop standards of quality in collaboration with health professionals and others and stimulate healthcare organizations to meet or exceed the standards through accreditation and the teaching of quality improvement concepts" (JCAHO, 1992, p. ii)
   B. CARF: "To serve as the preeminent standards-setting and accrediting body promoting quality services to people with disabilities" (CARF, 1993, p. vii)

II. Benefits of Accreditation
   A. JCAHO: Fulfills all or portions of state and/or federal licensure and certification requirements; expedites third-party payment; provides guidelines to improve care, services, and programs; enhances community confidence; affects staff recruitment
   B. CARF: Defines organizations that have met national standards specifically designed to meet the needs of persons with disabilities, provides organizations with a blueprint for operations and an internal tool to evaluate their programs, and offers confidence to consumers that a monitoring system is in place that is concerned with their best interests

III. Historical Perspectives
   A. Evolution of JCAHO
      1. By the turn of the 20th century, the internship model of postgraduate medical education had arisen to meet the needs of medical school graduates seeking clinical experiences in preparation for state license examinations; many believed, however, that the existing system was flawed
         a. There was great variability in the quality of educational experiences, with large university-affiliated hospital internships deemed superior, both in status and degree, to posts at small unaffiliated rural facilities
         b. Conflict also existed between the interests of local medical societies, which viewed interns as an essential component of the hospital work force, and the American Medical Association Council of Medical Education, which conceptualized the hospital as a laboratory for medical education
      2. In 1917, the American Medical Association and the American College of Surgeons worked together to improve the quality of care
         a. They agreed to certify practitioners and ensure quality internships
         b. They established a system for keeping adequate hospital case records
         c. They required the presence of X-ray and pathology departments in hospitals
         d. They established an organized medical staff
      3. In 1918, the American College of Surgeons' document, *Minimum Standard for Hospitals*, became widely accepted as the standard by which hospitals were judged
      4. Voluntary accreditation accepted as integral part of American medical scene by 1951 (Stevens, 1989), when Joint Commission on Accreditation of Hos-

pitals (JCAH) was formed as a direct outgrowth of American College of Surgeons' accreditation movement

a. JCAH originally represented perspectives of American College of Physicians, American Medical Association, American Hospital Association, American College of Surgeons, and Canadian Medical Association—all known as corporate members
    1) Canadian Medical Association withdrew in 1959
    2) American Dental Association was added in 1980
b. As health care diversified, the Joint Commission expanded its services into long-term care, ambulatory health care, home care, hospice care, mental health care, and managed care
c. In 1987, the organization changed its name to Joint Commission on Accreditation of Healthcare Organizations, reflecting its broadening base of activity

5. In 1993, JCAHO streamlined and combined standards, placing greater emphasis on ongoing improvement in the systems and processes that most influence patient care and outcomes

B. Evolution of CARF
1. Formed in 1966
2. Private, not-for-profit organization that has the benefit of a broad base of support from and involvement of consumers, providers, and purchasers of specialized services for people with disabilities
3. Assumed leadership in promoting outcome-oriented data collection and action to improve rehabilitation patient outcomes; in 1973, convened a conference on rehabilitation and the measurement of its results
4. Implemented specific standards related to special rehabilitation programs (e.g., spinal cord injury) in the mid-1980s
5. Began "Target 2000" in the early 1990s, an ongoing initiative to shape CARF's future in partnership with a wide variety of individuals and organizations concerned with people with disabilities

IV. Joint Commission on Accreditation of Healthcare Organizations

A. Organizational aspects
1. JCAHO is governed by 22 commissioners, almost all of whom are appointed by the five corporate member organizations
2. Commissioners' meetings are held several times a year to assess the changing healthcare environment and plan a response to those changes

B. Recent changes
1. Accreditation cycle
    a. In 1982, accreditation cycle was set at 3 years
    b. Contingencies were introduced to allow organizations to focus on areas in which they were having difficulties without losing accreditation
    c. Thus, JCAHO serves two functions: regulatory and educational
2. In 1987, the commission announced its "Agenda for Change," an ongoing and comprehensive research and development project that focuses on better methods of measuring and monitoring clinical and organizational effectiveness related to patient care outcomes (JCAHO, 1988)
3. The commission expanded its educative and consultative role to give healthcare organizations support in understanding the issues of providing quality care (JCAHO, 1990)
4. In 1991, the JCAHO standards for nursing were revised to become outcome-based, rather than process-based, representing a fundamental change in approach to standards development
5. In 1992, as part of JCAHO's ongoing "Agenda for Change," the revision and reorganization of standards shifted the focus from department-specific structure and processes to the effective performance of important organization-wide functions; by focusing performance improvement activities on these functions, hospitals ultimately should achieve improved patient outcomes (JCAHO, 1992)
6. In 1993, JCAHO announced that an organization could be surveyed at any time, with or without notice; continuous compliance with all standards is an expectation

C. The accreditation process
1. Process begins when an organization submits an application to the commission requesting that a survey be performed
2. Survey then is conducted to assess a given facility's compliance with the appropriate commission standards; the organization is notified of survey dates 4 to 6 weeks in advance
3. The survey team can include an administrator, a nurse, and/or a physician
4. Components of survey
    a. Initial conference with organizational leaders to set schedules
    b. Direct and indirect observations of organization's functioning—for example, observing activity on various nursing units and reviewing documentation in medical records
    c. Public information interview in which anyone requesting an interview with the commission can address the facility's compliance with standards
    d. Summation conference open to all hospital staff to announce findings and offer suggestions for correcting deficiencies, if there are any
    e. Modified or tailored surveys available to multi-institutional systems as well as hospitals offering multiple services, for which there are separate accreditation standards within JCAHO (e.g., a modified survey for physical rehabilitation services)

D. The accreditation decision
1. The accreditation decision is made on the basis of compliance with standards
    a. Organizational standards

b. Quality assessment and improvement standards
c. General nursing standards in the areas of patient care, nursing practice and competence, staffing, and nursing's role in hospital leadership
d. Nursing standards specifically related to physical rehabilitation services in the areas of physical and psychosocial nursing assessments and interventions, individualized nursing care goals, and participation in the interdisciplinary team process

2. Survey results are reported to the JCAHO Department of Survey Validation, which applies JCAHO-approved decision rules to render an accreditation decision
3. Accreditation decision
   a. Accreditation with commendation
   b. Accreditation with or without recommendations
   c. Conditional accreditation

V. Commission on Accreditation of Rehabilitation Facilities

A. Organizational aspects
1. Membership
   a. There are two categories of membership, sponsoring and associate
   b. Membership is broad-based and consists of representatives of those with disabilities, healthcare providers, and third-party financial organizations
   c. ARN is a sponsoring member; therefore, may appoint one voting member to the CARF Board of Trustees
2. Board of trustees
   a. Consists of individuals appointed by the sponsoring members (one appointee each) and an equal number of appointees chosen by board of trustees
   b. Is responsible for managing the commission and makes final decision on awarding accreditation

B. The accreditation process
1. Organization must first complete a self-study before the formal accreditation process can begin
2. Three months prior to accreditation survey and after completion of self-study, institution applies to the commission
3. A site survey, typically conducted by an administrator, a nurse, and a physician, then is scheduled and conducted
4. Components of the survey
   a. Opening orientation meeting with administrators, which is followed by a tour of the facility
   b. Interview with staff members and at least one user of facility's services
   c. Review of facility's documentation, including administrative policies, fiscal reports, minutes of meetings, and case records
   d. Exit conference summarizing survey team's findings

C. The accreditation decision
1. Results of the survey are communicated to the CARF Board of Trustees, which then will make a determination of accreditation
2. Accreditation decision is made on basis of compliance with standards
   a. Areas addressed by standards
      1) Organizational standards: Administration, information management systems, program evaluation, consumer-based planning, personnel administration and staff development, fiscal management, physical plant, and safety
      2) Overall program standards: Admission and orientation, assessment of clients' needs, individual program planning and management referral, discharge planning and follow-up, documentation, and assessment of program quality
      3) Specific program variables relating to the clinical program offered by the facility (e.g., comprehensive inpatient rehabilitation, spinal cord injury, brain injury, chronic pain management, work hardening, and vocational evaluation programs)
   b. Although similarity exists between CARF and JCAHO standards, CARF places greater emphasis on a number of factors
      1) Accessibility (e.g., architectural, attitudinal, and employment barriers)
      2) Comprehensiveness and continuity in individual treatment plan
      3) Input from persons served regarding overall organization and decision-making processes
      4) Safety—including, for example, fire and disaster drills and evacuation of persons with disabilities
      5) Outcomes after discharge
3. The applying institution receives notification of the decision as well as specific suggestions for improvement, if any are necessary
4. Accreditation decisions
   a. Three-year: Accreditation criteria met and substantial fulfillment of standards demonstrated
   b. One-year: Accreditation criteria met but deficiencies in relation to the standards
   c. Nonaccreditation: Accreditation criteria not met or major deficiencies related to standards
5. Any negative determinations can be reviewed at the request of the organization that is undergoing accreditation

Healthcare Quality Improvement

Activities that improve the delivery of health care, enhance the effectiveness of patient care, and result in attainment of expected outcomes are components of a quality improvement program. Standards for determining the quality of care come from external regulatory bodies, such as JCAHO and CARF, and from the nursing profession, through organizations such as the

American Nurses Association (ANA) and the Association of Rehabilitation Nurses (ARN).

Within the healthcare arena, a progressive movement from quality assurance to continuous quality improvement has occurred, placing greater emphasis on prospective problem resolution rather than retrospective problem identification (Patterson, 1993). JCAHO (1992) recently published standards based on the following quality improvement principles: (a) a hospital can im-prove patient care quality and patient satisfaction by assessing and improving governance, managerial, clinical, and support processes that affect patient outcomes; (b) these processes are carried out jointly by more than one of these groups, meaning they are cross-disciplinary and cross-departmental; (c) these processes must be coordinated and integrated; and (d) employees must be motivated and competent to carry them out. Hospital leaders will be increasingly responsible for integrating quality improvement processes throughout the organization. Mechanisms for accomplishing these goals will involve increased team quality improvement activities (Hamilton & Morales, 1988; Oie & Recker, 1992) and consumer participation in defining the parameters of quality care (Frost, 1992).

The delivery of quality patient care has always been a fundamental aspect of rehabilitation nursing practice. Rehabilitation nurses are prepared to be leaders in quality improvement activities by virtue of their tradition of collaborative practice with the rehabilitation team and commitment to patient and family participation in the rehabilitation process.

I. Definitions of Quality
   A. "Degree to which patient care services increase the probability of desired patient outcomes and reduce the probability of undesired outcomes given the current state of knowledge; potential components of quality include accessibility, appropriateness, continuity, effectiveness, efficacy, efficiency, patient perspective issues, safety of the care environment, and timeliness" (JCAHO, 1992, p. 234)
   B. "The sum of all activities to ensure that patients receive the best possible nursing care" (ANA & ARN, 1986, p. 13)
   C. The elements of quality that take priority for health caregivers are responsiveness to perceived care needs, level of communication, concern and courtesy, quality of facilities and support services, degree of symptom relief, and level of functional improvement (JCAHO, 1988)
   D. Any formal, systematic monitoring program that identifies problems in patient care delivery, designs activities to overcome these problems, and performs follow-up monitoring to ensure that no new problems have been introduced and that corrective steps have been effective (Kibbee, 1990)
   E. Meeting the needs of the customer with process costs being reduced as quality improves (Martin, 1991)
   F. Conformance to a standard, the quality standard being zero defects; a system of prevention is the best method for achieving zero defects; one of the measures of quality is the cost of doing things wrong (Crosby, 1979)

II. Historical Perspectives (see Figure 24.1)

Figure 24.1. History of Quality Monitoring in Health Care

1856 *Notes on Nursing: What It Is and What It Is Not* by Florence Nightingale (1856) provided the first description of nursing standards for noise levels, food consistency, type of mattress to be used, and positioning of the bed in relation to windows.

1912 Outcome-oriented medical audits were implemented to improve the quality of medical practice (Vail & Jacobs, 1986).

1918 American College of Surgeons' accreditation body was formed to review educational and practitioner performance standards.

1946 Minimum standards for nursing in hospitals were identified by the American College of Surgeons' *Manual of Hospital Standardization.* These standards describe the nursing organization within the hospital, personnel records, and educational records.

1953 The Joint Commission on Accreditation of Hospitals (JCAH) published the first *Standards for Hospital Accreditation.*

1967 Evaluation was defined as one of the four functions of the nursing process by Yura and Walsh (1967).

1973 Generic *Standards of Nursing Practice* that provided direction for determining the quality of nursing care given a client was published by the American Nurses' Association (ANA) (1973).

1974 Outcome standards for specific patient populations were written under the direction of Zimmer and Lang (1974).

1974 The Lang Model for Quality Assurance was adopted by the ANA.

1977 ANA published *Standards of Rehabilitation Nursing Practice* (1977).

1980 JCAH introduced quality assurance standards, which focused on problem resolution rather than numerical audits.

1986 ANA and ARN (1986) jointly published *Standards of Rehabilitation Nursing Practice.*

1990 The Agency for Health Care Policy and Research (AHCPR) was created to enhance the quality, access, appropriateness, and effectiveness of healthcare services (Lang and Marek, 1991).

1990 The Joint Commission on Accreditation of Healthcare Organizations (JCAHO) revised its nursing standards to reflect the increased emphasis on unit-based quality improvement activities and competency evaluation.

1991 ANA (1991) published generic *Standards of Clinical Nursing Practice,* which includes standards of care and standards of professional performance along with measurement criteria.

1992 JCAHO published quality assurance and improvement standards focusing on organizational and leadership efforts directed at improved patient outcomes.

Sources Consulted

American Nurses' Association (ANA). (1973). *Standards of nursing practice.* Kansas City, MO: Author.

American Nurses' Association. (1977). *Standards of rehabilitation nursing practice.* Kansas City, MO: Author.

American Nurses Association. (1991). *Standards of clinical nursing practice.* Kansas City, MO: Author.

American Nurses' Association & Association of Rehabilitation Nurses (ARN). (1986). *Standards of rehabilitation nursing practice.* Kansas City, MO: American Nurses' Association.

Lang, N.M., & Marek, K.D. (1991). The policy and politics of patient outcomes. *Journal of Nursing Quality Assurance, 5*(2), 7-12.

Nightingale, F. (1856). (1969 reprint). *Notes on nursing: What it is and what it is not.* New York: Dover Publications.

Vail, J.D., & Jacobs, M.E. (1986). Quality assurance: The pieces of the puzzle. *Journal of the Association of Nurse Anesthetists, 54*(2), 171-176.

Yura, H., & Walsh, M.B. (1967). *The nursing process.* Washington, DC: The Catholic University of America Press.

Zimmer, M.J., & Lang, N.J. (1974). *Development of sets of patient health outcome criteria by panels of nurse experts: Final report.* Madison, WI: Regional Medical Program, University of Wisconsin.

Figure 24.2. Quality Concepts and Definitions

Aspects of care: Diagnostic, preventive, therapeutic, rehabilitative, supportive, and/or palliative patient care activities within the scope of care that are of greatest significance to the quality of patient care; these activities are high-volume activities, high-risk activities (through omission or commission), and/or activities prone to be problems for patients and/or providers (e.g., bowel and bladder management, pain management, medication administration, discharge planning, patient safety)
Audit: Chart review, generally performed retrospectively
Compliance: Degree of achievement of identified thresholds for an indicator
Continuous quality improvement: Style of management that continuously improves the quality of all products and services while focusing shared responsibility on all employees for the service or the product produced; this concept differs from quality assurance in that it uses problem-solving management strategies to focus on the process instead of the people (Patton & Stanley, 1993)
Criteria: Expected levels of achievement by which care or performance can be evaluated
Critical paths: Plans of care that reflect patterns for a specific problem or diagnosis and delineate the care to be given by time intervals
Indicator: Measurable statement that reflects a clinical, administrative, or risk-related aspect of care and is related to structure, process, or outcome
Monitor: A data collection tool
Monitoring: Planned, systematic and ongoing collection, compilation, and organization of data about an indicator of quality of an important aspect of care, and the comparison of those data to an established level of performance to determine the need for evaluation
Outcome: The results of the performance or nonperformance of a function or process
Peer review: Process by which healthcare professionals appraise the quality of care delivered by members of their profession in accordance with established standards of practice
Performance: The ability of an individual, group, or organization to carry out processes that increase the probability of desired outcomes
Process: A goal-directed, interrelated series of actions, mechanisms, or steps
Quality assessment and improvement: "The ongoing activities designed to objectively and systematically evaluate the quality of patient care and services, pursue opportunities to improve patient care and services, and resolve identified problems" (JCAHO, 1992, p. 234)
Risk management: Process of making and carrying out decisions that will minimize the adverse effects of accidental losses
Sample: Segment of the total population being reviewed (e.g., all patients who fall; 40% of the patients discharged from the unit); sample size should be large enough to represent the total population
Scope of care and/or services: Range of care or services provided by a unit, department, or organization
Standard: A statement of expectation that defines the structure and processes that must be substantially in place in an organization to enhance the quality of care
Threshold: Established level of performance
Total quality management (TQM): Style of management that incorporates a value system composed of the mission, philosophy, goals, and policies of an organization
Values: Attributes that signify worth, merit, and usefulness

Sources Consulted

Patton, S., & Stanley, J. (1993). Bridging quality assurance and continuous quality improvement. *Journal of Nursing Care Quarterly, 7*(2), 15-23.

III. Quality Concepts (see Figure 24.2)

IV. Models for Quality Improvement Programs

A. Models relevant to nurses: There are two quality assurance models of particular value to nurses involved with quality improvement at the unit level; one is the ANA's conceptual model and the other is the JCAHO 10-step model
   1. *ANA conceptual model*: Promotes quality improvement using a cyclic process that is compatible with the nursing process and includes the following steps
      a. Identify values: Values form the basic underlying framework for quality improvement
      b. Identify standards; that is, standards developed by professional nursing organizations such as ANA or ARN
      c. Identify criteria to evaluate standards: Criteria are related to structure, process, or outcome (Donabedian, 1980)
         1) Structure criteria: Describe the environment and its resources, such as equipment or numbers of staff—for example, "All patients identified at risk for alteration in skin integrity will have an eggcrate mattress"
         2) Process criteria: Describe the specific activities of healthcare providers—for example, "The nurse will assess the patient's skin integrity at a minimum of every 8 hours or more frequently, if indicated"
         3) Outcome criteria: Describe the expected and/or actual results of the delivery of care (e.g., "95% of all patients on the rehabilitation unit will not develop a pressure ulcer during hospitalization")
      d. Obtain measurements to determine if standards and criteria were met
         1) Measurements to identify areas of concern and facilitate their investigation are obtained through data collection
         2) Data can be collected through audits, interviews, observations, or questionnaires
      e. Interpret the strengths and weaknesses of the measurements obtained
         1) Strengths indicate which standards and criteria are being met
         2) Weaknesses indicate inadequate compliance
      f. Determine courses of action after analyzing strengths and weaknesses—for example, holding in-service educational sessions, modifying policies and procedures, developing new policies and procedures, changing staffing mix, repairing defective equipment, and performing research
      g. Select appropriate courses of action
         1) Decision may be either to implement action to resolve the problem or to continue tracking the problem
         2) Target dates for the completion of activities should be set, and goals for problem resolution should be established

h. Take action: Institute the plan designating the persons involved and the time frames for reevaluation
i. Evaluate results: Evaluate effectiveness of action plan
   1) If it is effective, reevaluate it in the future
   2) If it is ineffective, consider the possibilities
      a) The action plan is unrealistic and requires revision
      b) The time frame is too short
      c) A new action plan is needed
j. Document the findings: All quality assurance activities should be documented, as should the steps taken to inform and gain input from the nursing staff

2. *JCAHO 10-step operational model*
   a. JCAHO expanded its model with the "Agenda for Change" (Patterson, 1988)
   b. This current model can be used to establish an effective quality assessment and improvement process that focuses on monitoring, evaluating, and problem solving (Bassett, 1993)
   c. It includes a 10-step process
      1) Assign responsibility
         a) Director of nursing is ultimately responsible for nursing quality assurance
         b) Responsibility typically is delegated to nurse managers, who then delegate aspects of the program to staff nurses
      2) Determine scope of care
         a) Information such as types of clients served
         b) Clients' age group
         c) Clients' types of disabilities
         d) Rehabilitative services provided
         e) Procedures performed
         f) Hours of care
         g) Staffing mix
      3) Identify important aspects of care, which have specific characteristics
         a) High volume: Affects many patients and occurs frequently
         b) High risk: Results in serious consequences
         c) Problem-prone: Tends to produce problems for patients and staff
         d) High cost, which may become important as costs and reimbursement become critical issues (Bassett, 1993)
      4) Decide on the indicator(s) that is (are) formulated for each aspect of care
      5) Establish a threshold based on information from facility data, national norms, consensus from experts, and research
      6) Collect data
         a) Data are collected, analyzed, acted upon, and communicated in accord with a monitoring schedule that ensures a systematic evaluation of identified aspects of care
         b) Data source, sample size, and time frame are specified
      7) Evaluate data, comparing them with the established thresholds; problems exist when deficiencies in care are repeated, widespread, or serious
      8) Take necessary actions to resolve problems and to improve care; problem resolution also can include refinement of indicators, thresholds, data collection, or evaluation techniques
      9) Follow up with an assessment to determine the current compliance with threshold following corrective action
      10) Communicate findings at the unit, departmental, and organizational levels using a format that includes a summary of collected data, recommendations, actions taken, and evaluation of changes

B. Organizational quality improvement model: Deming's (1982) 14-point plan for quality improvement
   1. W. Edwards Deming, an engineer and statistician who developed the quality improvement plan used in Japan following World War II, emphasized the process of quality through a 14-point plan that focuses primarily on the leadership roles of top management and improvement of organizational processes and structure
   2. Deming's model is the foundation for the total quality management (TQM) movement (Walton, 1986)
      a. TQM has been defined as doing the right thing right the first time, on time, all the time, and to strive always for improvement and customer satisfaction (Masters & Schmele, 1991)
      b. Although originally designed for the manufacturing industry, the model is now widely used by managers in the healthcare industry

V. Unit-Based Rehabilitation Nursing Quality Improvement: Research Opportunities
   A. The goal of rehabilitation nursing is the promotion of cost-effective care that prevents complications of physical disability, restores optimal functioning, and helps the individual adapt to an altered lifestyle
   B. Quality assurance programs at the unit level provide the opportunity to meet this goal (Mills, 1989) (see Figure 24.3)
   C. Unit-based quality assurance projects can serve as a springboard for nursing research, as both processes have the common aim of improving patient care using systematic inquiry (Acorn, Love, & Mills, 1990)
   D. As nursing moves into an era demanding a clearer definition of quality, the need to develop methods to measure quality care and the outcomes of quality care is pressing (Frost, 1992)

Program Evaluation

Program evaluation enables the organization to identify the results of services and the effects of the program on the persons served (CARF, 1993) and is a recognized method of determining

Figure 24.3. Application of the JCAHO 10-Step Model to a Unit-Based Indicator

JCAHO 10-Step Process	Unit-Based Quality Assurance Indicator: Patients' Falls
1. Assign responsibility	Nurse manager, day charge RN, evening staff RN, night staff RN
2. Determine the scope of care	Types of clients served demonstrate (a) functional loss or loss of previous gains, (b) a need for 24-hour-per-day rehabilitation nursing, (c) medical and physical stability and cognition sufficient for participation in 3 hours of intensive therapy per day Age: 65 and older Types of disabilities: Stroke and amputation Staffing mix: RNs, licensed practical nurses (LPNs), nursing assistants
3. Identify the important aspects of care	Patient safety
4. Decide on the indicator(s)	During hospitalization, the patient will not experience falls that result in an altered treatment plan or increased length of stay.
5. Establish a threshold	The number of falls resulting in an injury that alters the treatment plan or increases length of stay will be fewer than 1 per 1,000 patient days.
6. Collect data	Data are obtained from incident reports and then documented on a tracking tool developed to monitor falls as to their incidence, location, and lack or extent of nursing assistance and injury. Data collection is done on a quarterly basis.
7. Evaluate data	A total of 26 falls occurred during 2,385 patient days, yielding a fall rate of 10.9 per 1,000. Of these falls, 23 (88%) occurred in patients' rooms and 24 (91%) occurred while the patient was unattended. Six (25%) were experienced by one patient. The threshold was met, with all falls resulting in only a minor injury. No alterations in the treatment plan or length of stay were necessary. Although the threshold was met, data collection identified the problem that one patient was repeatedly falling and the related issues of availability and affordability of sitters. A sitter eventually was hired for the patient. The patient fell two additional times during a 24-hour period when a sitter was unavailable.
8. Take necessary action	Based on these findings, the action plan included the following: (a) Focus initial and ongoing nursing assessments on patient risk factors associated with increased incidence of falls (e.g., impaired sensory function, impaired mobility, fecal incontinence, urinary urgency and incontinence, and the effects of polypharmacy); (b) perform nursing interventions as indicated; (c) assess patients who fall frequently to determine if they need a private sitter (if a sitter is unavailable, the nurse caring for the patient will be assigned significantly fewer patients); (d) hold in-service training for staff on patient safety and fall prevention; and (e) develop and implement a fall prevention protocol.
9. Follow up with an assessment	Continue to monitor and evaluate for another quarter.
10. Communicate findings	The nurse manager discusses the findings with nurses at staff meetings and also shares information with the quality improvement department representative, who will then communicate the findings at the administrative level. As a result, issues regarding patient safety, adequate and available staffing, the need for new protocol development and implementation, and the appropriateness of patient admission are communicated, thus promoting increased awareness and prevention of the problem.

Source Consulted

Ruckstuhl, M.C., Marcionada, E.E., Salmons, J., & Larrabee, J.H. (1991). Patient falls: An outcome indicator. *Journal of Nursing Care Quality, 6*(1), 25-29.

Figure 24.4. Design Elements of Program Evaluation

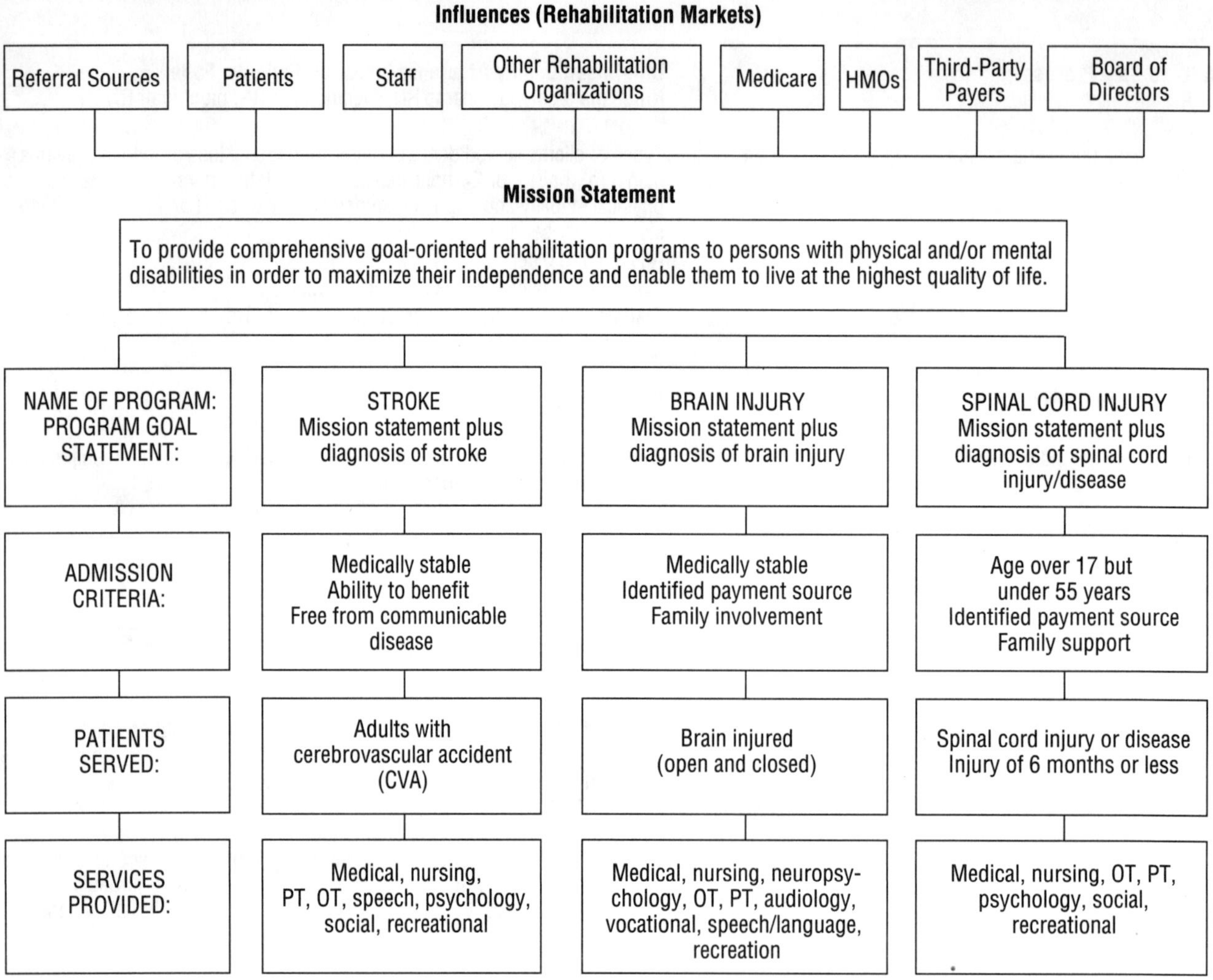

Reprinted with permission of American Hospital Publishing, Inc., from Glass, R.M. (1989). Program evaluation. In B. England, R. Glass, & C. Patterson (Eds.), *Quality rehabilitation: Results-oriented patient care* (p. 29). Chicago: American Hospital Publishing, Inc. Copyright © 1989 American Hospital Publishing, Inc.

quality, effectiveness, and efficiency of rehabilitation services (England, Glass, & Patterson, 1989). Within rehabilitation nursing, program evaluation is an organized method to evaluate the merit of nursing interventions directed toward improving patient outcomes.

The primary impetus for program evaluation is the need for accountability in clinical practice. Government regulations require documentation of rehabilitation program effectiveness as part of the accreditation process. For example, in 1978, CARF adopted the accreditation criterion that required policy statements committing institutions seeking approval to initiate formal program evaluation. Since 1982, CARF standards have emphasized integrating program evaluation methodologies and analyses to generate reports using outcome criteria (CARF, 1982).

Another major thrust for program evaluation has been the 1989 establishment of the federal Agency for Health Care Policy and Research (AHCPR). This agency mandates outcome assessment in all medically related fields with functional measurements as a primary outcome measure. Nursing process documentation has become an integral part of this process.

I. Scope and Purpose of Program Evaluation
   A. Purpose of program evaluation: To document effects of specific programs in relation to stated goals (Weiss, 1972)
      1. It provides a systematic means to judge decision making for treatment, program parameters, and future programming needs (Keith, 1982)
      2. By establishing measurable objectives at admission, an institution and/or specific service (e.g., stroke rehabilitation) can demonstrate cumulative client progress and functional gains through rehabilitation
      3. Program evaluation enhances quality assurance programs by defining indicators, problem identifiers, and thresholds in need of review

Figure 24.5. Characteristics of Selected Activities of Daily Living (ADL) Scales

Scale	Items Included	Type of Scale	Evaluation
Katz Index of ADL	Bathing, dressing, toileting, transferring, continence, feeding; order of items reflects natural progression in loss and acquisition of function	Dichotomous rating of independence or dependence on each item; forms a six-level Guttman Scale	By professional raters
Kenny Self-Care Evaluation	Seventeen activities in six categories: bed activities, transfers, locomotion, personal hygiene, dressing, and feeding	Each activity rated on a four-point scale (0= complete dependence, 4= complete independence); an average score is created for each of six categories, allowing a possible total score of 24	By rehabilitation staff; scores constructed on the basis of observations
Barthel Index	Feeding, transferring, grooming, toileting, bathing, walking, or propelling a wheelchair; climbing stairs, bladder control, bowel control	Partial scores for performing ADLs with help, full score for independent performance; items weighted; full score of 100 signifies ability to do all tasks independently	By rehabilitation staff

Sources Consulted

Jacelon, C.S. (1986). The Barthel Index: A review of the literature. *Rehabilitation Nursing, 11*(4), 9-11.

Katz, S., Lord, A.B., Moskowitz, R.W., Jackson, B.A., & Jaffe, M.W. (1963). Studies of illness in the aged. The index of ADL: A standardized measure of biological and psychological function. *Journal of the American Medical Association, 185*, 914-919.

4. Program evaluation is a systematic procedure for measuring results of services after a client leaves rehabilitation, by providing an overview of program performance and outcome (Forer, 1981)

B. General guidelines for program evaluation systems
   1. Data should be collected on a regular and continuous basis
   2. Outcomes should be results-oriented
   3. Outcome criteria should be used in decision making

C. Components and activities of program evaluation
   1. Vary with the type of institution and overall aims of the interventions
   2. Most evaluation systems form a circular feedback model in which information gathered throughout process can be used to modify program in relation to stated aims and goals of the service

D. Wilkerson (1991) identified three important features of thorough program evaluation
   1. Compliance evaluation, or program monitoring: Ensuring that a program is functioning within a set of defined standards
   2. Efficiency evaluation: Judging whether a program is productive and/or cost-effective
   3. Effectiveness evaluation: Gathering data and using information in a way that demonstrates how well a program meets its goals

II. Program Evaluation Model: Design Elements and Application to Practice

A. Design elements: Glass model (Glass, 1989)—program evaluation has external influences that regulate the need for measuring impact of a specific program (see Figure 24.4)
   1. Examples of some of these external influences
      a. Referral sources
      b. Government agencies
      c. General rehabilitation market
   2. Mission statement: Integral design element that identifies established goals of the institution
   3. Within each program, four major areas need to be addressed to help a facility fulfill its stated mission
      a. Program goals
      b. Admission criteria
      c. Identification of patients to be served
      d. Services and care to be provided

B. Application to practice
   1. Program evaluation provides a measure of efficiency and cost-effectiveness based on consumers' experience with a rehabilitation facility or program
   2. Information derived from program evaluation can justify the following changes, spending, and community support for action in the future
      a. Program modification as needed
      b. Assessment of quality of services
      c. Creation of individual care plans
      d. Collection of outcome data for research purposes
      e. Long-range planning for programs
      f. Marketing of positive results

III. Preliminary Considerations in Choosing a Program Evaluation System

A. Basic overall considerations to take into account when deciding on a program evaluation protocol
   1. Some institutions develop their own system to meet their unique and specific needs
   2. Others employ commercially available systems standardized within each discipline

B. System characteristics to consider when choosing a system
   1. Group versus individual measures of function and/or outcome
   2. Specific parameters to be measured
   3. Sources for measurement data
   4. Reliability and validity of tools to be employed
   5. Day-to-day performance versus tested functional capacity
   6. Criteria for client selection
   7. Reporting techniques that best present information

Figure 24.6. Characteristics of Selected Global Evaluation Scales

Name of Scale	Items Included	Type of Scale	Evaluator
Functional Independence Measure (FIM)	Eighteen items included in the following six categories: self-care, sphincter control, mobility, locomotion, communication, and social cognition	A seven-level scale, with a rating of 1 indicating a need for total assistance and 7 equaling complete independence, for inpatient and outpatient assessment	Trained professional disciplines as determined by facility
Level of Rehabilitation Scale (LORS)/LORS American Data System (LADS)	Nursing evaluation in following categories: ADL, mobility, verbal communication, and memory	A four-level scale for assessing capabilities of inpatients and outpatients	Evaluation by nurse and by appropriate discipline for each domain of measurement
Patient Evaluation Conference System (PECS™)	Nursing evaluation of bowel, urinary, skin care, self-care, interdisciplinary activities, patient education, resocialization, and safety awareness	A seven-level scale wherein a rating of 1 equals total dependence and 7 indicates abilities are within normal limits and no program is needed	Professional discipline responsible for each category

Sources Consulted

Formations in Health Care, Inc. (1992). *The LORS American Data System (LADS) evaluations by nursing staff.* (Available from Formations in Health Care, 1144 W. Wrightwood Avenue, Chicago, IL 60614)

Patient Evaluation and Conference System, Inc. (PECS™). (Available from Marianjoy Rehabilitation Hospital and Clinics, PO Box 795, Wheaton, IL 60189)

Uniform Data System for Medical Rehabilitation. (1990). *Guide for the use of the Uniform Data Set for Medical Rehabilitation in the Functional Independence Measure.* Buffalo, NY: State University of New York, Buffalo.

a. Statistics
b. Graphs, matrices
c. Narrative description
d. Patient's and/or family's comments

8. Collection of data regarding program effectiveness after discharge
   a. Telephone interview
   b. In-person evaluation and/or observation
   c. Survey by mail
   d. Long-term follow-up

IV. Functional Status Measurement: The Central Component of Program Evaluation

A. Measurement of physical functioning
   1. Most common method of documenting rehabilitation gains
   2. Assessment of effectiveness and quality of rehabilitation depends on reliability and sensitivity of assessment instruments
      a. Instrument development included measurement of basic activities of daily living (ADLs)
      b. Today, more global measures of assessment serve as basis of evaluation of outcomes

B. Focus of rehabilitation nursing interventions
   1. Restoration of function
   2. Maintenance of recovery gains
   3. Prevention of secondary complications

C. Purpose of functional assessment: At present, is a basic methodology used to obtain information on which goal attainments are measured

D. Functional assessment methodology
   1. Has evolved over the past three decades with the development of more than 40 measurement tools to document function
   2. Almost all scales include some combination of dressing, bathing, toileting, transferring, mobility, feeding, and continence
   3. Several ADL scales are still used in some rehabilitation settings (see Figure 24.5)
      a. Katz Index of ADL
      b. Kenny Self-Care Evaluation
      c. Barthel Index
   4. Global scales measuring functional abilities are widely used in rehabilitation practice and research (Granger, Cotter, & Hamilton, 1993) (see Figure 24.6)
      a. Functional Independence Measure (FIM) (Uniform Data System for Medical Rehabilitation, 1990) (see Figure 24.7)
      b. Level of Rehabilitation Scale (LORS)/LORS American Data System (LADS) (Formations in Health Care, Inc., 1992) (see Figure 24.8)
      c. Patient Evaluation and Conference System (PECS™) (see Figure 24.9)

E. Evaluation of a functional assessment instrument should be determined by several guiding principles
   1. Measurement tool should be a valid measure of the function being tested
   2. Previous studies should document the tool's having adequate reliability
   3. Tool should be sensitive enough to identify clinically important changes in status
   4. Method of administering the test can affect the

Figure 24.7. Functional Independence Measure

LEVELS		
	7 Complete Independence (Timely, Safely) 6 Modified Independence (Device)	NO HELPER
	Modified Dependence 5 Supervision 4 Minimal Assist (Subject = 75%+) 3 Moderate Assist (Subject = 50%+) Complete Dependence 2 Maximal Assist (Subject = 25%+) 1 Total Assist (Subject = 0%+)	HELPER

Self Care	ADMIT	DISCHG	FOL-UP
A. Eating	☐	☐	☐
B. Grooming	☐	☐	☐
C. Bathing	☐	☐	☐
D. Dressing—Upper Body	☐	☐	☐
E. Dressing—Lower Body	☐	☐	☐
F. Toileting	☐	☐	☐
Sphincter Control			
G. Bladder Management	☐	☐	☐
H. Bowel Management	☐	☐	☐
Mobility			
Transfer:			
I. Bed, Chair, Wheelchair	☐	☐	☐
J. Toilet	☐	☐	☐
K. Tub, Shower	☐	☐	☐
Locomotion			
L. Walk/wheel Chair	w ☐ c ☐ ☐	w ☐ c ☐ ☐	w ☐ c ☐ ☐
M. Stairs	☐	☐	☐
Communication			
N. Comprehension	a ☐ v ☐ ☐	a ☐ v ☐ ☐	a ☐ v ☐ ☐
O. Expression	v ☐ n ☐ ☐	v ☐ n ☐ ☐	v ☐ n ☐ ☐
Social Condition			
P. Social Interaction	☐	☐	☐
Q. Problem Solving	☐	☐	☐
R. Memory	☐	☐	☐
Total FIM	☐	☐	☐

NOTE: Leave no blanks; enter 1 if patient not testable due to risk.

Reprinted with permission of Uniform Data Management Service from Uniform Data System for Medical Rehabilitation. (1990). *Guide for the use of the Uniform Data Set for Medical Rehabilitation in the Functional Independence Measure* (Version 3.1). Buffalo, NY: State University of New York, Buffalo.

Figure 24.8. Level of Rehabilitation Scale (LORS) American Data System (LADS) Evaluations by Nursing Staff

Patient ______________________ Rater ______________

Admission Date ______________ Discharge Date ________

Major surgical procedure during or within 60 days before rehabilitation? Yes ☐ No ☐

These ratings are for:
Admission________ or Discharge________ Date of Rating____

Activities of Daily Living — **Rating**

A. Dressing ____

B. Grooming ____

C. Washing/Bathing: Rate focus of program at admission. If unknown, rate all appropriate areas and determine focus at discharge.
Bedbath ☐ Sink ☐ Tub/Shower ☐ ____

D. Toileting: Rate focus of program at admission. If unknown, rate all appropriate areas and determine focus at discharge.
Bedpan ☐ Commode ☐
Toilet ☐ Colostomy/Catheter ☐ ____

E. Feeding: Rate focus of program at admission. If unknown, rate all appropriate areas and determine focus at discharge.
Oral ☐ Enteral ☐ Parenteral ☐ ____

Mobility Rate focus of program at admission. If unknown, rate all appropriate areas and determine focus at discharge.

A. Ambulation ____

B. Wheelchair Management ____

Verbal Communication

A. Auditory Comprehension ____

B. Oral Expression
Language Impairment ☐ or
Neuromuscular Impairment ☐ ____

Alternate Communication ____

Short-Term Memory ____

Long-Term Memory ____

Reprinted with permission of Formations in Health Care, Inc., from Formations in Health Care. (1992). *The LORS American Data System (LADS) evaluations by nursing staff.* Chicago: Author. (Available from Formations in Health Care, Inc., 1144 W. Wrightwood Avenue, Chicago, IL 60614)

Figure 24.9. Listing of Patient Evaluation and Conference System (PECS™) Items and Item Groupings

I. Rehabilitation Medicine (MED)
1. Motor Loss
2. Spasticity/Involuntary Movement
3. Joint Limitations
4. Autonomic Disturbance
5. Sensory Deficiency
6. Perceptual & Cognitive Deficits
7. Associated Medical Problems
8. Postural Deviations

II. Rehabilitation Nursing (NSG)
1. Performance of Bowel Program
2. Performance of Urinary Program
3. Performance of Skin Care Program
4. Assumes Responsibility for Self-care
5. Performs Assigned Interdisciplinary Activities
6. Patient Education
7. Safety Awareness

III. Physical Mobility (PHY)
1. Performance of Transfers
2. Performance of Ambulation
3. Performance of Wheelchair Mobility
4. Ability to Handle Environmental Barriers (e.g., stairs, rugs, elevators)
5. Performance of Car Transfer
6. Driving Mobility
7. Assumes Responsibility for Mobility
8. Position Changes
9. Endurance
10. Balance

IV. Activities of Daily Living (ADL)
1. Performance in Feeding
2. Performance in Hygiene/Grooming
3. Performance in Dressing
4. Performance in Home Management
5. Performance of Mobility in the Home Environment (including utilization of environmental adaptations for communication)
6. Bathroom Transfers

V. Communication (COM)
1. Ability to Comprehend Spoken Language
2. Ability to Produce Language
3. Ability to Read
4. Ability to Produce Written Language
5. Ability to Hear
6. Ability to Comprehend and Use Gesture
7. Ability to Produce Speech
8. Ability to Swallow
12. Impairment in Thought (Verbal Linguistic) Processing (NP4)

VI. Medications (DRG)
1. Knowledge of Medications

VII. Nutrition (NUT)
1. Nutritional Status—Body Weight
2. Nutritional Status—Lab Values
3. Knowledge of Nutrition and/or Modified Diet
4. Skill with Nutrition & Diet (Adherence to Nutritional Plan)
5. Utilization of Nutrition & Diet (Nutritional Health)

VIII. Assistive Devices (DEV)
1. Knowledge of Assistive Mobility Devices
2. Skill with Assuming Operating Position of Assistive Mobility Devices
3. Utilization of Assistive Mobility Devices

IX. Psychology (PSY)
1. Distress/comfort
2. Helplessness/self-efficacy
3. Self-directed Learning Skills
4. Skill in Self-management of Behavior and Emotions
5. Skill in Interpersonal Relations
6. Ability to Participate in the Rehabilitation Program
7. Acceptance/understanding of Disability

X. Neuropsychology (NP)
1. Impairment of Short-term Memory
2. Impairment of Long-term Memory
3. Impairment in Attention-concentration Skills
4. Impairment in Verbal Linguistic Processing
5. Impairment in Visual Spatial Processing
6. Impairment in Basic Intellectual Skills
7. Orientation
8. Alertness/Coma State

XI. Social Issues (SOC)
1. Ability to Problem Solve and Utilize Resources
2. Family: Communication/Resources
3. Family: Understanding of Disability
4. Economic Resources
5. Ability to Live Independently
6. Living Arrangements

XII. Vocational/Educational Activity (V/E)
1. Active Participation in realistic Voc/Ed Planning
2. Realistic Perception of Work-related activity
3. Ability to Tolerate Planned Number of Hours of Voc/Ed
4. Vocational/Educational Placement
5. Physical Capacity for Work

XIII. Therapeutic Recreation (REC)
1. Participation in Group Activities
2. Participation in Community Activities
3. Interaction with Others
4. Participation and Satisfaction with Individual Leisure Activities
5. Active Participation in Sports

XIV. Pain (PAI)
1. Pain Behavior
2. Physical Activity
3. Social Interaction
4. Pacing
5. Sitting Tolerance
6. Standing Tolerance
7. Walking Tolerance
8. Use of Body Mechanics
9. Use of Relaxation Techniques
10. Performance of Medication Program

XVI. Pastoral Care (PC)
1. Awareness of Spiritual Dimensions of Illness/Disability
2. Knowledge of Spiritual Resources
3. Skill in Self-management of Spirituality
4. Utilization of Spiritual Resources

quality of information obtained

5. Test administrator should distinguish between capacity to perform and actual performance of an activity
6. Tool should provide a numerical measure of dependence as an indicator of severity of disease

V. Summary: Demand for quality rehabilitation services has been a major impetus for the documentation of outcomes related to nursing interventions; through implementation of program evaluation methodologies, institutions and rehabilitation nurses can measure the effectiveness, efficiency, and quality of care delivered

References

Acorn, S., Love, S., & Mills, W. (1990). Implementation of unit-based quality assurance projects in a rehabilitation hospital. *Rehabilitation Nursing, 15*, 10-12.

American Nurses' Association (ANA). (1973). *Standards of nursing practice.* Kansas City, MO: Author.

American Nurses' Association. (1977). *Standards of rehabilitation nursing practice.* Kansas City, MO: Author.

American Nurses Association. (1991). *Standards of clinical nursing practice.* Washington: Author.

American Nurses' Association & Association of Rehabilitation Nurses (ARN). (1986). *Standards of rehabilitation nursing practice.* Kansas City, MO: American Nurses' Association.

Bassett, S.S. (1993). Quality assurance/quality improvement. In M.W. Koch & T.M. Fairly (Eds.), *Integrated quality management: The key to improving nursing care quality* (pp. 56-72). St. Louis: The C.V. Mosby Company.

Commission on Accreditation of Rehabilitation Facilities (CARF). (1982). *Program evaluation: A guide to utilization.* Tucson, AZ: Author.

Commission on Accreditation of Rehabilitation Facilities (CARF). (1993). *Standards manual for organizations serving people with disabilities.* Tucson, AZ: Author.

Crosby, P.B. (1979). *Quality is free.* New York: New American Library.

Deming, W.E. (1982). *Out of the crisis.* New York: New American Library.

Donabedian, A. (1980). *The definition of quality and approaches to its assessment.* Ann Arbor, MI: Health Administration Press.

England, B., Glass, R.M., & Patterson, C. (1989). *Quality rehabilitation: Results-oriented patient care.* Chicago: American Hospital Publishing, Inc.

Forer, S.K. (1981). Integrating program evaluation and quality assurance. *Journal of the Organization of Rehabilitation Evaluators, 2*, 15-21.

Formations in Health Care, Inc. (1992). *The LORS American Data System (LADS) evaluations by nursing staff.* Chicago: Author. (Available from Formations in Health Care, Inc., 1144 W. Wrightwood Avenue, Chicago, IL 60614)

Frost, M.H. (1992). Quality: A concept of importance to nursing. *Journal of Nursing Care Quality, 7*(1), 64-69.

Glass, R.M. (1989). Program evaluation. In B. England, R.M. Glass, & C. Patterson (Eds.), *Quality rehabilitation: Results-oriented patient care* (pp. 19-37). Chicago: American Hospital Publishing, Inc.

◆Granger, C.V., Cotter, A.C., & Hamilton, B.B. (1993). Functional assessment scales: A study of persons after stroke. *Archives of Physical Medicine and Rehabilitation, 72*, 133-138.

Hamilton, S., & Morales, B.J. (1988). Unit level quality assurance: Essential for success. *Rehabilitation Nursing, 13*, 76-78, 92.

Jacelon, C.S. (1986). The Barthel index: A review of the literature. *Rehabilitation Nursing, 11*(4), 9-11.

Joint Commission on Accreditation of Healthcare Organizations (JCAHO). (1992). *1993 accreditation manual for hospitals.* Oakbrook Terrace, IL: Author.

Joint Commission on Accreditation of Healthcare Organizations (JCAHO). (1988). *A guide to quality assurance.* Chicago: Author.

Joint Commission on Accreditation of Healthcare Organizations (JCAHO). (1990). *Accreditation manual for hospitals.* Oakbrook Terrace, IL: Author.

Katz, S., Lord, A.B., Moskowitz, R.W., Jackson, B.A., & Jaffe, M.W. (1963). Studies of illness in the aged. The index of ADL: A standardized measure of biological and psychological function. *Journal of the American Medical Association, 185*, 914-919.

Keith, R.A. (1982). *Functional assessment in program evaluation for rehabilitation medicine.* Baltimore: Williams & Wilkins.

Kibbee, P.E. (1990). *Quality assurance utilization and risk management.* Deerfield, IL: National Association of Quality Assurance Professionals, Inc.

Lang, N.M., & Marek, K.D. (1991). The policy and politics of patient outcomes. *Journal of Nursing Quality Assurance, 5*(2), 7-12.

Martin, C.A. (1991). National Association of Quality Assurance Professionals position paper: The role of quality improvement in health care quality assurance. *Journal of Quality Assurance, 12*(5), 12-19.

Masters, F., & Schmele, J.A. (1991). Total quality management: An idea whose time has come. *Journal of Nursing Quality Assurance, 5*(4), 7-16.

Mills, W.C. (1989). Unit-based outcomes developed through nursing diagnoses. *Journal of Nursing Quality Assurance, 4*(1), 10-17.

Nightingale, F. (1856). (1969 reprint). *Notes on nursing: What it is and what it is not.* New York: Dover Publications.

Oie, M., & Recker, D. (1992). Empowerment through collaboration: Implementing a team quality assurance model. *Journal of Nursing Care Quality, 6*(2), 32-40.

Patient Evaluation and Conference System, Inc. (PECS™). (Available from Marianjoy Rehabilitation Hospital and Clinics, PO Box 795, Wheaton, IL 60189)

Patterson, C.H. (1988). Standards of patient care: The Joint Commission focus on nursing quality assurance. *Nursing Clinics of North America, 23*, 625-638.

Patterson, C.H. (1993). Joint Commission nursing care standards: The framework for a comprehensive program to assess and improve quality. *Journal of Nursing Care Quality, 7*(2), 1-14.

Patton, S., & Stanley, J. (1993). Bridging quality assurance and continuous quality improvement. *Journal of Nursing Care Quality, 7*(2), 15-23.

Ruckstuhl, M.C., Marcionada, E.E., Salmons, J., & Larrabee, J.H. (1991). Patient falls: An outcome indicator. *Journal of Nursing Care Quality, 6*(1), 25-29.

Stevens, R. (1989). *In sickness and in wealth: American hospitals in the twentieth century.* New York: Basic Books.

Uniform Data System for Medical Rehabilitation. (1990). *Guide for the use of the Uniform Data Set for Medical Rehabilitation in the Functional Independence Measure.* Buffalo, NY: State University of New York, Buffalo.

Vail, J.D., & Jacobs, M.E. (1986). Quality assurance: The pieces of the puzzle. *Journal of the Association of Nurse Anesthetists, 54*(2), 171-176.

Walton, M. (1986). *The Deming management method.* New York: Dodd, Mead & Company, Inc.

Weiss, C.H. (1972). *Evaluation research.* Englewood Cliffs, NJ: Prentice Hall, Inc.

Wilkerson, D.L. (1991). Program and outcome evaluation: Opportunity for the 1990s. *Occupational Therapy Practice, 2*, 1-15.

Yura, H., & Walsh, M.B. (1967). *The nursing process.* Washington,

DC: The Catholic University of America Press.

Zimmer, M.J., & Lang, N.J. (1974). *Development of sets of patient health outcome criteria by panels of nurse experts: Final report.* Madison, WI: Regional Medical Program, University of Wisconsin.

Suggested Readings

Arikian, V. (1991). Total quality management: Applications to nursing services. *Journal of Nursing Administration, 21*(6), 46-50.

Avillion, A.E., & Mirgon, B.B. (1989). *Quality assurance in rehabilitation nursing: A practical guide.* Rockville, MD: Aspen Publishers, Inc.

Burwick, D.M. (1989). Continuous improvement as an ideal in health care. *The New England Journal of Medicine, 320*(1), 53-56.

Carey, R.G., & Prosavac, E.J.. (1982). Rehabilitation program evaluation using a revised level of rehabilitation scale (LORS-II). *Archives of Physical Medicine and Rehabilitation, 63*, 367-370.

Carey, R.G., & Seibert, M.A. (1988). Integrating program evaluation, quality assurance, and marketing for inpatient rehabilitation. *Rehabilitation Nursing, 13*, 66-70.

Commission on Accreditation of Rehabilitation Facilities (CARF). (1988). *Standards manual for organizations serving people with disabilities.* Tucson, AZ: Author.

Courts, N.F. (1988). A patient satisfaction survey for a rehabilitation unit. *Rehabilitation Nursing, 13*, 79-81.

Do, H.K., Sahagian, D.A., Schuster, L.C., & Sheridan, S.E. (1988). Head trauma rehabilitation: Program evaluation. *Rehabilitation Nursing, 13*, 71-75.

Granger, C.V., Hamilton, B.B., & Sherwin, F.S. (1986). *Guide for use of the Uniform Data Set for Medical Rehabilitation.* Buffalo, NY: Buffalo General Hospital.

Gresham, G.E., & Labi, M.L.C. (1984). Functional assessment instruments currently available for documenting outcomes in rehabilitation medicine. In C.V. Granger & G.E. Gresham (Eds.), *Functional assessment in rehabilitation medicine* (pp. 65-85). Baltimore: Williams & Wilkins.

Gresham, G.E., Phillips, T.F., & Labi, M.L.C. (1980). ADL status in stroke: Relative merits of three standard indexes. *Archives of Physical Medicine and Rehabilitation, 61*, 355-358.

Hamilton, B.B., Granger, C.V., Sherwin, F.S., Zielezny, M., & Tasham, J.S. (1987). A uniform national data system for medical rehabilitation. In M.J. Fuhrer (Ed.), *Rehabilitation outcomes: Analysis and measurement* (pp. 137-147). Baltimore: Paul H. Brookes Publishing Company.

Hamilton, B.B., Laughlin, J.A., Granger, C.V., & Kayton, R.M. (1991). Interrater agreement of the seven level functional independence measure (Abstract from the Scientific Meeting of the 1991 American Academy of Physical Medicine and Rehabilitation and the American Congress of Rehabilitation, October 27-31, 1991, Washington, DC). *Archives of Physical Medicine and Rehabilitation, 71*, 790.

Isaac, D.N. (1983, March). Suggestions for organizing a quality assurance program. *Quality Review Bulletin*, pp. 68-72.

Kane, R.A., & Kane, R.L. (1981). *Assessing the elderly: A practical guide to measuring.* Lexington, MA: Lexington Books.

◆Kelly-Hayes, M., Jette, A., Wolf, P.A., D'Agostino, R.A. & Odell, P. (1992). Functional limitations and disability among elders in the Framingham study. *American Journal of Public Health, 82*(6), 841-845.

Mahoney, F.I., & Barthel, D. (1965). Functional evaluation: The Barthel index. *Maryland State Medical Journal, 14*, 61-65.

McCourt, A. (1987). Implementation of nursing diagnoses through integration with quality assurance. *Nursing Clinics of North America, 22*, 899-904.

McCourt, A. (1986). Nursing diagnoses: Key to quality assurance. In M. Hurley (Ed.), *North American Nursing Diagnosis Association: Proceedings of the Sixth Conference on Classification of Nursing Diagnosis* (pp. 133-138). St. Louis: The C.V. Mosby Company.

Nadzam, D.M. (1991). The Agenda for Change: Update of indicator development and possible implications for the nursing profession. *Journal of Nursing Quality Assurance, 5*(2), 18-22.

Ricciardi, E., & Kuck, A.W. (1992). Improving patient outcomes: The role of the clinical nurse specialist in quality assurance. *Journal of Nursing Care Quality, 6*(2), 46-50.

◆Rondinelli, R.D., Murphy, J.R., Wilson, D.H., & Miller, C.C. (1991). Predictors of functional outcome and resource utilization in inpatient rehabilitation. *Archives of Physical Medicine and Rehabilitation, 72*, 447-453.

Rowland, H.S., & Rowland, B.L. (1992). *The manual of nursing quality assurance.* Gaithersburg, MD: Aspen Publishers, Inc.

Stenvig, T.E., & Karpuik, K. (1991). A nursing care monitoring and evaluation system: Making it work in differentiated practice. *Nursing Forum, 26*(1), 27-34.

◆Wilkerson, L.L., Bativia, A.I., & De Jong, G. (1992). Use of functional status measures for payment of medical rehabilitation services. *Archives of Physical Medicine and Rehabilitation, 73*, 111-119.

◆ indicates a research-based work

Section V
Community Reentry

As rehabilitation nurses, our commitment to our clients extends beyond the facility and beyond acute care management of the disability; therefore, our responsibility is to be aware of community resources for care and promote access to these services. Serving as an advocate for our clients with disabilities requires an understanding of their needs for care as well as the federal, state, and private organizations and agencies that provide a wide array of healthcare services.

Nurse case management has evolved historically to be a very efficient and comprehensive method of helping clients gain access to healthcare services and of allocating available funding. This section will discuss the nurse case manager's role in rehabilitation, the life skills and community resources necessary for clients to live in the community, and the issues regarding access to these healthcare services. It is the rehabilitation nurse who, through clinical expertise and knowledge about community services, promotes community living for clients with a disability and enhances their quality of life.

CHAPTER 25

Nurse Case Management in Rehabilitation

Escalating healthcare costs have given rise to the development of new and more effective approaches to the delivery of healthcare services. One such approach, that of case management, has emerged as a significant trend in managed health care. Rehabilitation nurses, with their specialized knowledge and skills in caring for persons with disabilities, are in a unique position to serve as case managers for clients in acute, rehabilitation, and community settings. The objectives of this chapter are to describe the role functions of the rehabilitation nurse case manager and identify the impact of the rehabilitation nurse case manager on the quality and cost-effectiveness of healthcare services.

Case management is the process of planning, organizing, coordinating, and monitoring the services and resources needed to respond to a client's healthcare needs (Association of Rehabilitation Nurses [ARN], 1991). Case management does not usually involve hands-on nursing care of clients. By assessing, planning, implementing, coordinating, and evaluating, the rehabilitation nurse case manager ensures the delivery of cost-effective, quality healthcare services that help the client move toward optimal health following a disabling illness or injury.

Rehabilitation nurse case managers practice in a variety of acute, rehabilitation, and community settings. These settings include, but are not limited to, rehabilitation facilities, acute care hospitals, long-term care facilities, home health agencies, insurance carriers, governmental agencies, and private rehabilitation companies. Many rehabilitation nurse case managers are self-employed and function as independent case managers. Those practicing in insurance, private rehabilitation, community, and independent practice settings are commonly referred to as *external case managers*, while those practicing in hospitals and facilities are known as *internal case managers*.

Case management has become an accepted—even preferred—method of managing the multiple, often complex aspects of health care. As case management continues to develop as a primary healthcare delivery system, the opportunities for rehabilitation nurses to provide case management services will expand. While much research on client and system outcomes is needed, rehabilitation nurse case managers will continue to facilitate a client's optimal functioning and independence, while minimizing healthcare costs.

Historical Perspectives on Case Management

The development of rehabilitation nursing practice in the insurance, private rehabilitation, and independent practice settings over the past three decades has greatly influenced the role of the rehabilitation nurse case manager. The Association of Rehabilitation Nurses formally recognized this in 1991 by publishing a role description for rehabilitation nurse case managers. In facility-based settings, the role has evolved due to the influence of primary nursing as a nursing care delivery system as well as because of the interdisciplinary nature of rehabilitative care.

In the 1950s, the first rehabilitation nurses were employed by large national insurance carriers to assist persons with work-related injuries in their return to work as quickly as possible (Latus, 1982). By the 1960s, rehabilitation nurses were involved in the management of not only workmen's compensation claims but also liability and long-term disability claims; the primary focus of this rehabilitation nurse consultant role was that of cost control through the coordination and monitoring of services.

The 1970s marked the beginning of private rehabilitation companies that provided case management services on a fee-for-service basis. These proprietary companies primarily managed workmen's compensation claims; case management in workmen's compensation included the coordination of vocationally oriented services aimed at returning the client to work. These companies employed both rehabilitation nurses and vocational rehabilitation counselors. Soon thereafter, rehabilitation nurses with experience in insurance and/or private rehabilitation settings began entrepreneurial efforts in independent practice (Mumma, 1987). In addition to workers' compensation, liability, and long-term disability claims, accident and health claims involving catastrophic illnesses or injuries associated with long-term consequences and potentially high costs recently have become a focus of external case management.

Facility-based case management has its roots in primary nursing. First introduced in the 1970s, primary nursing was based on the concept of 24-hour accountability for nursing care. Over the past decade, nursing case management models have evolved from this delivery system, expanding upon the concept of accountability to encompass outcomes of care. Case management models vary depending upon the healthcare setting, and many new models are emerging as case management evolves.

Zander and associates (Center for Nursing Case Management, New England Medical Center, 1989) developed and implemented one such model at the New England Medical

Center in Boston; the model promotes a collaborative approach among disciplines, emphasizing both quality and the cost-effectiveness of care delivery from hospital admission to discharge. Critical pathways have been developed that standardize appropriate services and treatment within an appropriate length of stay and identify expected client and care delivery outcomes. Carondelet St. Mary's Hospital and Health Center in Tucson, AZ, developed a similar model expanding the provision of case management services from discharge into the community setting and providing internal case management services on a fee-for-service basis (Etheridge & Lamb, 1989).

Facility-based case management in rehabilitation nursing also has developed as a result of the interdisciplinary team approach used in rehabilitative care. In many settings, rehabilitation nurses are being recognized for their ability to assess the client from a holistic perspective and to coordinate services delivered by rehabilitation team members. Thus, more and more rehabilitation nurses in these settings are stepping into case manager roles, and more and more healthcare providers and funding sources are recognizing the rehabilitation nurse's expertise as they function as case managers.

I. Case Management Goals

- A. The rehabilitation nurse case manager uses a goal-oriented approach emphasizing both quality and cost-effectiveness of services; goals include the following
  1. Outcomes of care
     - a. Optimal functioning and independence in the least restrictive environment
     - b. Prevention of complications
     - c. Effective coping with the disability
     - d. A successful return to work, school, and community
  2. System outcomes: Provision of timely, appropriate services by qualified service providers
  3. Minimization of healthcare costs
- B. The rehabilitation nurse case manager facilitates outcomes of case management
  1. As a *coordinator*, the case manager facilitates client access to healthcare services and coordinates and monitors all health care provided to the client; timely provision and continuity of services are essential to effective coordination
  2. As a *collaborator*, the rehabilitation nurse case manager collaborates with the facility-based and community-based rehabilitation teams through ongoing communication
  3. As an *educator*, the case manager promotes or provides the education of clients regarding their health status and prevention of complications or further disability; emphasis is placed on self-management and responsibility for healthcare needs
  4. As an *advocate*, the rehabilitation nurse case manager strives to promote the client's optimal functioning and independence in the community

II. Client Characteristics and Referral Considerations

- A. Early identification of clients is essential to successful case management and subsequent achievement of outcomes; ideally, this should occur at the onset of disability
  1. Internal, or facility-based, case managers typically serve all clients receiving care and initiate services upon a client's admission
  2. External case managers receive referrals primarily from insurance carriers and other third-party payers
     - a. These referrals are usually based on predetermined criteria used by the referral source and encompass clients with catastrophic illnesses or injuries, those at high risk for the long-term consequences of disability, and those with work-related illnesses or injuries
     - b. External case managers often can facilitate early identification of clients needing case management through ongoing education of referral sources and reviews of claim files
- B. Clients of all ages are served by rehabilitation nurse case managers; those who provide services to children and older adult client populations need additional specialized knowledge
  1. Children served by case managers include those with disabilities at birth, those with developmental disabilities, and those with acquired catastrophic illness or injury
  2. Community reintegration of children with an emphasis on education is a major focus of the rehabilitation team and case manager
  3. Older adult clients include those who, through the case manager's coordination of appropriate services, can continue to function independently in their community
  4. The case manager facilitates placement when a client's remaining at home is no longer feasible
- C. Considerations in referring clients for case management
  1. The nature and severity of the illness or injury
     - a. Catastrophic illness or injuries: Multiple trauma, burns, head injury, spinal cord injury, stroke, cancer, and AIDS
     - b. Workers' compensation cases: Back injury, chronic pain, soft tissue or joint injury, or repetitive motion disorder
     - c. Presence of secondary disability
  2. Type of treatment received or recommended
  3. Emotional and/or behavioral status
  4. Age
  5. Available social support systems

III. Role Functions of the Rehabilitation Nurse Case Manager: Correspond to the Phases of the Nursing Process

- A. Assessment
  1. A comprehensive assessment is completed upon referral to the case manager; authorization, if necessary, is obtained prior to the assessment that is performed in the client's home, whenever possible
  2. Assessment data are collected from a variety of sources
     - a. Interview with client and client's family
     - b. Attending physician and other healthcare disciplines involved in client's care
     - c. Review of medical records and school reports

d. Employer contact in workers' compensation cases

3. Areas of emphasis during assessment
   a. Present illness or injury as well as health status
      1) Diagnosis, prognosis, current treatment, and future treatment recommendations
      2) Functional abilities and/or activities of daily living
   b. Psychosocial status
      1) Emotional and/or behavioral response to illness or injury
      2) Roles and relationships and/or family functioning
   c. Financial status
      1) Income sources
      2) Eligibility for additional funding sources
   d. Home environment
      1) Accessibility
      2) Safety
   e. Educational and vocational assessment (Mumma, 1987)
      1) Educational
         a) Current ability to read and write
         b) Level of education completed; degrees held
         c) Specialized training obtained in military service
         d) Eligibility for Department of Veterans Affairs training benefits
      2) Vocational
         a) Past employment
            (1) Jobs held
            (2) Duration of employment
            (3) Reason(s) for leaving job(s)
            (4) Special skills attained
            (5) Union involvement
            (6) Client's verbalized or demonstrated attitude toward employer, coworkers, union
         b) Transferable skills
            (1) Help determine client's vocational potential
            (2) Are determined by analyzing client's past work history
            (3) Can be determined by using various resources
               (a) Vocational Diagnosis and Assessment of Residual Employability (VDARE) worksheet (Sink & Field, 1981)
               (b) *Dictionary of Occupational Titles* (U.S. Department of Labor, Employment and Training Administration, 1991)
         c) Job analysis
            (1) Formalized process for observing a job as it is performed and describing its characteristics, including its physical demands, working conditions, prerequisite general education, training time, and required aptitudes (Sink & Field, 1981)
            (2) A means to compare job characteristics with postinjury abilities
            (3) A method for observing and/or measuring a job's physical demands
               (a) Lifting
               (b) Carrying
               (c) Bending
               (d) Reaching
               (e) Grasping
               (f) Standing
               (g) Walking
               (h) Talking
               (i) Hearing
               (j) Seeing
            (4) Classifying physical demands as described in the *Dictionary of Occupational Titles* (U.S. Department of Labor, Employment and Training Administration, 1991)
               (a) Sedentary (0 to 10 lbs lifted frequently)
               (b) Light (10 lbs lifted frequently; 20 lbs lifted occasionally)
               (c) Medium (20 lbs lifted frequently; 50 lbs lifted occasionally)
               (d) Heavy (50 lbs lifted frequently; 100 lbs lifted occasionally)
               (e) Very heavy (more than 100 lbs lifted frequently)

B. Planning
   1. Problems or nursing diagnoses are formulated from assessment data
   2. Rehabilitation plan is developed in partnership with the client, family, and facility-based and/or community-based rehabilitation team members
      a. Rehabilitation plan has several features
         1) Short- and long-term goals and/or expected outcomes that are patient-centered
         2) Recommendations for care, treatment, and services
         3) Target dates for achievement of goals and/or outcomes
         4) Costs of services
         5) Treatment alternatives and associated costs
         6) Available community resources and/or alternate funding sources
         7) Discharge plans, when appropriate
      b. Community-based rehabilitation team members include those described in Chapter 22 as well as the following
         1) Rehabilitation nurse case manager
         2) Rehabilitation counselor
         3) Claims representative for client's insurance carrier, third-party payer, or private funding source
         4) Employer or volunteer supervisor for noncompetitive placement
         5) School personnel
         6) Client's attorney

7) Discharge planner
8) Community health nurse

3. Service providers are evaluated according to whether they offer quality services at reasonable cost
4. Authorization for services usually is obtained through client's insurance carrier or third-party payer
5. Long-term planning for catastrophic cases is done through development of life care plans
   a. Life care plans involve projection of comprehensive needs and costs over the course of the lifetime of the person with a catastrophic illness or injury
   b. Life care plans are often used in litigation of catastrophic cases; however, most importantly, they serve to provide a framework for the long-term care needs of clients and families (Deutsch & Sawyer, 1989)
   c. Life care plans include projections of future rehabilitation interventions and costs as the client ages, experiences a change in medical status, or requires periodic reinitiation of healthcare services
6. In workers' compensation cases, the primary goal is return to work
   a. A return-to-work hierarchy is used to determine an appropriate vocational goal (Rubin & Roessler, 1987)
   b. Hierarchy includes return-to-work alternatives
      1) Same job and same employer
      2) Same job (modified) and same employer
      3) Different job and same employer
      4) Same job but different employer
      5) Same job (modified) but different employer
      6) Different job and different employer
      7) Different job involving retraining; employer could be either same or different
      8) Self-employment

C. Implementation
1. Involves procurement and coordination of monitoring of the care, treatment, and/or services provided to the client
2. Services can include various options
   a. Medical or surgical treatment
   b. Inpatient, outpatient, day treatment, or community reintegration rehabilitation programs
   c. Specialized rehabilitation programs for persons with head injuries, spinal cord injuries, burns, chronic pain
   d. Skilled, intermediate, or long-term nursing care
   e. Home health care
   f. Attendant care and/or assistance with behavioral management
   g. Home evaluation services and home modification
   h. Orthotic and prosthetic devices
   i. Durable medical equipment and supplies
   j. Psychological services
   k. Outpatient or home-based physical, occupational, speech, or cognitive therapy; community skills or life skills training
   l. Independent or transitional living centers
   m. Hospice care
   n. Transportation services
   o. Meal programs
   p. Support groups
   q. Vocational services
      1) Work hardening
      2) Vocational evaluation
      3) Vocational counseling
      4) Job placement or supported employment
      5) Job modifications
      6) Work adjustment
      7) On-the-job training or job coaching
      8) Formal training
      9) Volunteer or noncompetitive placement
      10) Referral to vocational rehabilitation office
3. Community reintegration is addressed
   a. Access to community agencies is obtained
   b. Reentry to the home or an alternative living site is facilitated
4. Costs of services are negotiated, whenever possible, taking into account preferred provider organization (PPO) networks and mandated fee schedules
5. Services are coordinated through ongoing communication and collaboration among rehabilitation team members
   a. Case manager attends team staff meetings, whenever possible, in all settings
   b. Client progress is communicated by and to rehabilitation team members

D. Evaluation
1. Outcomes are evaluated and progress toward goal achievement is identified
2. Goals are modified when necessary
3. Successful goal achievement ideally determines the discontinuation of case management services or case closure; cases can be closed for various other reasons as well
   a. Client is unwilling to participate in services
   b. Attending physician is not receptive to case management
   c. Client's attorney is not receptive to case management
   d. Closure is requested by insurance carrier or third-party payer
   e. Funding has been exhausted
4. If goals are unable to be met or funding is exhausted, case manager must refer client to community agencies
5. Case closure in external case management includes a cost-benefit analysis
6. Case closure should also identify circumstances under which the case will be reopened
   a. Change in medical status
   b. Impact of aging
   c. Progression of illness
   d. Change in family structure
   e. Change in placement
   f. Reinitiation of rehabilitation services

IV. Legislative and Regulatory Influences on Case Management

A. The rehabilitation nurse case manager must have knowledge of federal, state, and local governmental regulations and legislation and their impact on healthcare services

B. The rehabilitation nurse case manager will encounter regulatory and service systems that require knowledge of the benefits provided
   1. Medicare
   2. Medicaid
   3. Private healthcare insurance
   4. Social Security disability
   5. Veterans Administration disability
   6. Workers' compensation
   7. State vocational rehabilitation programs
   8. Other federal, state, and local agencies
   9. Community groups

C. Much legislation at the federal, state, and local levels affects case management practice
   1. Economic Opportunity Acts of 1964 and 1974: Initiated Head Start program; included children with disabilities in 1974
   2. Rehabilitation Act of 1973 and the amendments of 1978: Provided funding for variety of efforts
      a. Vocational rehabilitation
      b. Affirmative action efforts to employ qualified persons with disabilities
      c. Accessibility of federally funded building and transportation systems
      d. Funding for independent living
   3. Education for All Handicapped Children Act of 1975 and the amendments of 1986: Provided funding for educational assistance and early intervention programs for children with disabilities
   4. Americans with Disabilities Act of 1990: Mandated nondiscrimination in the employment of persons with disabilities and barrier-free transportation systems and buildings

V. Current Issues in Case Management

A. Quality assurance for case management practice
   1. Essential component of rehabilitation case management services
   2. Provides a mechanism for the case manager to evaluate the case management provided; aspects to be evaluated include the following
      a. Client outcomes
      b. System outcomes based on accepted standards of practice
      c. Client satisfaction
   3. Quality assurance data are used to strengthen ongoing provision of case management services

B. Governmental regulation of practice that includes scope of nurse case managers, state nurse practice acts, educational preparation, and referral or funding source guidelines

C. Legal and ethical issues influencing practice
   1. Many insurance claims involve litigation and, thus, attorneys are often actively involved in cases; attorneys are considered members of the rehabilitation team and should be kept informed of services provided to clients as well as the benefits of each service
   2. Complete and accurate documentation of all case management services provided is essential, because these records are admissible as evidence in a court of law
   3. When funding for case management services is terminated, referrals to community and government-supported agencies should be initiated

D. Accountability to clients
   1. In external case management (services are provided on a fee-for-service basis): Rehabilitation nurse case manager's services usually are retained by the insurance carrier or third-party payer, but may be retained by the family directly or by the attorney, trustee, or court-appointed guardian
      a. Case manager's primary responsibility is to the client
      b. Case manager's level of responsibility to the referral source should be defined prior to initiation of case management services; goals and outcomes of the case management services expected by the referral source and case manager should be identified in measurable terms
   2. In internal case management: Rehabilitation nurse case manager has a responsibility to all rehabilitation team members to ensure that all services provided are in the best interest of the client and directed toward discharge goals

E. Funding
   1. Claim dollars available for services to the client are often limited due to parameters of the policy
   2. The rehabilitation nurse case manager should be aware of a client's insurance policy limits because insurance carriers set aside reserves to pay claim costs
   3. Often the case manager is required to provide funding of services within the policy limits and, thus, must be proactive and creative in developing a rehabilitation plan for the client
   4. When funding is from a reinsurance source, the case manager must be familiar with monies available (e.g., trusts, annuities, estate funds) and recommend services accordingly throughout the client's life span

F. Regulation of case management practice
   1. Federal and state governments are beginning to determine some aspects of case management practice
   2. Credentialing of case managers: Professional bodies are also attempting to determine recommended education, experience, and certification
      a. A baccalaureate education
      b. A minimum of 2 years of clinical experience in rehabilitation or a related specialty
      c. Certification in rehabilitation nursing (Certified Rehabilitation Registered Nurse [CRRN] credential)
   3. Rehabilitation nurse case managers must take a strong leadership role in influencing future regulatory efforts

References

Association of Rehabilitation Nurses (ARN). (1991). *The rehabilitation nurse case manager: Role description.* Skokie, IL: Author.

Center for Nursing Case Management, New England Medical Center. (1989). *Collaborative care: Nursing case management.* Chicago: American Hospital Publishing, Inc.

Deutsch, P., & Sawyer, H. (1989). *A guide to rehabilitation.* New York: Matthew Bender & Company, Inc.

Etheridge, P., & Lamb, G. (1989). Professional nursing case management improves quality, access and costs. *Nursing Management, 20*(3), 30-35.

Latus, M.J. (1982). The role of the insurance rehabilitation nurse. *Rehabilitation Nursing, 7*(3), 26-29.

Mumma, C.M. (Ed.). (1987). *Rehabilitation nursing: Concepts and practice—A core curriculum* (2nd ed.). Evanston, IL: Rehabilitation Nursing Foundation.

National Head Injury Foundation. (1992). *Selecting and monitoring head injury rehabilitation.* (Available from National Head Injury Foundation, 1776 Massachusetts Avenue NW, Suite 100, Washington, DC 20036)

Rubin, S., & Roessler, R. (1987). *Foundations of the vocational rehabilitation process* (3rd ed.). Austin, TX: PRO-ED, Inc.

Sink, J., & Field, T. (1981). *Vocational assessment planning & jobs.* Athens, GA: VSB, Inc.

U.S. Department of Labor, Employment and Training Administration. (1991). *Dictionary of occupational titles* (4th ed., rev.). Lanham, MD: Bernan Press.

Suggested Readings

American Nurses' Association (ANA). (1988). *Nursing case management.* Kansas City, MO: Author.

Applebaum, R.A., & Austin, C.D. (1986). *A guide to the evaluation of long-term care case management.* Seattle: University of Washington Press.

Austin, C.D. (1983). Case management in long-term care: Options and opportunities. *Health and Social Work, 8*(1), 16-30.

Brewer, E.J., McPhearson, M., Magrot, P.R., & Hutchins, V.L. (1989). Family-centered community-based coordinated care for children with special health care needs. *Pediatrics, 3*, 1055-1061.

Capitman, J.A., Haskins, B., & Bernstein, J. (1986). Case management approaches in coordinated community-oriented long term care demonstrations. *Gerontologist, 26*, 398-404.

Donahue, M. (1985). Advocacy. In G. Bulechek & J. McCloskey, *Nursing interventions: Treatments for nursing diagnoses* (pp. 338-351). Philadelphia: W.B. Saunders Company.

Kaufman, J. (1991). An overview of public sector financing for pediatric home care: Part I. *Pediatric Nursing, 17*, 280-281.

Kaufman, J. (1991). An overview of public sector financing for pediatric home care: Part II. *Pediatric Nursing, 17*, 380-381, 422.

Loveridge, C., Cummings, S., & O'Malley, J. (1988). Developing case management in a primary nursing system. *Journal of Nursing Administration, 18*(10), 36-38.

MacAdam, M., & Capitman, J. (1989, July-August). Case management for elders expands hospital boundaries. *Continuing Care*, p. 26.

McKenzie, C., Torkelson, N., & Holt, M. (1989). Care and cost: Nursing case management improves both. *Nursing Management, 20*(10), 30-33.

Managed care: Special report. (1989, January 13). *Modern Healthcare*, pp. 27-54.

Mullahy, C.M. (1991). Making case management count. *The Case Manager, 2*(3), 40-48.

Olivas, G., Del Togno Armanasco, V., Erickson, J., & Harter, S. (1989). Case management: A bottom-line care delivery model. Part I. *Journal of Nursing Administration, 19*(11), 16-20.

Olivas, G., Del Togno Armanasco, V., Erickson, J., & Harter, S. (1989). Case management: A bottom-line care delivery model. Part II. *Journal of Nursing Administration, 19*(12), 12-17.

Peck, N. (1990, January). Case management partnerships link hospitals to payers. *Continuing Care*, pp. 29-34.

Wahlstedt, P., & Blaser, W. (1986). Nurse case management for the frail elderly. *Home Healthcare Nurse, 4*(2), 30-35.

Wiener, S.M. (1983). Rehabilitation nursing in the private sector. *Rehabilitation Nursing, 8*(2), 31-32.

Winder, P. (1988, July). Case managements by nurses at a county facility. *Quality Review Bulletin*, pp. 215-219.

Zander, K. (1988). Managed care within acute care settings: Design and implementation via nursing case management. *Health Care Supervisor, 6*(2), 27-43.

Zander, K. (1987). Nursing case management: A classic. *Definition, 2*(2), 1-4. (Available from New England Medical Center Department of Nursing, 750 Washington Street, Boston, MA 02111)

Zawadski, R.T. (1983). Community based system of long term care. *Home Health Care Services Quarterly, 4*(3-4), entire issue.

CHAPTER 26

Life Skills and Community Living

The purpose of rehabilitation is to help persons with disabilities adapt to living with the disability and to promote independent functioning in their own environment. There are a number of life skills that the person with a disability must develop to successfully complete the transition from institution to community. Environmental modifications and a variety of support services are also essential to promote independent living.

This chapter addresses issues related to safe and accessible housing, transportation, vocational rehabilitation, disability management in the workplace, educational programs, adaptive equipment to facilitate community living, support services and advocacy groups, and community resources.

I. Housing: Selection and Assessment
   A. Factors and alternatives to consider in selecting housing
      1. Be aware that many alternatives are available, depending upon the client's functional ability, support systems, needs, and goals
      2. Secure an appropriately adapted residence; if necessary, make adaptations
         a. Build access ramp(s)
         b. Widen doors
         c. Modify the kitchen and bathroom so that all facilities and appliances are easily accessible
         d. Make parking available
      3. Consider moving client into congregate housing with or without attendant services
      4. Encourage client to join an independent living program that allows people with disabilities to remain in their own dwellings while offering, but not managing, provision of support services
         a. Support services related to ADLs
            1) Training in communication techniques
            2) Communal meals
            3) Training in homemaking skills
            4) Supervision of and guidance in transportation skills
            5) Recreational opportunities
            6) Emergency procedures
            7) Housing options
         b. Support services related to personal health management
            1) Training in communication techniques
            2) Counseling regarding sexuality and family relationships
            3) Management of attendants
         c. Support services related to counseling assistance
            1) Advocacy services
            2) Peer counseling
            3) Consumer and legal information
            4) Personal business management
      5. Be aware of laws governing housing availability and accessibility
         a. The Housing Act of 1959: Provided funding for mortgage loans to developers to build housing for the elderly and the handicapped
         b. The Architectural Barriers Act of 1968: Mandated physical accessibility to any federally funded building being constructed
         c. The Rehabilitation Act of 1973: Prohibited discrimination against the disabled when they rented or purchased federally subsidized property
         d. The Housing and Community Development Act of 1974: Subsidized rent payments to low-income families
         e. The Rehabilitation, Comprehensive Services, and Developmental Disabilities Amendment of 1978: Issued grants for housing
         f. The Americans with Disabilities Act of 1990: Established new laws governing physical access to the community; these laws need to be evaluated in relation to access to services and ways to implement them in communities in order to ensure access
      6. Consider alternative housing situations for clients who are unable to remain in their previous residence
         a. Independent living programs (see I.A.4. on this page)
         b. Residential living: An arrangement in which a group of people with disabilities live in the same building or geographic area and share support services; can involve several challenges
            1) Finding accessible housing
            2) Securing attendant assistance
            3) Providing accessible transportation
            4) Obtaining rent subsidies
         c. Extended-care facilities (e.g., subacute rehabilitation or neurobehavioral programs, skilled care facilities)
   B. Factors to consider in assessing a home
      1. Availability of occupational therapy, physical therapy, and nursing evaluations to assist in determining safety, access, interventions, and the patient's ability to function in his or her own environment

2. Definition of the type of living quarters; design of the building
3. Lighting of the residence and its entrance, heating, running water, electrical outlets, and toilet facilities
4. Access to the residence and the need for wider doors, assistance with door opening, and handrails; bathroom and kitchen modifications
5. Assistive devices needed to facilitate mobility and safe participation in community environments
6. Availability of support systems to assist with mobility
7. Patient's level of independence regarding transfers, homemaking skills, personal care, food procurement and preparation, and household maintenance
8. Availability and adequacy of communications devices
9. Clutter in the environment—for example, scatter rugs, cords, carpets, toys, animals that might pose safety risks
10. Presence and accessibility of an elevator, availability of adaptive equipment (e.g., braille buttons, an elevator bell to indicate floor for visually impaired), automatic door timing for opening and closing
11. Furniture: Arrangement, functionality, client's ability to use it safely, the need for adaptive equipment (e.g., chair with a seat lift)
12. Type of floor surface and ability to maneuver assistive device(s) on it
13. Storage of a vehicle and access to residence from the storage area
14. Ability to hear the telephone, fire alarms, doorbells, and availability of required adaptive equipment

II. Transportation
  A. Legislative mandates for public transportation systems and buildings: Designed to guarantee all persons two basic rights
    1. Equal access to public transportation
    2. Completion of required modifications of airplanes, terminals, buses, subways, and public railroad systems
      a. Space to accommodate wheelchairs
      b. Wider doors and aisles, shorter or tiered steps
      c. Ramp or lift systems, elevators
  B. Issues related to modifications for vehicles for people with disabilities
    1. Hand controls, lifts, seating, and transfer mechanisms
    2. Funding for vehicle modification
    3. Travel programs and clubs for the disabled
  C. Adapted driver education and evaluation procedures
  D. Considerations regarding public transportation for those with disabilities
    1. Transportation services should be contacted prior to use to ensure that assistive services and/or accommodations are available
      a. Chambers of commerce in many cities can provide booklets with information regarding community accessibility
      b. The U.S. Department of Transportation has information regarding highways and airports
    2. It is vital that people with disabilities have access to the workplace, medical services, shopping, support services, recreational facilities, churches, public buildings, banks, clinics, post offices, grocery stores, and clothing stores, among other places, in order to increase independence in self-care and community participation
    3. Other transportation factors to be considered for people with disabilities
      a. Distance from residence to public transportation
      b. Cost of both public transportation and privately owned, specially adapted vehicles
      c. Availability of assistance
      d. Amount of assistance required

III. Vocational Rehabilitation
  A. Federal law mandates that each state have a public agency that provides vocational rehabilitation (Office of Vocational Rehabilitation [OVR])
  B. Funding is provided for various aspects of vocational rehabilitation to facilitate a return to competitive work or supported employment
    1. Vehicle and home modifications
    2. Work hardening programs; assessment of work capacities
    3. Assessment of training facilities, equipment, and transportation
    4. Determination of each individual's vocational limitations
    5. Identification of vocational interests, previous work experience, and current abilities
    6. Assessment of the job market
    7. Employer education and development
    8. Matching the disabled person's functional, cognitive, and emotional abilities with job placement options
      a. Job training
      b. Job modification
      c. Job placement
  C. Supported employment integrates people with disabilities into work settings
    1. History
      a. Rehabilitation Act Amendments of 1986 describe the content of supported employment programs
      b. Traditional vocational rehabilitation programs have served individuals with disabilities primarily in sheltered environments
    2. Foci of supported employment settings
      a. Providing services to the severely disabled is a priority
      b. Workers are paid
      c. Work settings are integrated (persons with disabilities work in settings with able-bodied workers)
      d. Ongoing support is provided

1) Supervision
2) Job adaptations
3) Personal care
4) Money management
5) Social skills
6) Transportation

IV. Disability Management Programs in the Workplace
A. Emphasize early identification of disabled workers; focus on prevention of work-related injuries
B. Identify conditions in the work environment that result in worker disability
C. Provide evaluations to identify the medical, social, and psychological assistance that would enable the worker to return to work
D. Provide case management services in the form of job analysis, job modifications, and job placement
E. Monitor services to address problems that arise after job placement occurs
F. Motivate businesses to develop these programs due to the cost of worker disabilities and subsequent healthcare costs
G. Develop work-hardening programs
H. May result in favorable outcomes
1. Lower workers' compensation costs
2. Reduced absenteeism
3. Reduced costs of rehabilitation services
4. Reduced medical costs
5. Employee retention

V. Educational Program Considerations
A. Availability of institutions offering programs for the disabled (e.g., residential schools for hearing-impaired, blind, and/or head-injured persons)
B. Special services offered for the disabled to facilitate access to educational services
1. Services related to the learning process
a. Adaptation of educational materials (e.g., talking books, braille books, textbook recordings, cognitive software, computer-assisted learning programs)
b. Equipment (e.g., reading machines, audiology services, communication augmentation devices, voice-activated computers)
c. Tutors, interpreters, or note-takers
2. Other access issues
a. Access to classrooms, including parking
b. Access to cafeteria, library, bookstore, dorms, chapel
c. Access to social activities
d. Access to entertainment, recreation, or sports activities
e. Access to adapted bathrooms and shower facilities
C. Availability of support services
1. Financial assistance
2. Attendant services for students residing on campus
3. Healthcare services
4. Career planning and placement services
5. Accessibility of programs for persons with disabilities
6. Programs that take into consideration each individual's functional and cognitive abilities
7. Vocational or guidance counseling
D. Adapted driver evaluation and education: Modification of existing driver education program within the school system or referral to a rehabilitation facility for adapted driver training (e.g., for a teenager with a spinal cord injury who has never driven)

VI. Adaptive Equipment to Facilitate Community Reintegration: Considerations
A. Devices for ADLs and mobility
1. Specific type needed for physical mobility (e.g., wheelchair, walker, crutches, commode, braces, scooter, sliding board)
2. Adaptive equipment needed for independent functioning (e.g., for personal hygiene, dressing, cooking)
a. Need for and availability of amplification systems, assistive listening devices, telecommunication devices, vibrator for alarm clock, visual alert systems, telephone amplifiers
b. Provision of round-the-clock relay services by telephone companies that is mandated by the Americans with Disabilities Act of 1990 (effective as of June 26, 1993) for individuals who have telecommunication devices for the deaf (TDDs) so they can communicate with those who do not
c. Communication boards, speech synthesizers
d. Hearing-ear dogs for the hearing-impaired, guide dogs for the visually impaired, independence dogs
3. Devices needed to prevent medical sequelae after a disability (e.g., wheelchair cushion, equipment for self-catheterization)
B. Funding needed for equipment and/or devices
C. Availability of vendor and repair contracts
D. Client and/or family education regarding use, repair, and replacement of equipment

VII. Support and/or Advocacy Groups (see Appendix B)
A. Associations established and composed of individuals with disabilities (e.g., National Head Injury Foundation, Paralyzed Veterans of America)
B. Self-help organizations that assist the disabled by providing a variety of services (e.g., Easter Seal Society, Variety Clubs)
1. Offer mutual assistance
2. Assist with development of coping strategies
3. Foster abilities and skills to combat isolation and alienation
4. Develop information networks and counseling
C. National Institute on Disability and Rehabilitation Research
1. Oversees comprehensive rehabilitation service programs under the supervision and auspices of the U.S. Department of Education
2. Participates in research and data collection; provides research grants
3. Emphasizes community reentry

D. Client assistance programs: Are federally mandated and require states to provide information to all persons with disabilities regarding benefits available under the Rehabilitation Act of 1973 and its amendments

VIII. Community Resource Delivery

A. Definition of community resources: New or existing support services that fulfill the health and social needs of the community's residents (Furukawa & Shomaker, 1982)

B. Factors affecting community resource delivery

1. Number and extent of public services available in individual communities to persons with disabilities
2. Commitment of the community to ensuring the rights of the disabled
3. Payer source (e.g., insurance, funding sources); financial resources (e.g., community fund raising, personal assets)
4. Geographical location (e.g., urban or rural, region of the country)
5. Length of time that services and/or equipment are needed
6. Availability of caregivers who are able and willing to learn the care required (i.e., caregivers who are not associated with community agencies)
7. Healthcare needs and related plan of care, including caregivers, equipment, transportation, and home environment

References

Furukawa, C., & Shomaker, D. (1982). *Community health services for the aged.* Rockville, MD: Aspen Publishers, Inc.

Suggested Readings

Gottlieb, A., Vandergoot, D., & Lutsky, L. (1991). The role of the rehabilitation professional in corporate disability management. *Journal of Rehabilitation, 57*(2), 23-28.

◆Greenwood, R., Schriner, K.F., & Johnson, V. (1991). Employer concerns regarding workers with disabilities and the business-rehabilitation partnership: The PWI practitioners' perspective. *Journal of Rehabilitation, 57*(1), 21-25.

Grossi, T.A., Test, D.W., & Keul, P.K. (1991). Strategies for hiring, training and supervising job coaches. *Journal of Rehabilitation, 57*(3), 37-42.

Hirsch, S.W. (1989). Meeting the vocational needs of individuals with psychiatric disabilities through supported employment. *Journal of Rehabilitation, 55*(4), 26-31.

◆LeRoy, B.W., & Hartley-Malivuk, T. (1991). Supported employment staff training model. *Journal of Rehabilitation, 57*(2), 51-54.

Resources for Rehabilitation, Inc. (1991). *Resources for people with disabilities and chronic conditions.* Lexington, MA: Author.

Roessler, R.T., & Schriner, K.F. (1991). Partnerships: The bridge from disability to ability management. *Journal of Rehabilitation, 57*(1), 53-58.

Rogan, P., & Hagner, D. (1990). Vocational evaluation in supported employment. *Journal of Rehabilitation, 56*(1), 45-51.

Rogan, P., & Murphy, S. (1991). Supported employment and vocational rehabilitation: Merger or misadventure? *Journal of Rehabilitation, 57*(2), 39-45.

Spencer, J.C. (1990). An ethnographic study of independent living alternatives. *The American Journal of Occupational Therapy, 45*(3), 243-251.

United States Architectural and Transportation Barriers Compliance Board. (1991). Accessibility guidelines for buildings and facilities. *Federal Register, 56*(144), 35,408.

◆ indicates a research-based work

CHAPTER 27

Access to Healthcare Services

Access to health care historically has been a challenge to those with disabilities. Healthcare providers must be able to define strategies for obtaining healthcare services, identify the available financial resources, be knowledgeable regarding public laws governing access to healthcare services, and assist those with disabilities in securing and using healthcare services. This chapter will address access to health care and to community resources; funding options through various governmental, private, and public agencies; and rehabilitation nurses' roles in promoting access to health care for their clients.

I. Access to Health Care for People with Disabilities

A. Obstacles to healthcare services

1. Geographic location
   a. Availability and transportation issues related to access to healthcare facilities and community resources
   b. Access to home-based care services
   c. Prohibitive cost of transportation services
   d. Limited public funds for assistance with obtaining vehicle modifications or purchasing a vehicle (e.g., a van with hand controls), which decreases access to healthcare services, especially in rural areas
2. Architectural issues related to accessibility (including buildings and grounds)
   a. Parking lot accessibility and design
   b. Sidewalk accessibility
   c. Office building accessibility and design
   d. Healthcare facility accessibility and design
3. Attitudes: Discrimination by healthcare providers toward older clients
   a. Age can impose additional limits on healthcare access secondary to payer source limits (e.g., Medicare coverage for home care services, equipment, and outpatient services)
   b. Elderly people often have additional and more complex health problems
   c. Discrimination can lead to poor self-esteem due to increased physical, social, and psychological stressors
   d. Ageism may bring about job discrimination or loss of a job, with a subsequent loss of medical benefits
4. Lack of information about care needs of those with disabilities
5. Economic constraints
   a. Personal finances
      1) Loss of medical benefits, Supplemental Security Income (SSI), or Social Security Disability Insurance (SSDI) if a disabled person is employed and earns more than the allowable amount
      2) Possible reduction in Social Security benefits and medical benefits if a person with a disability marries
      3) Medical benefits that are now tied to income criteria and encourage disabled persons to be dependent on the system
   b. Unavailability of medical benefits for people with disabilities under Medicare until 2 years after the onset of the disability
      1) Discourages persons with disabilities from seeking healthcare services
      2) Raises possibility of disabled persons being without any medical benefits if they do not qualify for state assistance or Medicaid and, thus, contributes to increased numbers of indigent persons seeking healthcare services
      3) Raises possibility that people with disabilities will seek healthcare services only when healthcare needs are well advanced and require hospitalization
      4) Begins a cycle that increases the burden on healthcare providers to supply free care and contributes to an increase in the overall cost of healthcare services
   c. Limited eligibility for funding for attendant care
      1) Funding that is usually tied to eligibility for income assistance
      2) Long waiting periods that frequently last for 1 or 2 years
      3) Minimal reimbursement for attendants, which makes it difficult to recruit and retain qualified attendants
      4) Programs that require the clients to be able to manage their own workers independently and to handle training and payroll, which may not be possible for persons with severe disabilities and/or the elderly
      5) Strict definitions of what constitutes a disability that may disqualify many of those who need the services
   d. Ability to obtain needed equipment, supplies, and medications
      1) Dependence on insurance coverage

        2) Possible requirement of a down payment (in cash)
        3) Frequent limits on additional equipment covered by insurance
        4) Possible inability to obtain the necessary equipment (e.g., a padded commode chair with removable arms for a spinal cord injured person)
    6. Limited funding for independent living arrangements (residential and nonresidential models)
        a. Continued limitation of funds for independent living centers (ILCs) despite their having been mandated by the Rehabilitation, Comprehensive Services and Developmental Disabilities Amendments of 1978 (Public Law 95-602)
        b. Some support through Medicaid Title XIX (state) funding for attendant assistance and community support services
        c. The rarity of ILC programs in rural areas
    7. Issues in attendant training
        a. On-the-job training
        b. Lack of regulations regarding worker qualifications
        c. No supervision of work performance
        d. Lack of public funding that would allow control over worker qualifications and performance
        e. Lack of availability of attendants able to meet the specialized needs of the pediatric population
B. Limited healthcare services: Limits might arise due to attitudes, architectural designs, and/or reimbursement limits
    1. Limited counseling services
        a. Medical social worker services are usually available only through home care agencies
        b. Few psychiatrists and psychologists make home visits
        c. Reimbursement for counseling is limited
    2. Special healthcare needs of people with disabilities
        a. Obstetric and gynecological services
            1) Exam tables that are accessible to women with disabilities
            2) Healthcare providers knowledgeable in obstetric and gynecological areas
            3) Specialized training for personnel (e.g., how to care for a spinal cord injured person who has had a baby)
        b. Dental services
            1) Offices that are architecturally accessible
            2) Accessible, comfortable office chairs
            3) Elimination of financial obstacles to preventive care (e.g., insurance such as Medicare or Medicaid that does not cover preventive care)

II. Obtaining Access to Community Resources and Healthcare Services (see Figure 27.1)

A. Contact local governmental disability office, city commission, or city departments to determine public services available to persons with disabilities
    1. Accessible housing
        a. Established referral system in place
        b. Technical assistance
        c. Development, design, and building assistance
        d. Home mortgage loans
        e. Availability of accessible public housing
        f. Funding for adaptations in private residences
    2. Transportation
        a. Designated parking
        b. Private transportation services
        c. Public transportation (e.g., availability, accessibility)
        d. Reduced bus passes
        e. Paratransit
        f. Parking stickers
    3. Advocacy
        a. Established advisory council
        b. Involvement of advocacy groups with community agencies
        c. Funding for programs
        d. Information exchange regarding disability issues (e.g., legislation)
        e. Appointment of persons with disabilities to governmental boards and commissions
        f. Legal assistance
        g. Public education regarding disability issues
    4. Employment
        a. Affirmative action for hiring the disabled
        b. Training and placement assistance; supported employment services
        c. Funding for environmental modifications
    5. Recreation
        a. Accessible community centers and leisure programs
        b. Special events focused on population with disabilities (e.g., wheelchair division of marathon races)
    6. Supportive services
        a. Information and referral
        b. Counseling
        c. Personal care assistance programs
        d. Telecommunication devices for the deaf; sign language interpreters (e.g., at public hearings)
        e. Homemaker services
        f. Augmentative communication aids, adaptive toys, assistive technology
        g. Health screening services
        h. Funding for rehabilitation technology services and adaptive equipment
        i. Access to electronic bulletin-board systems (Fullmer & Majumder, 1991)
    7. Education
        a. Availability of educational opportunities
        b. Funding
        c. Building accessibility
        d. Programs for disadvantaged children
        e. Therapy services available in school systems (e.g., occupational therapy, speech and language therapy, physical therapy)
        f. Head Start program; early intervention programs
        g. Bilingual education

Figure 27.1. Gaining Access to Community Resources

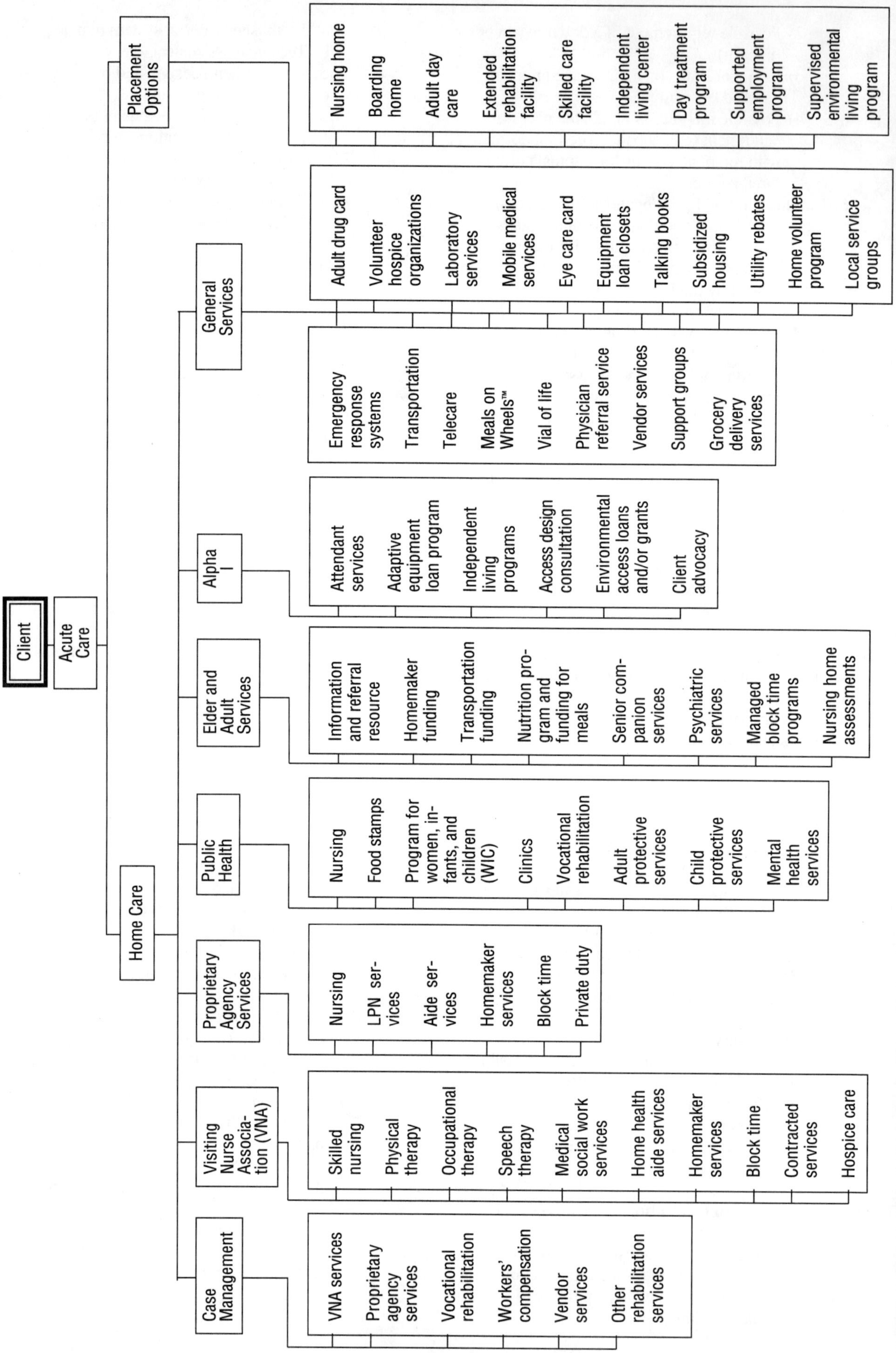

h. Acquisition of equipment to supplement special education and related services; training in computer technology
i. Self-help groups
j. Playground accessibility; school environment modifications
k. Specialized buses, cars, vans to meet the needs of school children

B. Contact other local agencies or healthcare professionals
1. Social workers in hospitals, rehabilitation centers, extended-care facilities, government bureaus
2. Department of health and human services
3. Visiting nurse associations (VNAs)
4. Case managers at private insurance companies
5. Physicians' referral services
6. Local bureau of elder and adult services
7. Vendors
8. Mental health department
9. American Association of Retired Persons
10. Department of Veterans Affairs

C. Contact public affairs departments of local media

III. Funding Sources for Gaining Access to Rehabilitation and Supportive Services in the Community

A. Agencies and sectors receiving state funding through appropriation of monies or grants or through direct reimbursement
1. VNAs and private not-for-profit home care agencies
2. Alpha I (member of National Council on Independent Living)
a. Is funded through state and federal monies
b. Provides services to people with disabilities
1) Peer support, attendant services, client advocacy
2) Access to design consultation
a) Education of design professionals and the public regarding legal requirements for creating accessible environments
b) Building product information
c) Design review
d) Assessments of home after occupancy
3) Environmental access grants and loans
4) Loan program for adaptive equipment
a) Low-interest loans
b) Loans available to citizens and businesses to purchase technological aids that enhance independence in the home, workplace, or other environment
5) Independent living programs: Provide instruction on and hands-on experience in transitional living skills
6) Adapted vehicle driving evaluation and education
7) Monitoring of access issues
a) Watchdog project to correct building code violations and publicize standards for accessible design
b) Statewide network of grassroots advocacy
c) Group that informs the design and construction industries about legal requirements for building or remodeling public buildings and public housing
d) Group that files complaints or litigation if corrective action is not taken
3. Proprietary (for-profit) agencies
4. Public health services
a. Nursing services
1) Home visits for health teaching and screening
2) Clinics for blood pressure, screening, child immunizations, and flu vaccines
b. Vocational rehabilitation (see Chapter 25, page 207)
c. Adult and child protective services
5. Elder and adult services
6. Transportation resources
a. Public transportation
b. Private organizations receiving state funds to purchase vans with lifts and to serve the elderly, those with disabilities, and those who have state benefits (e.g., Medicaid, paratransit)
7. Independent living programs
a. Services vary according to locality and program
1) Referral to housing and training in independent living skills
2) Permanent residential, transitional residential, or temporary housing
3) Attendant referral, training, and/or management training
4) Client and system advocacy
5) Disability awareness among community
6) Equipment repair and referral
7) Reduction of environmental barriers
8) Promotion of consumer involvement in community activities and information and referral services
b. Program components vary with each independent living program
8. Extended rehabilitation facilities, skilled nursing facilities, boarding homes
9. Vendor services
a. Durable medical equipment
b. Intravenous therapy: Hydration, total parenteral nutrition, antibiotics, blood and blood products, pain management
c. Chemotherapy
d. Medical supplies
e. Oxygen and/or ventilator services
f. Nutrition-related services
g. Enteral feedings
10. Selective professional services
a. Physicians' visits (office and home)
b. Inpatient and outpatient hospital services
c. Counseling services
d. Outpatient phlebotomy services
e. Mobile medical services (e.g., X rays, EKGs in the home)
f. Eye care cards (e.g., funding for eye exams, eyeglasses)

11. Programs
    a. Adult day care
    b. Day treatment programs (e.g., for those with a head injury or with Alzheimer's disease)
    c. Supervised environmental living program
    d. Hospice
    e. Prosthetic and orthotic devices

B. Agencies and sectors receiving federal funding through appropriation of monies, grants, or direct reimbursement to agencies for services that they provide
   1. VNAs and private not-for-profit agencies providing home care services
   2. Vendor services
   3. Some independent living programs
   4. Outpatient phlebotomy services
   5. Physicians' visits (office and home)
   6. Extended rehabilitation facilities
   7. Hospice care
   8. Prosthetic and orthotic devices
   9. Mobile medical services
   10. Inpatient and outpatient hospital services (acute and rehabilitation)
   11. Outpatient rehabilitation services (e.g., hospital-based, VNA, private)

C. Department of Veterans Affairs services
   1. Inpatient and outpatient hospital services
   2. Pharmacy services
   3. Vocational rehabilitation services
   4. Nursing home care
   5. Home health care
   6. Orthotic and prosthetic devices
   7. Durable medical and adaptive equipment
   8. Services for the visually impaired
   9. Home modifications for people with disabilities
   10. Mortgage loans

D. Federal or state-subsidized assistance based upon income, age, or disability
   1. Adult drug cards
   2. Subsidized housing
   3. Utility and telephone rebates
   4. Eye care cards
      a. Provide reimbursement for eye examinations and glasses
      b. Are unavailable for those holding state medical cards, as they would duplicate some coverage
   5. Healthcare services at public clinics (e.g., immunizations, flu vaccines)
   6. Meals on Wheels™ program
   7. Talking books

E. Elder and adult services
   1. Services funded primarily for those over the age of 62 years
   2. Age and income are the two main criteria for determining eligibility for programs
   3. Services provided by typical senior companion program
      a. Respite care
      b. Running errands
      c. Taking clients out to do errands
      d. Light housekeeping

IV. Rehabilitation Nursing Interventions to Help Clients Gain Access to Healthcare Resources

A. Coordinating referrals to not-for-profit and private home care agencies

B. Identifying agencies that provide free care or sliding scale fees for services based on income and the duration of needed services

C. Arranging for social work services to assist with access to community systems for obtaining subsidized housing, Medicaid applications, SSI, SSDI, counseling services, advocacy assistance, equipment needs, and transportation and to find organizations that provide community services (see Chapter 25, pages 207-208)

D. Contacting the local department of human services regarding services available for rehabilitation care needs

E. Contacting legislators to support funding for transferring client to an ILC and for attendant training, as well as for supplemental funding that allows those with disabilities to work without a drastic reduction in or termination of medical benefits

F. Attending public hearings on issues affecting people with disabilities

G. Acting as a community advocate to promote increased environmental accessibility, decreased architectural barriers, increased access to public transportation, decreased cost of services to elderly clients on fixed incomes, and increased access to healthcare services

H. Making referrals to rehabilitation counselors, peer counselors, and those providing psychological services

I. Contacting state disability office, commission(s), or department(s) for assistance

J. Promoting the education of healthcare providers and caregivers within facilities and the community
   1. Providing in-service education
   2. Consulting one-on-one with providers regarding healthcare issues, ways to manage individual clients' healthcare needs, and ways to promote access to healthcare services
   3. Encouraging family involvement early in the rehabilitation process and teaching about equipment, procedures, medications, and ways to manage emergencies
   4. Coordinating a home visit by the rehabilitation team to evaluate the need for home modifications, equipment, and ways to improve safety
   5. Making referrals to appropriate community resources
   6. Promoting interagency communication regarding rehabilitation needs, follow-up teaching needs, and previous nursing interventions in the event of a transfer to a different environment
   7. Periodically reassessing and evaluating the client's ability to perform ADLs, changes in level of independence, healthcare needs, and barriers to gaining access to required services
   8. Contacting healthcare providers in the community to determine access to buildings, cost of services, insurance coverage, ways to modify the office environment, and the availability of transportation

K. Speaking at service club meetings

L. Actively participating in professional organizations

Figure 27.2. Laws Governing Access to Rehabilitation Services

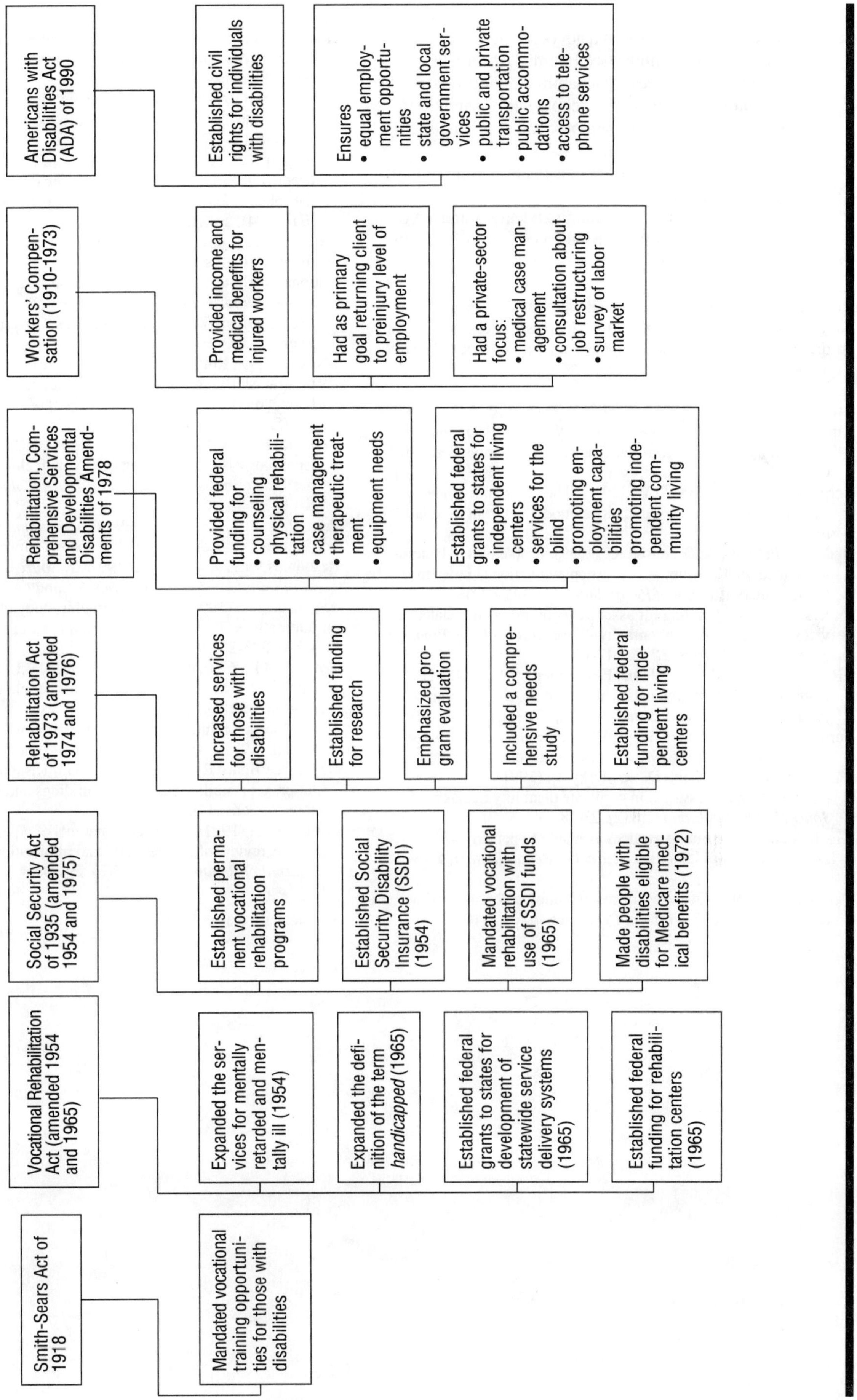

that support legislation and advocacy activities for people with disabilities (see Figure 27.2 for a list of laws governing access to rehabilitation services)

M. Promoting appointment of people with disabilities to public offices and commissions, and to private-sector industry and business boards

N. Helping clients with disabilities prepare testimony for legislative hearings

O. Participating in health planning endeavors and advocating for services that meet the needs of children and adults

References

Fullmer, S., & Majumder, R.K. (1991). Increased access and use of disability related information for consumers. *Journal of Rehabilitation, 57*(3), 17-22.

Suggested Readings

American Hospital Association. (1987). *Directory of national self-help and mutual aid resources.* Evanston, IL: Illinois Self-Help Center.

Bergland, M.M., & Clark, D.W. (1991). The community independent living program: An educational model. *Journal of Rehabilitation, 57*(3), 43-46.

Budde, J., Petty, C.R., & Nelson, C. (1989). Problems and benefits associated with consumer satisfaction evaluation at independent living centers. *Journal of Rehabilitation, 55*(4), 62-68.

Enders, A. (1990). Funding for assistive technology and related services: An annotated bibliography. *Physical and Occupational Therapy in Pediatrics, 10*(2), 147-173.

◆Fanning, R.A., Judge, J., Weihe, F., & Emener, W.G. (1991). Housing needs of individuals with severe mobility impairments: A case study. *Journal of Rehabilitation, 57*(2), 7-13.

Furukawa, C., & Shomaker, D. (1982). *Community health services for the aged.* Rockville, MD: Aspen Publishers, Inc.

◆Gottlieb, A., Vandergoot, D., & Lutsky, L. (1991). The role of the rehabilitation professional in corporate disability management. *Journal of Rehabilitation, 57*(2), 23-28.

Groch, S.A. (1991). Public services available to persons with disabilities in major U.S. cities. *Journal of Rehabilitation, 57*(3), 23-26.

Hedman, G. (1990). Overview of rehabilitation technology. *Physical and Occupational Therapy in Pediatrics, 10*(2), 1-10.

Holmes, G.E., & Karst, R.H. (1990). The institutionalization of disability myths: Impact on vocational rehabilitation services. *Journal of Rehabilitation, 56*(1), 20-27.

Mann, W.C. (1991). State-wide planning for access to technology applications for individuals with disabilities. *Journal of Rehabilitation, 57*(1), 17-20.

Middleton, R.A., & McDaniel, R.S. (1990). The (re)habilitation needs of the older non-disabled handicapped person: Expanding the role of the rehabilitation professional. *Journal of Rehabilitation, 56*(4), 23-27.

Molnar, G.E. (Ed.). (1992). *Pediatric rehabilitation* (2nd ed.). Baltimore: Williams & Wilkins.

National Institute of Handicapped Research. (1986). *Directory of national information sources on handicapping conditions and related services.* Washington, DC: U.S. Government Printing Office.

◆Nosek, M.A., Roth, P.L., & Zhu, Y. (1991). Independent living programs: The impact of program age, consumer control, and budget on program operation. *Journal of Rehabilitation, 56*(4), 28-35.

◆Parette, H.P., & VanBiervliet, A. (1991). Rehabilitation assistive technology issues for infants and young children with disabilities: A preliminary examination. *Journal of Rehabilitation, 57*(3), 27-36.

Pratt, P.N., & Allen, A.S. (1989). *Occupational therapy for children* (2nd ed.). St. Louis: The C.V. Mosby Company.

Resources for Rehabilitation. (1991). *Resources for people with disabilities and chronic conditions.* Lexington, MA: Author.

◆Spencer, J.C. (1991). An ethnographic study of independent living alternatives. *The American Journal of Occupational Therapy, 45*(3), 243-251.

Teague, M.L., Cipriano, R.E., & McGhee, V.L. (1990). Health promotion as a rehabilitation service for people with disabilities. *Journal of Rehabilitation, 56*(1), 52-56.

United States Architectural and Transportation Barriers Compliance Board. (1991). Architectural and Transportation Barriers Compliance Board Rules: Americans with Disabilities Act implementation accessibility guidelines, buildings and facilities. *Federal Register, 56*(144), 35,408.

Ziolko, M.E. (1991). Counseling parents of children with disabilities: A review of the literature and implications for practice. *Journal of Rehabilitation, 57*(2), 29-34.

◆ indicates a research-based work

Section VI
Legislative and Economic Issues

Rehabilitation nurses often are involved in activity that takes them outside the strictly clinical realm—activity such as participation in the legislative process and involvement in the economic issues of rehabilitation. This section provides a brief overview of the rehabilitation nurse's role in both of these areas.

The legislative process presents an opportunity for rehabilitation nurses to share their expertise with local, state, and federal government agencies and legislators. Rehabilitation nurses' special knowledge of the long-term care needs of clients with disabilities puts them in a position to advocate for healthcare policy and healthcare system reform. Chapter 28 describes the ways in which rehabilitation nurses can do this (including involvement in the ARN Health Policy Committee).

The economic aspects of rehabilitation require the rehabilitation nurse to be aware of the various possible sources of funding for healthcare and/or rehabilitation programs. Chapter 29 identifies the funding resources available in the federal, state, and private sectors for healthcare insurance, workers' compensation, income support, and vocational rehabilitation.

CHAPTER 28

Legislative Issues in Rehabilitation Nursing

The legislative process presents an opportunity for rehabilitation nurses to share their expertise with local, state, and federal government agencies and legislators. The rehabilitation nurse's involvement can range from conducting prevention programs related to unsafe or unhealthy behaviors in schools to lobbying legislators to pass helmet and seatbelt legislation and to holding political rallies and letter-writing campaigns to garner support for proposed bills. Rehabilitation nurses' unique knowledge and understanding of the long-term care needs of clients with disabilities positions them to advocate for healthcare policy and reform. By doing so, they inform those from the public sector, including government representatives, about the special healthcare needs of rehabilitation clients. The ARN Health Policy Committee is the mechanism for coordinating the rehabilitation nurses' position with regard to pending legislation and serves as the members' resource for political action and policy making.

I. Reasons for Nursing's Involvement in the Political and Legislative Arenas
   A. Participation in decisions relating to the future of the profession and of health care
   B. Positive effect on the healthcare delivery system
   C. Ability to supply input at the policy-making and healthcare-planning levels
   D. Commitment to maintaining healthcare standards

II. Current Political and Legislative Issues Related to Health Care
   A. Access to health care: The major issue of the 1990s
      1. Healthcare entitlement programs
      2. Medicare and Medicaid rules and regulations for implementation
      3. Health care for the disadvantaged
      4. Development of healthcare delivery alternatives
   B. Reimbursement for nursing services, including reimbursement for rehabilitation nursing
   C. Nursing's scope of practice (as defined by state licensure laws and regulatory bodies)
   D. Funding for nursing education and research
   E. Social issues related to the populations that rehabilitation nurses serve
      1. Availability of vocational rehabilitation services
      2. Disincentives for people with disabilities to return to work
      3. Community accessibility
      4. Discrimination against people with disabilities in hiring practices or in the workplace
   F. Environmental health issues
      1. Occupational health hazards—for example, neurotoxicity from chemicals in the workplace
      2. Testing of food and drugs
   G. Prevention of catastrophic injuries
      1. Mandating seatbelts, inflatable restraints, and helmets for on-road vehicles, bicycles, and off-road recreational vehicles
      2. Providing education about substance abuse, particularly as a cause of accidents that can result in spinal cord injury and traumatic brain injury
   H. Women's issues
      1. Equal rights for women, including research on women's health concerns
      2. Economic equity (including child support)
      3. Child care and/or elder care
      4. Employers' support of family health
      5. Vocational training for women newly forced into the workplace because of circumstances such as divorce or death of a spouse

III. The Legislative Process (see Figure 28.1) and Nursing's Involvement
   A. Citizens urge members of Congress to introduce a bill
      1. Any citizen, including a professional nurse, can bring an issue to a legislator's attention; if a nursing-related issue is being researched already, nurses can offer their expertise to legislators and their staffs (see Figure 28.2)
      2. Nurses can obtain names and addresses of legislators from their states through their local libraries, through state nursing associations, and/or by contacting their local government offices; the American Nurses Association (ANA) has been very involved in the legislative process and has guidelines for participation (ANA, 1993)
   B. A congressional aide draws up draft of bill
   C. Bill is introduced by a representative or a senator and assigned to an appropriate committee
   D. Lobbyists work to pass or defeat the bill
      1. Organized groups or individual nurses can contact their elected representatives and request that they cosponsor the bill
      2. If legislators are unwilling to cosponsor a bill,

Figure 28.1. The Path of Legislation in the U.S. Congress: A Typical Example

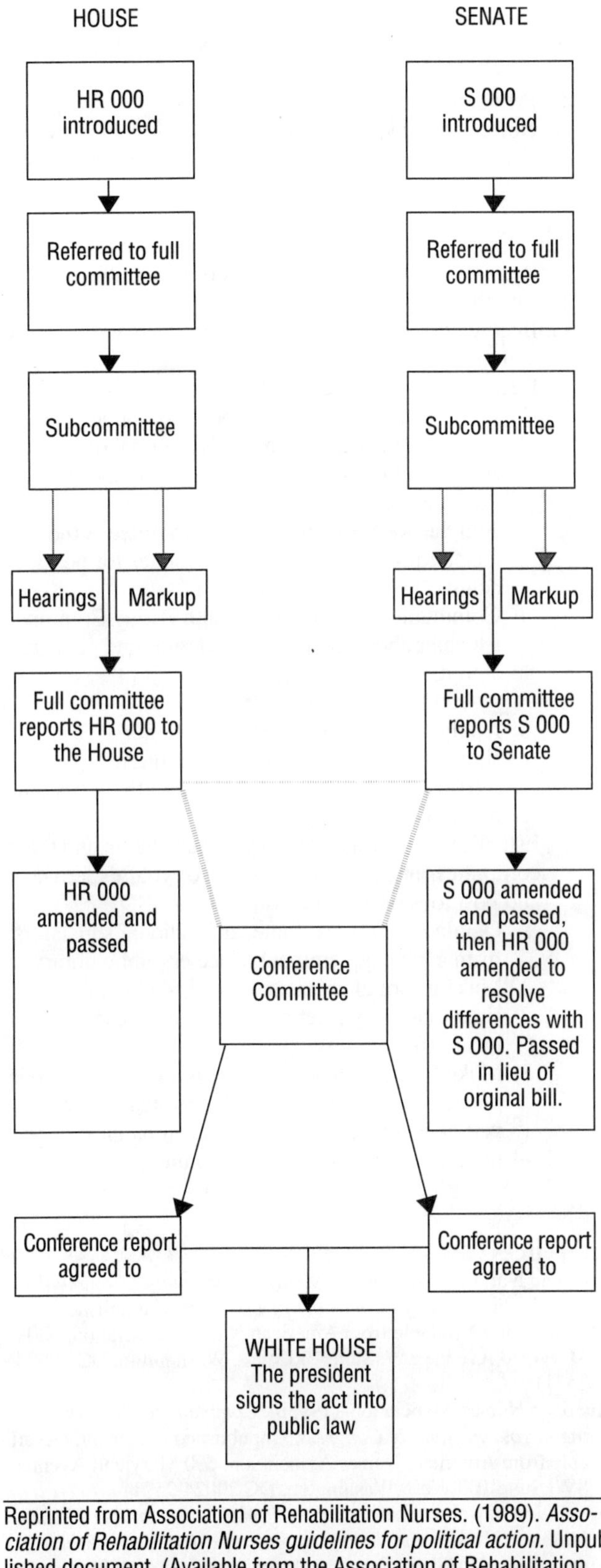

Reprinted from Association of Rehabilitation Nurses. (1989). *Association of Rehabilitation Nurses guidelines for political action.* Unpublished document. (Available from the Association of Rehabilitation Nurses, 5700 Old Orchard Road, First Floor, Skokie, IL 60077-1057)

Figure 28.2. American Nurses Association Tips on Writing to Your Member of Congress

- Use personal or business stationery with a return address. If you are a constituent, tell the member.
- State the purpose of your letter in the first paragraph. When the letter pertains to a specific piece of legislation, identify it (for House bills, HR____; for Senate bills, S____).
- Keep your letter concise; try to convey your message in one page.
- Whenever possible, include data and sources of information to support your position.
- Maintain a positive attitude throughout the letter. Congressional offices are strongly influenced by the correspondence they receive from their constituents.

Recommended Forms of Salutation
Dear Senator____: or Dear Representative____:

When writing to the chair of a committee or the speaker of the House:
Dear Mr. Chairman or Madam Chairwoman:
or Dear Mr. Speaker:

Addressing Correspondence
To a Senator
The Honorable (Senator's name)
United States Senate
Washington, DC 20510

To a Member of the House of Representatives
The Honorable (Member's name)
U.S. House of Representatives
Washington, DC 20515

Reprinted with permission of the American Nurses Association from American Nurses Association. (1993b). *Communiqué: Tips on writing to your member of Congress.* Unpublished document. (Available from American Nurses Association, 600 Maryland Avenue SW, Suite 100 West, Washington, DC 20024-2571)

nurses can alert legislators to nursing's interest in a particular component of legislation

E. Witnesses testify at committee hearings
   1. Committee can hold hearings before taking action on a bill; nurses can use this opportunity to testify and bring nursing's viewpoint to committee
   2. Nurses can individually visit committee members to brief them on selected issues (see Figure 28.3)
F. House or the Senate debates bill, makes amendments, if desired, and votes
G. If bill is passed by one chamber, it moves to the other, and legislators hear from citizens about bill that was passed in the originating chamber
H. Senate or House committee may rewrite or amend bill or may pass it in form in which it was received
I. Senate or House may pass an amended version of bill or pass it in form in which it was received
J. If bill has been changed, it goes to conference commit-

Figure 28.3. American Nurses Association Tips for Communicating Effectively with Your Member of Congress

Effective communication between constituents and their legislators begins at home with a strong, well-coordinated grassroots lobbying effort. Lawmakers need first-hand input from voters to make sound decisions. As few as 30 letters from constituents in a congressional district or state can impact the votes of undecided legislators. Making nurses' viewpoint known not only promotes nursing interests, but it is also a vital part of citizen participation. You, as a nurse and a constituent, can be the most effective lobbyist.

Suggestions for a Successful Visit with Your Member of Congress

Plan your visit. Decide what you want to achieve from this visit. Determine which members you want to visit and know the committees they serve on.

Make an appointment. Call your member's office and indicate that you would like to schedule a meeting when the member is home during a recess. Tell the staff person the subject you want to discuss.

Be prompt. Be on time for your appointment.

Be patient. Due to votes or caucuses, members often run behind schedule. Be patient. Interruptions will occur; allow extra time in your schedule. You may have to wait a long period of time, reschedule the meeting, or agree to meet with staff in order to be heard.

Introduce yourself. Open the meeting with a comment to establish a tie between you and the legislator. Next, if appropriate, state how many of the member's constituents you represent and what your mission is. If you are not from the member's congressional district, demonstrate the connection between your position and the interests of the member's constituency.

Be prepared. If you are meeting to discuss a particular piece of legislation, state the bill number. Members are very busy and are not likely to know all the details of every piece of legislation; therefore they value personal examples that demonstrate positive or negative impacts associated with a piece of legislation. Indicate precisely what action you want the member to take, whether it be co-sponsorship or voting for or against the bill. Leave a one- or two-page fact sheet with the member summarizing the issue and your positions, along with names and telephone numbers of contact people.

Be concise. Discuss the issue at hand. Do not become too technical in the examples and background materials you use to justify your position. Also, avoid using technical jargon; you will lose the member and your lobbying efforts will be lost.

Be responsive. Follow up the meeting with a letter thanking the member, reiterating your position, and including any information requested during the meeting.

Reprinted with permission of the American Nurses Association from American Nurses Association. (1993a). *Communiqué: Communicating effectively with your member of Congress.* Unpublished document. (Available from American Nurses Association, 600 Maryland Avenue SW, Suite 100 West, Washington, DC 20024-2571)

tee of Senate and House

1. If House version of bill is different from Senate version, bill is sent to conference committee composed of members of both houses to resolve their differences; revised bill is then sent back to both houses for approval
2. Nurses can contact their senators to urge them to support nursing's position

K. Congress agrees on revised bill and sends bill to president

L. President signs bill into law

M. Nurses still have an opportunity to be involved by assisting in the process of writing regulations that make statutes clear, concise, and enforceable

IV. Guidelines for Political Action in Health Policy

A. Register and vote for candidates of your choice

B. Be informed on all issues

C. Become involved in professional nursing associations and their legislative task forces

D. Become aware of ARN health policy

1. Be informed about ARN's positions on legislation
2. Obtain information from ARN national office, ARN Health Policy Committee chair, and ARN publications
3. Join the ARN Health Policy Committee at the chapter level and use ARN guidelines for political action
4. Communicate with ARN Health Policy Committee chair about local and state issues and personal activities
5. Attend legislative seminars
6. Apply for the Malcom Maloof Memorial Scholarship to the Nurse-in-Washington Internship (NIWI) (information available from the ARN national office)

E. Establish a relationship with your legislators and their committees and make them aware of your expertise and positions on specific issues

1. Obtain lists of local, state, and national legislators from a local government office or public library
2. Make informal contacts with legislators in social situations or by offering to serve as a resource to local officials
3. Make formal contacts with legislators through telephone calls, letters, personal meetings, written or verbal testimony, and personal campaign support (e.g., monetary donations or volunteering)

References

American Nurses Association. (1993a). *Communiqué: Communicating effectively with your member of Congress.* Unpublished document. (Available from American Nurses Association, 600 Maryland Avenue SW, Suite 100 West, Washington, DC 20024-2571)

American Nurses Association. (1993b). *Communiqué: Tips on writing to your member of Congress.* Unpublished document. (Available from American Nurses Association, 600 Maryland Avenue SW, Suite 100 West, Washington, DC 20024-2571)

Association of Rehabilitation Nurses. (1989). *Association of Rehabilitation Nurses guidelines for political action.* Unpublished document. (Available from the Association of Rehabilitation Nurses, 5700 Old Orchard Road, First Floor, Skokie, IL 60077-1057)

Suggested Readings

Barry, C.T. (1990). Profiles of nurses professionally involved in public policy. *Nursing Economics, 8*(3), 174-176.

Buresh, B., Gordon, S., & Bell, N. (1991). Who counts in news coverage of health care? *Nursing Outlook, 39*(5), 204-208.

Burke, M. (1991, January). Congressional leaders outline their health agendas. *Hospitals*, pp. 20-26.

Equal Employment Opportunity Commission and U.S. Department of Justice. (1992). *A technical assistance manual on the employment provisions of the Americans with Disabilities Act.* Washington, DC: U.S. Government Printing Office.

Equal Employment Opportunity Commission and U.S. Department of Justice. (1991). *The ADA handbook.* Washington, DC: U.S. Government Printing Office.

Fagin, C.M. (1990). Nursing's value proves itself. *American Journal of Nursing, 90*(10), 16-18, 22-29.

Griffith, H.M., Thomas, N., & Griffith, L. (1991) M.D.'s bill for these routine nursing tasks. *American Journal of Nursing, 91*(1), 22-25, 27.

Harris, M. (1988). The changing scene in community health nursing. *Nursing Clinics of North America, 23*, 559-568.

Milburn, L., Hayes, K., & Griffith, H. (1988, June). The information seekers guide to health policy news. *Nursing and Health Care*, pp. 307-309.

Schaeffer, F. (1988). DRGs: A new era for health care. *Nursing Clinics of North America, 23*, 453-463.

Sharp, N. (1990). What will physician payment reform mean for nurses? *Nursing Management, 21*(10), 14-15.

Sharp, N., Biggs, S., & Wakefield, M. (1991). Public policy. *Nursing and Health Care, 12*(1), 16-22.

Skydell, B., & Arndt, M. (1988). The price of nursing care. *Nursing Clinics of North America, 23*, 493-501.

Thompson, J., & Deits, D. (1988). Management of nursing intensity. *Nursing Clinics of North America, 23*, 473-491.

Wakefield, M.K. (1990). Prospectives on health policy. *Nursing Economics, 8*(3), 188-190.

Zander, K. (1988). Nursing case management: Resolving the DRG. *Nursing Clinics of North America, 23*, 503-520.

CHAPTER 29

Economic Considerations in Rehabilitation

The rehabilitation nurse needs to be aware of the various programs that are available as possible resources for funding healthcare and/or rehabilitation programs and income support programs for people with disabilities. These resources can affect the rehabilitative care the client receives as well as the client's outcomes.

The purpose of this chapter is to identify the funding resources available in the federal, state, and private sectors that provide benefits to cover rehabilitation through healthcare insurance programs; to recognize that workers' compensation programs, whatever the funding source, provide both medical care and income support; to identify the funding resources that provide income support; and to identify the programs that include vocational rehabilitation benefits through either job placement or vocational training.

The following information is intended as a general overview of the resources available through the federal, the state, and the private sector.

I. Funding Resources for Healthcare and/or Rehabilitation Programs (see Table 29.1)
  A. Federal programs
    1. Medicare—Title XVIII, Social Security Act of 1965; a federal health insurance program under authority of U.S. Department of Health and Human Services
      a. Includes three types of health insurance plans
        1) Part A: Compulsory program of hospital insurance
        2) Part B: Voluntary program of supplementary medical insurance
        3) Part C: Special programs (e.g., end-stage renal disease)
      b. Managed by the Health Care Financing Administration (HCFA), which designates intermediaries on a regional basis to process claims (e.g., Blue Cross plans)
      c. Eligibility
        1) Retired workers (and spouses) over the age of 65
        2) Workers disabled for 2 years or more
    2. Medicaid—Title XIX, Social Security Act of 1965, which provides federal grants to states for medical assistance programs
  B. State programs
    1. Medicaid
      a. Administration: Within broad federal guidelines, each state develops and administers its own program
      b. Eligibility: Those determined by states to be "medically needy"; federal guidelines designate mandatory groups (e.g., children from age 1 to 6 years, people enrolled in state's Aid to Families with Dependent Children [AFDC] program)
      c. Reimbursement: States are reimbursed at a rate between 50% and 78.5% of actual costs
    2. Workers' compensation systems
      a. Administration: Each state designates an agency that will administer program
      b. Eligibility: Workers disabled by injury or families of worker whose death "arose out of and in the course of employment"
      c. Coverage: Provides both medical care related to the compensable injury and income benefits through the following sources
        1) Private commercial insurance companies
        2) Self-insurance (corporations able to carry their risk)
        3) State fund
        4) State's second injury fund
      d. Medical care provisions
        1) Treatment and rehabilitative programs for the work-related injury
        2) Reimbursement in full or, in certain states, according to a medical fee guide
      e. Vocational rehabilitation benefits: The majority of states have provisions for job retraining, education, and job placement
      f. Administration of each state's workers' compensation law (includes administration of workers' compensation in the District of Columbia, Puerto Rico, and the Virgin Islands)
        1) State department of labor (26 states)
        2) Independent workers' compensation agency (23 states)
        3) Court administration (4 states)
  C. Private healthcare insurance
    1. Financial considerations
      a. Employer pays full or partial premiums
      b. Individual pays premium

Table 29.1. Funding Resources for Healthcare and Rehabilitation Programs

	Programs			
	Medicare (Federal)	**Medicaid** (State)	**Workers' compensation**	**Private health insurance**
Eligibility Requirements	Must be over the age of 65 or have been disabled for 2 years	Categories include the medically needy (e.g., AFDC recipients, blind people)	Workers injured in the course of employment	Policyholders
Benefits	Part A—hospital Part B—supplemental medical insurance (individual must enroll) Part C—miscellaneous (e.g., for those with end-stage renal disease)	Hospital costs and visits to a physician Care in a skilled nursing facility	Medical care related to a compensable injury Income support during period of disability	Hospital costs and outpatient treatment, as specified in policy Physicians' visits, as specified in policy May or may not cover rehabilitation therapies

Sources Consulted

Pell, A.E. (1990). *Making the most of Medicare: A guide through the Medicare maze.* Minneapolis: DCI Publishing.
Social Security programs in the United States. (1989). *Social Security Bulletin, 52*(7), 2-79.

2. Various types of health service plans
   a. Contractual plans with variable deductibles (e.g., Blue Cross/Blue Shield)
   b. Health maintenance organizations (HMOs)
   c. Preferred provider organizations (PPOs)
   d. Medicare Supplemental Benefits Plan (Medigap)
   e. Auto liability policy that covers medical care needed as a result of an auto accident

D. Programs for special groups
   1. Benefits for veterans of the armed forces
      a. Administered by the Veterans Benefits Administration
      b. Coverage provided either for treatment of a service-connected disability or for needy veterans who have nonservice-connected disabilities
   2. Federal government civilian employee workers' compensation programs
   3. Railroad Retirement Act Program
   4. Black Lung Benefits Act of 1972
   5. Longshoreman and Harbor Workers' Compensation Act

II. Funding Resources for Income Support Programs (see Table 29.2)
   A. Social Security: Consists of two programs—Old-Age and Survivors Insurance and Disability Insurance
      1. Old-Age and Survivors Insurance (OASI)
         a. Eligibility
            1) Must be retired worker who is 65 (by 2009, the minimum age will be 66); reduced benefits are available to workers retiring at age 62 or to a widow(er) or a surviving divorced spouse
            2) Must have reached "fully insured" status—that is, must have worked under the program for a minimum of 10 years (1 year equals 4 credits and 40 credits are needed)
         b. Benefits: No means test is required; benefits are paid as an earned right; no minimum income amount required during active working years; no limit on other sources of income, including savings, pensions, insurance
      2. Disability Insurance
         a. Eligibility
            1) Must be a disabled worker below the age of 65; "a disabling condition is one in which the worker is so severely impaired physically or mentally, that he or she is not able to perform substantial gainful work" (Jehle, 1992, p. 33)
               a) Regulations established by U.S. secretary of health and human services
               b) Disability determination service in each state agency
            2) Must have "fully insured" status and have 20 quarters of coverage in the 40-quarter period ending with the quarter of disability
         b. Benefits: Applicants are referred to state departments and/or agencies for vocational rehabilitation services benefits that vary according to each state
   B. State income support programs
      1. Workers' compensation
         a. Eligibility: Condition must be work-related
         b. Benefits: Usually calculated as a percentage of worker's weekly earnings at time of injury or death
            1) Restrictions
               a) Frequently at two-thirds of gross salary; each state designates a maximum amount
               b) There may be a waiting period
               c) Some states may stipulate a maximum

Table 29.2. Income Support Programs Pertinent to Rehabilitation

	Programs		
	Social Security Disability Insurance	**State workers' compensation**	**Private and/or individual disability insurance**
Population	Workers disabled before the age of 65 years and "fully insured" under covered work	Injured workers who meet state criteria for work-related conditions	Injured workers with a nonoccupational disability who are defined as unable to perform either the work related to their own occupation or any reasonable occupation
Benefits	Amount payable in retirement	Temporary total benefits that are calculated by a state formula, which is usually two-thirds of salary	A percentage of previous earnings
Time Period	For as long as person is disabled; trial work period may be stipulated	Variable; could be for person's lifetime; some states stipulate a maximum number of weeks (e.g., 500)	Policy may have a maximum benefit period (e.g., 2 years)

Sources Consulted

Pell, A.E. (1990). *Making the most of Medicare: A guide through the Medicare maze.* Minneapolis: DCI Publishing.
Social Security programs in the United States. (1989). *Social Security Bulletin, 52*(7), 2-79.

number of weeks for benefits (e.g., 500 weeks)

2) Types of benefits
   a) Temporary total disability: Worker is disabled for temporary period, but is expected to recover
   b) Permanent total disability: Worker is disabled permanently and unable to perform any type of work
   c) Temporary partial disability: Worker is able to work, but has a diminished capacity
   d) Permanent partial disability: Person is able to work, but has a ratable partial impairment
   e) Survivor (death): Payments made to spouse until remarriage and to children until age 18

2. State or federal income programs
   a. Aid to Families with Dependent Children
   b. Food stamps
   c. Supplemental food for Women, Infants, and Children (WIC) Program
   d. Public housing and subsidized housing
   e. State general assistance or welfare programs

C. Types of insurance and benefits available from the private sector
   1. Retirement plans and/or disability income insurance
      a. Purchased by individual
      b. Purchased by employer
      c. Purchased by union and/or association
   2. Types of automobile insurance benefits
      a. No-fault
      b. Automobile liability
   3. General liability insurance for personal injury or wrongful death
   4. Accidental death and dismemberment insurance
   5. Hospital indemnity insurance benefits
   6. Travel accident insurance benefits
   7. Mortgage and credit disability insurance benefits

References

Jehle, F.F. (1992). *The complete and easy guide to Social Security and Medicare* (9th ed.). Charlotte, VT: Williamson Publishing Company.

Pell, A.E. (1990). *Making the most of Medicare: A guide through the Medicare maze.* Minneapolis: DCI Publishing.

Social Security programs in the United States. (1989). *Social Security Bulletin, 52*(7), 2-79.

Suggested Readings

Landay, E. (Ed.). (1990). *The complete Medicare handbook.* Rocklin, CA: Prima Publishing.

Pope, A., & Tarlov, A.R. (Eds.). (1991). *Disability in America.* Washington: National Academy Press.

Tucker, B.P., & Goldstein, B.A. (1991). *Legal rights of persons with disabilities: An analysis of federal law.* Horsham, PA: LRP Publications.

Section VII
Ethics in Rehabilitation Nursing

Ethical principles and concepts, and their attendant legal considerations, are gaining increasing importance in the practice of rehabilitation. Chapter 30 presents an overview of the basic ethical principles of health care and reproduces important ethical statements such as the American Nurses Association's Code for Nurses and the Patient's Bill of Rights set forth by the American Hospital Association. The chapter also deals with legal considerations such as living wills, advance directives, and patient self-determination. In addition, it offers a brief outline of emerging related public policy issues that rehabilitation professionals, the public at large, and the government must address.

CHAPTER 30

Ethical and Legal Considerations

Ethical dilemmas, perpetuated in part by the technological advances of science and rises in the incidence of catastrophic injury and new disease processes, continue to confront rehabilitation nurses. Ethical issues rarely are settled by institutional policies and established legal parameters. In fact, the attempted resolution of ethical issues often results in more questions and more issues. In addition, financial and healthcare resources are not always available to persons with permanent disabilities. "Because rehabilitation is based on the belief that clients should participate in the decision-making process, rehabilitation nurses face the dilemma of caring for individuals whose decisions may not reflect the values of independence and wellness. Conflicts may arise among rights of individuals, rights of families, and what is available, accepted scientific and technological treatment. In such cases, the rehabilitation nurse should seek legal and/or ethical consultation to determine the best course of action" (American Nurses' Association [ANA] & Association of Rehabilitation Nurses [ARN], 1988, p. 6). This chapter provides an overview of ethical issues and legal considerations frequently encountered in rehabilitation practice and reflected in the following questions:

- Does a rehabilitation client have the right to refuse recommended treatments but still receive funding for his or her choice of services?
- Does everyone have a right to rehabilitation or should there be exceptions (e.g., illegal aliens, those disabled in the perpetration of a violent crime)?
- Who on the rehabilitation team should decide that services are to be discontinued due to lack of progress toward goals or lack of funding?
- If a client informs the rehabilitation staff that he or she does not want to be treated or rehabilitated and, in fact, wants to die, should the team accept his or her decision and discontinue treatment?
- What should the rehabilitation team do when discharge is indicated and the client has no acceptable disposition (e.g., a homeless person who has had a stroke)?
- Where should ventilator-dependent patients go after acute hospitalization when funding for long-term care is not available?
- When should staff discontinue gastrostomy/tube feedings for a comatose patient?
- When should chemical and physical restraints be implemented?
- Should healthcare dollars be spent for organ transplants for a patient in a persistent vegetative state following traumatic brain injury?
- If an adolescent with a disability requests information on sex education, should parental consent be requested?

I. Ethics

A. Definitions
1. Ethics: Study of the nature and justification of general ethical principles that can be applied to special areas where moral problems are presented
2. Morality: Traditions of belief about right and wrong human conduct
3. Bioethics: Ethics applied to health care; involves moral rules, principles, and values that guide relationships among healthcare professionals and their clients

B. Ethical principles and theories
1. Principles and concepts related to ethical issues
   a. Respect
      1) Relates to the idea that individuals are members of a human community
      2) Involves the consideration that most decisions that people make will affect others
      3) Acknowledges the interconnectedness and interdependence of individuals
   b. Beneficence
      1) Holds that people should not inflict evil or harm, should prevent evil and harm, and should remove evil
      2) Holds that people should do or promote good works
   c. Nonmaleficence: Holds that the prohibition of intentional harm, except in special circumstances, requires that risks be justified by the probable benefits to be gained
   d. Justice
      1) Relates to the balance between and the management of good and evil, of burdens and benefits
      2) Applies to any society in which resources are limited
   e. Confidentiality
      1) Relates to the obligation to preserve clients' privacy
      2) Relates to holding certain information in strict confidence
      3) Includes both written and verbal interaction

- f. Paternalism
    - 1) Restricts the liberty of individuals without their consent
    - 2) May be justified by either the prevention of harm others might otherwise do to themselves or by the production of some benefits they might otherwise not secure
- g. Autonomy
    - 1) The principle of self-determination or self-governance
    - 2) Includes the right to informed consent and the right to refuse treatment

2. Related theories of ethics
    - a. Utilitarian ethics
        - 1) Holds that the rightness or wrongness of an act is always a function of the extent to which it is being performed or omitted
        - 2) Contributes to the goal of maximizing the overall good, which is construed variously as the total or average happiness or welfare
    - b. Duty-based ethics: Establishes some particular duty or set of duties as fundamental (e.g., the Ten Commandments, Hippocratic Oath)
    - c. Rights-based ethics: Fundamental rights require fulfillment of certain corresponding duties (see Thomas Paine's *Common Sense*)
    - d. Intuitionist ethics
        - 1) Includes no prior ordering of basic social goals, duties, and rights
        - 2) Accords each ethical component the same prima-facie basic status
        - 3) Resolves dilemmas or conflicts on a case-by-case basis
        - 4) Compares the relative weights of the conflicting prima-facie goals, duties, and rights

C. Ethics committee

1. Characteristics
    - a. Is a multidisciplinary group of healthcare professionals
    - b. Operates in healthcare setting
    - c. Is established specifically to address the ethical dilemmas that occur within the setting
2. Responsibilities
    - a. To address issues of informed consent
    - b. To render decisions for incompetent or incapacitated patients when an emergency exists or an immediate decision is needed
    - c. To rule on difficult dilemmas that present a compelling case
    - d. To attempt resolution of treatment differences
    - e. To serve as a forum for discussion of such concerns and to act in an advisory capacity before judicial review occurs (ANA, 1988)
    - f. To educate staff
3. Composition
    - a. Physicians
    - b. Nurses
    - c. Social workers
    - d. Allied health professionals
    - e. Member(s) of the clergy
    - f. Ethicist
    - g. Hospital administrators
    - h. Community members (e.g., disabled persons or members of their families)
    - i. Attorney

D. Professional ethics codes and statements of rights

1. American Nurses Association
    - a. Code of ethics (see Figure 30.1)
    - b. Topics on which ANA has position statements and guidelines (ANA, 1988)
        - 1) The withdrawal or withholding of food and/or fluid with a special focus on circumstances when it is unclear whether food and fluid would be more beneficial or more harmful
        - 2) Risks versus responsibilities in providing nursing care, which is particularly relevant for nurses caring for clients with communicable or infectious diseases
        - 3) Safeguards for clients' health and safety, including specific attention to clients' rights and best interests
        - 4) Nurses' participation and leadership in their own institutions' ethical review processes
        - 5) Encouragement of the development of mechanisms by state nurses' associations to consider ethical issues and concerns
        - 6) The nonnegotiable nature of the ANA *Code for Nurses with Interpretive Statements* (1985) and its importance in defining the profession's standards
        - 7) Nurses' participation in capital punishment as a breach of the ethical tradition of nursing
        - 8) Support of the nurses' participation in multidisciplinary institutional review processes such as ethics committees and support of professional autonomy in a decision-making process that includes patients' families vis-a-vis government intervention in or control of healthcare decisions
    - c. Standard V from ANA's *Standards of Clinical Nursing Practice: Standards of Professional Performance* (1991b)
        - 1) Statement that says, "The nurse's decisions and actions on behalf of clients are determined in an ethical manner" (ANA, 1991b, p. 15)
        - 2) Guidelines for conduct (ANA, 1991b, p. 15)
            - a) The nurse's practice is guided by the *Code for Nurses with Interpretive Statements*
            - b) The nurse maintains the client's confidentiality
            - c) The nurse acts as a client advocate
            - d) The nurse delivers care in a nonjudgmental and nondiscriminatory manner that is sensitive to clients' diversity
            - e) The nurse delivers care in a manner that preserves and/or protects client's autonomy, dignity, and rights
            - f) The nurse seeks available resources to help formulate ethical decisions

Figure 30.1. American Nurses Association Code for Nurses

1. The nurse provides services with respect for human dignity and the uniqueness of the client, unrestricted by considerations of social or economic status, personal attributes, or the nature of health problems.
2. The nurse safeguards the client's right to privacy by judiciously protecting information of a confidential nature.
3. The nurse acts to safeguard the client and the public when health care and safety are affected by the incompetent, unethical, or illegal practice of any person.
4. The nurse assumes responsibility and accountability for individual nursing judgments and actions.
5. The nurse maintains competence in nursing.
6. The nurse exercises informed judgment and uses individual competence and qualifications as criteria in seeking consultation, accepting responsibilities, and delegating nursing activities to others.
7. The nurse participates in activities that contribute to the ongoing development of the profession's body of knowledge.
8. The nurse participates in the profession's efforts to implement and improve standards of nursing.
9. The nurse participates in the profession's efforts to establish and maintain conditions of employment conducive to high quality nursing care.
10. The nurse participates in the profession's effort to protect the public from misinformation and misrepresentation and to maintain the integrity of nursing.
11. The nurse collaborates with members of the health professions and other citizens in promoting community and national efforts to meet the health needs of the public.

Reprinted with permission of the American Nurses Association from American Nurses Association. (1985). *Code for nurses with interpretive statements* (p. 1). Washington, DC: Author.

2. The Association of Rehabilitation Nurses is currently developing a code of ethics
3. *A Patient's Bill of Rights* (American Hospital Association, 1992) (see Figure 30.2)
   a. Applies to all clients receiving services from healthcare providers
   b. Many providers have special adaptations and protect additional patient rights according to the healthcare setting or the type of service; as members of the healthcare team, nurses need to be aware of and respect the rights of the rehabilitation client

II. Legal Issues

A. Legal considerations
1. Informed consent
   a. Definition: Consent obtained from a patient or a subject in a study or experiment after the subject has been fully informed about the risks and consequences of either agreeing to or refusing to submit to an operation or procedure; any inherent risk of death or serious bodily injury that the patient might not know about or an instance when the probability of success in a medical procedure is low are examples of situations when informed consent of the patient is needed (Goldstein, Perdew, & Pruitt, 1989)
   b. Responsibilities of the physician in informing a patient
      1) To describe a proposed procedure
      2) To disclose a procedure's risks of death and injury
      3) To disclose the benefits and alternatives
      4) To explain anticipated results
      5) To disclose the likely course of recuperation before subjecting a patient to a procedure that carries a risk of injury
2. Living will
   a. Generally allows clients to make their wishes known prior to hospitalization regarding medical care, illness, or conditions resulting in incompetency
   b. Is a recognized legal document in 40 states and the District of Columbia (as of 1992)
   c. Is defined by varying protocols within each state and healthcare setting
3. Natural death acts: State legislation that allows for the creation of documents that provide a legally recognized way for competent adults to express, in advance, their desires regarding crucial medical decisions in the event that they become terminally ill and death is imminent
4. Patient Self-Determination Act: Incorporated into the Omnibus Budget Reconciliation Act (OBRA) of 1990
   a. Requirements for institutional providers (Obade, 1990)
      1) Provide written notice to adult patients
         a) Is determined by state law regarding patients' rights to consent to and refuse care and to formulate advance directives—for example, California was first state to approve right-to-die bill
         b) Is determined by relevant policies of a particular institution
      2) Inquire whether patient has executed an advance directive and document response in the medical record; documentation policy is established by each healthcare setting
      3) Provide education about these issues
      4) Ensure compliance with any state law applicable to advance directives
      5) Maintain written policies and procedures that list requirements (Obade, 1990)
   b. Nursing's role in implementing the Patient Self-Determination Act (see Figure 30.3)
5. Guardianship: A position of responsibility given to

Figure 30.2. American Hospital Association: A Patient's Bill of Rights*

1. The patient has the right to considerate and respectful care.

2. The patient has the right to and is encouraged to obtain from physicians and other direct caregivers relevant, current, and understandable information concerning diagnosis, treatment, and prognosis.

   Except in emergencies when the patient lacks decision-making capacity and the need for treatment is urgent, the patient is entitled to the opportunity to discuss and request information related to the specific procedures and/or treatments, the risks involved, the possible length of recuperation, and the medically reasonable alternatives and their accompanying risks and benefits.

   Patients have the right to know the identity of physicians, nurses, and others involved in their care, as well as when those involved are students, residents, or other trainees. The patient also has the right to know the immediate and long-term financial implications of treatment choices, insofar as they are known.

3. The patient has the right to make decisions about the plan of care prior to and during the course of treatment and to refuse a recommended treatment or plan of care to the extent permitted by law and hospital policy and to be informed of the medical consequences of this action. In case of such refusal, the patient is entitled to other appropriate care and services that the hospital provides or transfer to another hospital. The hospital should notify patients of any policy that might affect patient choice within the institution.

4. The patient has the right to have an advance directive (such as a living will, health care proxy, or durable power of attorney for health care) concerning treatment or designating a surrogate decision maker with the expectation that the hospital will honor the intent of that directive to the extent permitted by law and hospital policy.

   Health care institutions must advise patients of their rights under state law and hospital policy to make informed medical choices, ask if the patient has an advance directive, and include that information in patient records. The patient has the right to timely information about hospital policy that may limit its ability to implement fully a legally valid advance directive.

5. The patient has the right to every consideration of privacy. Case discussion, consultation, examination, and treatment should be conducted so as to protect each patient's privacy.

6. The patient has the right to expect that all communications and records pertaining to his/her care will be treated as confidential by the hospital, except in cases such as suspected abuse and public health hazards when reporting is permitted or required by law. The patient has the right to expect that the hospital will emphasize the confidentiality of this information when it releases it to any other parties entitled to review information in these records.

7. The patient has the right to review the records pertaining to his/her medical care and to have the information explained or interpreted as necessary, except when restricted by law.

8. The patient has the right to expect that, within its capacity and policies, a hospital will make reasonable response to the request of a patient for appropriate and medically indicated care and services. The hospital must provide evaluation, service, and/or referral as indicated by the urgency of the case. When medically appropriate and legally permissible, or when a patient has so requested, a patient may be transferred to another facility. The institution to which the patient is to be transferred must first have accepted the patient for transfer. The patient must also have the benefit of complete information and explanation concerning the need for, risks, benefits, and alternatives to such a transfer.

9. The patient has the right to ask [about] and be informed of the existence of business relationships among the hospital, educational institutions, other health care providers, or payers that may influence the patient's treatment and care.

10. The patient has the right to consent to or decline to participate in proposed research studies or human experimentation affecting care and treatment or requiring direct patient involvement, and to have those studies fully explained prior to consent. A patient who declines to participate in research or experimentation is entitled to the most effective care that the hospital can otherwise provide.

11. The patient has the right to expect reasonable continuity of care when appropriate and to be informed by physicians and other caregivers of available and realistic patient care options when hospital care is no longer appropriate.

12. The patient has the right to be informed of hospital policies and practices that relate to patient care, treatment, and responsibilities. The patient has the right to be informed of available resources for resolving disputes, grievances, and conflicts, such as ethics committees, patient representatives, or other mechanisms available in the institution. The patient has the right to be informed of the hospital's charges for services and available payment methods.

**These rights can be exercised on the patient's behalf by a designated surrogate or proxy decision maker if the patient lacks decision-making capacity, is legally incompetent, or is a minor.*

A Patient's Bill of Rights was first adopted by the American Hospital Association (AHA) in 1973. This revision was approved by the AHA Board of Trustees on October 21,1992.

Figure 30.3. American Nurses Association Position Statement on Nursing and the Patient Self-Determination Act

Summary: The American Nurses Association (ANA) believes that nurses should play a primary role in implementation of the Patient Self-Determination Act, passed as part of the Omnibus Budget Reconciliation Act of 1990. It is the responsibility of nurses to facilitate informed decision-making for patients making choices about end-of-life care. The nurse's role in education, research, patient care and advocacy is critical to implementation of the Patient Self-Determination Act within all health care settings.

The Patient Self-Determination Act, passed as part of the Omnibus Budget Reconciliation Act of 1990, bec[ame] effective December 1, 1991. The federal law applies to all health care institutions receiving Medicaid funds and requires that all individuals receiving medical care must be given written information about their rights under state law to make decisions about medical care, including the right to accept or refuse medical or surgical treatment. Individuals must also be given information about their rights to formulate advance directives such as living wills and durable powers of attorney for health care. Patients must be made aware of their rights to make decisions about these issues upon admission (in the case of hospitals or skilled nursing facilities), enrollment (in the case of health maintenance organizations), on first receipt of care (in the case of hospices) or before the patient comes under an agency's care (in the case of home health personal care agencies) .

ANA supports the patient's right to self-determination and believes that nurses will and must play a primary role in implementation of the law. Ideally, decisions about advance directives should be made by the patient with the family and the primary provider prior to admission. The formation of advance directives is an important decision and will inevitably involve nurses, who are the most omnipresent professionals in health care facilities. It is imperative that the decision making that will fall to patients and their families as they make choices about end-of-life care be facilitated by nurses.

- Each nurse should know the laws of the state in which she/he is practicing pertaining to advance directives, and should be familiar with the strengths and limitations of the various forms of advance directive.
- The nurse is one of several health care professionals who has a responsibility for ensuring that the advance care directives initiated by the patient are current and reflective of the patient's choices. Facilitating self-determination of patients with respect to end-of-life decisions is a process that includes evaluating changes in the patient's perspective and health state.
- The nurse has a responsibility to facilitate informed decision making, including but not limited to advance directives.
- ANA recommends that these questions about advance directives be part of the nursing admission assessment: Do you have basic information about advance care directives, including living wills and durable power of attorney? Do you wish to initiate an advance care directive? If you have already prepared an advance care directive, can you provide it now? Have you discussed your end-of-life choices with your family and/or designated surrogate and health care team worker?
- The role of the nurse is critical in implementation of the Patient Self-Determination Act and includes public education, research, patient care, advocacy, education of the profession and inservice education of other health care providers.

someone by the court to make decisions for an incompetent person or on behalf of the incompetent person's estate; limited guardianship is granted by the court only if imminent danger to person or property of the ward is shown

6. Estate planning
   a. Providing for the consequences of the possibility of a catastrophic illness and/or injury requires long-term planning for future care and expense
   b. Structured financial plans allow for generation of additional monies over future years
   c. Future medical and rehabilitative care needs may be identified by rehabilitation nurses functioning as case managers or life-care planning consultants; establishing these needs is a component of estate planning
7. Durable power of attorney for health care: Enables a competent individual (the principal) to appoint a surrogate decision maker who will be empowered legally to make medical care decisions if the principal subsequently is incapacitated (e.g., becomes comatose) (Goldstein et al., 1989)
8. Incompetence
   a. A physician may render a clinical opinion regarding client's competence; a court decides if a person is legally incompetent and then authorizes another to act on his or her behalf (Goldstein et al., 1989)
   b. Court decisions regarding determination of incompetence vary, depending upon individual state procedures
9. Legal death: Brain death is the legal parameter that determines when life ceases; most states rely on this guideline in pronouncing death
10. Ethical issues related to withholding and/or withdrawal of treatment
    a. Withholding often is termed *omission*
    b. Withdrawal often is termed *commission*
    c. A consideration is whether either withdrawal or

withholding achieves the expected benefit

11. Research on human subjects
    a. Basic rules and requirements can be found in various codes and regulations
    b. Participating patients should comprehend purpose of research and what is expected of them
    c. Patients should be competent to make the decision to participate
    d. Policy regarding compensation for patients injured by research procedures should be formulated
12. Do-not-resuscitate order (DNR)
    a. Generally means that cardiopulmonary resuscitation measures will be withheld in the event of an acute cardiac or respiratory arrest
    b. Does not prohibit other forms of life-sustaining interventions (e.g., intravenous fluids, medications)
    c. Should not imply that the patient's care will be less aggressive or substandard or that the amount of nursing care will be reduced

B. Neurological conditions requiring medical and/or treatment decisions (Cranford, 1991)
1. Brain death: Irreversible loss of all brain functions in both the cerebral hemisphere and the brainstem
2. Persistent vegetative state: Irreversible loss of all neocortical functions, although brainstem functions are intact
3. Permanent locked-in state: Irreversible loss of motor functions to a severe degree
4. Dementia: Irreversible loss of neocortical functions to a variable degree

C. Effective communication
1. Intensity of medical care should be discussed with patients and families
    a. Determines how far the medical team should go to prolong life in light of expected outcomes
    b. Involves balancing the burdens of a particular therapy against benefits of that therapy to patient
2. Steps for communicating with families
    a. Encourage a dialogue to determine cultural and/or socioeconomic attitudes related to defining appropriate level of care
    b. Identify options
        1) Components of life support systems in current use
        2) Brief historical overview of recent legal decisions
        3) Policies of the particular healthcare setting
        4) Written information for further reflection
        5) Resources for support (e.g., professional nurse, social worker, pastoral counselor)
    c. Involve the entire rehabilitation team in family communication and discuss their concerns regarding treatment

III. Future Directions of Medical Ethics

A. Increased importance of issues in several areas
1. The continuing biomedical technical revolution
2. The maturation of biomedical ethics as a discipline
3. An increasing intersection of ethics and health policy
4. A broader engagement of the public in issues related to biomedical ethics
5. A change in the conceptual foundations of bioethics
6. Changes in the relationship between physician and patient (Pellegrino, Siegler, & Singer, 1991)

B. Prediction of increased government intervention in the decision-making process
1. Emergence of mandatory clinical guidelines and/or standards for physicians and other healthcare professionals
2. Mandates governing advance medical directives such as a living will and a durable power of attorney for health care
3. An increase in the number of states with natural death acts

C. Increased public involvement in ethical issues
1. Provision of public education concerning legal ramifications of treatment decisions and responsibility to patients themselves and family members (e.g., living will)
2. Analysis of research data as the basis for setting policy
3. Mechanisms for public participation—for example, awareness, legislative involvement, position statements of healthcare organizations

D. Rehabilitation professionals must continue to address issues such as those listed below
1. Balancing medical and rehabilitative needs that present a moral quandary to rehabilitation care providers (Haas, 1993)
2. Team contribution to decision making with regard to services for clients, as well as their progress and outcomes
3. Definition of quality-of-life issues as well as related involvement of decision-making bodies
4. Overall access to rehabilitation services regardless of disability and funding
5. Legal requirements, including guardianship, living wills, and durable power of attorney
6. Meeting standards and regulations as imposed by various entities without participation in the formulation of these standards or regulations
7. Client decisions to adhere or not adhere to recommended therapeutic regimens as defined by rehabilitation teams
8. Encouragement of the formation of ethics committees within rehabilitation settings

References

American Hospital Association (AHA). (1992). *A patient's bill of rights* [Management advisory]. Chicago: Author.

American Nurses Association (ANA). (1985). *Code for nurses with interpretive statements.* Washington, DC: Author.

American Nurses Association. (1988). *Ethics in nursing: Position statements and guidelines.* Kansas City, MO: Author.

American Nurses Association. (1991a). *American Nurses Association position statement on nursing and the Patient Self-Determination Act.* Kansas City, MO: Author.

American Nurses Association. (1991b). *Standards of clinical nursing practice: Standards of professional performance.* Kansas City, MO: Author.

American Nurses' Association & the Association of Rehabilitation Nurses (ARN). (1988). *Rehabilitation nursing: Scope of practice; process and outcome criteria for selected diagnoses.* Kansas City, MO: American Nurses' Association.

Cranford, R.E. (1991, July). Major neurological syndromes requiring life sustaining medical treatment decisions. *Medical Ethics Advisor*, p. 87.

Goldstein, A., Perdew, S., & Pruitt, S. (1989). *The nurse's legal advisor.* Philadelphia: J.B. Lippincott Company.

Haas, J. (1993). Ethical issues in rehabilitation medicine. In J. DeLisa & B. Gans (Eds.), *Rehabilitation medicine: Principles and practice* (2nd ed.) (pp. 28-39). Philadelphia: J.B. Lippincott Company.

Obade, C.C. (1990). Right church wrong pew. *The Journal of Clinical Ethics, 1*, 320-322.

Pellegrino, E.D., Siegler, M., & Singer, P. (1991). Future directions in clinical ethics. *The Journal of Clinical Ethics, 2*(1), 5-9.

Suggested Readings

Bandman, E., & Bandman, B. (1990). *Nursing ethics through the life span.* Norwalk, CT: Appleton-Century-Crofts.

Banja, J. (Ed.). (1989). Ethical and legal issues in traumatic brain injury. *Journal of Head Trauma Rehabilitation, 4*, 1.

Barth, J., Gideon, D., Sciara, A., Hulsey, P., & Anchor, K. (1986). Forensic aspects of mild head trauma. *Journal of Head Trauma Rehabilitation, 1*(2), 63-70.

Beauchamp, T.L., & Walters, L. (1985). *Contemporary issues in bioethics.* Belmont, CA: Wadsworth Publishing Company.

Benjamin, M., & Curtis, J. (1986). *Ethics in nursing.* New York: Oxford University Press.

Caplan, A.L. (1988). Informed consent and provider-patient relationships in rehabilitation medicine. *Archives of Physical Medicine and Rehabilitation, 69*, 312.

Caplan, A.L., Callahan, D., & Haas, J. (1987). Ethical and policy issues in rehabilitation medicine. *Hastings Center Report Special Supplement, 17*, 1-20.

Creighton, H. (1986). *Law every nurse should know.* Philadelphia: W.B. Saunders Company.

Cunningham, N., & Hutchinson, S. (1990). Myths in health care ethics. *Image, 22*(4), 235-238.

Davis, A., & Aroskar, M. (1991). *Ethical dilemmas and nursing practice.* Englewood Cliffs, NJ: Prentice Hall, Inc.

De Jong, G., & Batavia, A. (1989). Societal duty and resource allocation for persons with severe traumatic brain injury. *Journal of Head Trauma Rehabilitation, 4*(1), 1-12.

Fletcher, G., Banja, T., Tann, B., & Wolf, S. (1992). *Rehabilitation medicine: Contemporary clinical perspectives.* Philadelphia: Lea & Febiger.

Fry-Revere, S. (1990). Legal trends in bioethics. *The Journal of Clinical Ethics, 1*, 322-325.

Hardwig, J. (1991). Treating the brain dead for the benefit of the family. *The Journal of Clinical Ethics, 2*(1), 53-56.

Holthaus, D. (1989, November 20). Right-to-die: An executive report. *Hospitals*, pp. 33-35.

Kolpan, K. (1986). Medicolegal issues, amnesia and the law. *Journal of Head Trauma Rehabilitation, 1*(3), 81-82.

Miedema, J. (1991). Medical treatment after brain death: A case report and ethical analysis. *The Journal of Clinical Ethics, 2*(1), 50-52.

Obade, C. (1990). Cruzan and its sequelae: The Supreme Court decides its first "right-to-die" case. *The Journal of Clinical Ethics, 1*, 242-249.

President's Commission for the Study of Ethical Problems in Medicine and Biomedical Research. (1983). *Deciding to forego life sustaining treatment.* Washington, DC: U.S. Government Printing Office.

Purtilo, R.B. (1988). Ethical issues in teamwork: The context of rehabilitation. *Archives of Physical Medicine and Rehabilitation, 69*, 318-322.

Reed, M.E., & Olson, C.A. (1985). Proxy decision making for the terminally ill: Where are the guidelines? *American College of Surgeons Bulletin, 70*(6), 25-29.

Romano, M.D. (1989). Ethical issues and families of brain-injured persons. *Journal of Head Trauma Rehabilitation, 4*(1), 33-41.

Singer, P., Pellegrino, E., & Siegler, M. (1990). Ethics committees and consultants. *The Journal of Clinical Ethics, 1*, 263-267.

Sullivan, P.A., & Brown, T. (1991, October 21). Commonsense ethics in administrative decision making: Preparatory steps—Part I. *Journal of Nursing Administration*, pp. 21-23.

Sullivan, P.A., & Brown, T. (1991, November 21). Commonsense ethics in administrative decision making: Proactive steps—Part II. *Journal of Nursing Administration*, pp. 57-61.

Wold, J.L. (1992). The living will: Legal and ethical perspectives. *Journal of Neuroscience Nursing, 24*(1), 50-53.

Wurzbach, M. (1990). The dilemma of withholding or withdrawing nutrition. *Image, 22*(4), 226-230.

Section VIII
The Future of Rehabilitation Nursing

Rehabilitation has come an amazing distance in the 20th century; anyone who gauges today's practice against the beginnings of the specialty in the 1900s (see Chapter 2) will find that obvious. But there is much yet to be done and many challenges yet to face, because the population of people with disabilities continues to expand in changing and sometimes unpredictable ways. Chapter 31 addresses in a broad fashion some of the topics that rehabilitation nurses will confront in the last years of the 20th century: the growth of the population of people with disabilities, the expansion of the rehabilitation specialty in numbers and educational demands, the need for research, the implications of healthcare reform and alternative methods of delivering healthcare services, legislative issues, and emerging technology.

CHAPTER 31

Future Challenges for the Specialty Practice of Rehabilitation Nursing

Population trends, technological advances, and healthcare reform will shape and determine the changing and future roles of rehabilitation nursing. The demands placed upon the profession and its leadership will provide both a challenge and an opportunity. As the rehabilitation nursing discipline expands, rehabilitation nurses must continue to define their scope of practice, ensure adequate educational preparation for practitioners, conduct and use research, and maintain a strong professional organization to provide the specialty with a unified voice. This chapter provides an overview of the future of rehabilitation nursing in terms of two major influences: the demands of a growing population of people with disabilities, and the implications of healthcare reform in the United States.

Meeting the increased demand for rehabilitation nursing

As this century comes to a close, the need for medical rehabilitation services will continue to grow. This will have a number of implications, as detailed below, but it is occurring due to two primary causes: the aging of the U.S. population and the growth of the number of people with disabilities. The baby-boomers, the largest demographic segment of the U.S. population, are growing older. As they age, many will succumb to chronic disease and debilitating illnesses, necessitating more rehabilitation services. People will enjoy longer life expectancies as a result of improved health care and advances in medical technology and treatment. By the year 2000, there will be 118,000 people who are more than 100 years old (Celtron, 1992). Because of longer life spans, more people will have an increased chance of becoming disabled—thus, perhaps, changing the perception that disabilities are "something that happens to others."

As earlier chapters of this book have asserted, rehabilitation issues cover the entire life span—from pediatrics through adolescence and young and middle adulthood to old age. As the majority of the U.S. population reaches the age of 65 and older, rehabilitation professionals will need more knowledge about gerontological issues. In addition, medical advances now have made normal life spans possible for people with spinal cord injuries and brain injuries. As these people grow into adulthood and old age, health problems that have not had to be addressed before will arise. An increase in cases of dual disability, such as a patient with a spinal cord injury who also has a brain injury, will be seen in larger numbers among those in the older population. People with Parkinson's disease who have suffered a stroke or people with arthritis who also have had an amputation will not be uncommon.

What will this expansion in the disabled population mean to rehabilitation? It will give rise to a number of developments: alteration in practice settings, a greater demand for patient and family education, a need for increased recruitment and further education of nurses, an increased insistence on certification, an expansion of professional activities into consultation and research, and ensuring a unified voice for the specialty.

Alteration in practice settings: Rehabilitation practice settings already have expanded from inpatient units and freestanding rehabilitation hospitals to outpatient clinics, independent living centers, long-term care and skilled nursing facilities, home health agencies, and facilities managed by private industry and insurance companies. The emphasis in health care has been and will continue to be on outpatient and home care. In rehabilitation, more home health agencies are expected to focus on providing direct rehabilitation services in the home.

The range of practice settings for rehabilitation care is great, as is the range of disabilities and illnesses encountered in rehabilitation. Many rehabilitation programs treat not only people with strokes, orthopedic problems, spinal cord injuries, and brain injuries, but also those with pulmonary and cardiac conditions, pain, oncology, AIDS, burns, and chemical dependency problems. New diagnoses—for example, postpolio syndrome—and rehabilitation programs to deal with them will arise as medical advances are made.

Patient and family education: One challenge in rehabilitation that certainly will remain constant as the 20th century declines is the education of patients. Teaching is a key element of rehabilitation, and it will become more so as the length of stay on inpatient units continues to decrease. The average total length of stay for patients in freestanding hospitals and rehabilitation units in 1978 was 52.2 days; in 1980, the length of stay averaged 36.2 days, and in 1990, 29.1 days (S. Sonic, personal communication, March 23, 1993). In light of this, more efficient and more effective ways to teach patients and family members will become necessary. More research on effective educational programs will have to be done in this area. Educational sessions may need to be developed for ongoing outpatient or in-home programs and taught by rehabilitation nurses as an extension of inpatient programs.

Recruitment and education of nurses: The need for expanded rehabilitation services will require a greater number of rehabilitation nurses. Two of the major challenges for the specialty will be recruiting nurses into the field and educating them once they have been recruited. Because of the explosion of knowledge in the areas of medicine and nursing, colleges and universities are unable to cover all the existing specialty practice areas, so rehabilitation nursing frequently is not included in their curricula. At the national level, the Association of Rehabilitation Nurses (ARN) is working with the National Federation for Specialty Nursing Organizations (NFSNO) to address education and awareness issues concerning specialty practice at the basic level of preparation. To recruit staff, rehabilitation units and hospitals will need to involve more students in the area of rehabilitation by offering clinical and observational rotations and/or by providing in-service training on rehabilitation nursing concepts and practice.

More educational programs at the local and national levels will be needed. Nurses who are new to the field will need to be informed of new medical and nursing diagnoses as well as treatment techniques and approaches, and experienced rehabilitation nurses need up-to-date knowledge to continue to practice at an advanced level. As medical procedures such as the insertion of chest tubes, parenteral nutrition, patient-controlled analgesics, and dialysis are used more frequently, the emphasis on discharging patients sooner will create a greater challenge for rehabilitation nurses. Depending on their practice setting, rehabilitation nurses may need to expand their knowledge base.

This growing need for education has several implications. Because more employers in the healthcare sector may have increasingly less money for educational programs, ARN may face greater pressure to offer more scholarships. Qualified advanced practitioners and teachers of rehabilitation nursing will be necessary for the increased educational demands of the specialty. Currently, there are five graduate programs offering master's degrees in rehabilitation nursing (see Chapter 3, page 18); more will be needed.

Certification: The demand for Certified Rehabilitation Registered Nurses (CRRNs) will continue to increase as the specialty grows and as more employers and insurance providers realize the benefits of certification. An increased number of courses will be needed to help rehabilitation nurses validate their knowledge and skills for intermediate-level practice and to facilitate preparation for the certification examination. The American Board of Nursing Specialties (ABNS), which was established in 1991, sets criteria for certification programs. ABNS's goal is to establish national standards for specialty nursing certification programs. This will ensure that healthcare consumers receive the same quality of nursing care from all certified nurses in the various specialties. Membership in ABNS is open to certification programs and other national nursing organizations involved in credentialing, as well as to others whose interests are important in certification. The Rehabilitation Nursing Certification Board is a charter member. By the year 2000, those taking certification exams will be required to meet specific educational and degree criteria. Members of ARN and their employers will be challenged with providing scholarships and tuition reimbursement programs that will help nurses take courses and pursue degrees leading to certification. Another challenge may be the development of additional examinations for subspecialty or advanced practice certification.

Expansion of professional activities: As rehabilitation expands, so will the scope of rehabilitation nurses' professional activities. One area in which there will be a sizeable need for rehabilitation nurses is consultation. Nurses will be needed as expert witnesses for attorneys, as independent consultants for inpatient units, and as private insurance case managers; they also will be needed to provide expert testimony on healthcare issues related to rehabilitation before legislative bodies. Consultants who are experts in advanced rehabilitation nursing practice will be needed to assist with difficult patient care problems and to establish nursing criteria for quality assurance programs and program evaluation.

Research is another professional activity in which more rehabilitation nurses will and must become involved. More research needs to be conducted on treatments and patient outcomes. Nurses must participate in research on the cost-effectiveness of rehabilitation and rehabilitation nursing. Two questions must be addressed: Does rehabilitation nursing make a difference? If so, how much of a difference does it make in terms of patient outcomes? Providers are looking for successful patient outcomes—particularly those related to functional ability—that will prove that rehabilitation is an effective part of the continuum of care.

Ensuring a unified voice for the specialty: As rehabilitation practice expands into new settings with additional medical and nursing diagnoses, ARN must be prepared to meet the varied needs of its membership. At the beginning of this decade, the number of rehabilitation nurses was estimated to be approximately 44,000. Because there is strength in numbers, recruiting more members and keeping rehabilitation professionals together—rather than encouraging the development of various subspecialty groups—will continue to be of tremendous importance.

Dealing with the implications of healthcare reform

Healthcare reform is one of the major topics to be addressed in the United States over the next few years. Approximately 37 million people in the United States have no health insurance (Celtron, 1992). Furthermore, rehabilitation services have had limited visibility among the public and payer sources. A Stanford Research Institute (SRI)/Gallup market research study done in 1988 (sponsored by the National Association of Rehabilitation Facilities and The American Hospital Association Section for Rehabilitation Hospitals and Programs) to evaluate public awareness of medical rehabilitation revealed that 28 million Americans who could benefit from rehabilitation services were not receiving them. Only 35% of insurers encourage rehabilitation by including it as a benefit in their policies (National Association of Rehabilitation Facilities & The American Hospital Association Section for Rehabilitation Hospitals and Programs, 1988). It is imperative that ARN continue its active involvement with other organizations—such as the Agency for Health Care Policy and Research, the American Academy of Physical Medicine and Rehabilitation, the American Congress of Rehabilitation Medicine, the American Hospital Association, the American Nurses Association, the Commission on Accreditation for Rehabilitation Facilities, the Joint Commission on Accreditation of Healthcare Organizations, the National Association of Rehabilitation Facilities, the National Federation for Specialty Nursing Organizations, the National Rehabilitation Caucus, and the Nursing Organization Liaison Forum, among others—to promote a greater awareness of rehabilitation and its benefits to individuals and society as a whole. Such relationships also will help to ensure that rehabilitation services are provided as a core benefit of any proposed healthcare system reform.

Managed care: Managed care will continue to grow. California currently has one of the largest managed care markets; 35% of its insured population is part of either a health maintenance organization (HMO) or a preferred provider organization (PPO). This trend will continue to expand across the country. PPOs, having grown from 13% to 24% of the nation's total market from 1988 to 1991, are the fastest growing of the contract arrangements (Friedman, 1992). Many of the proposed national and state healthcare programs advocate a managed care system; if such a system is adopted, a need for experienced rehabilitation nurses to function as case managers will emerge. It will become increasingly important for ARN to advocate for the recognition of rehabilitation nurses as case managers to ensure that appropriate care and equipment are available for patients.

Cost containment: Cost containment will remain an issue as healthcare budgets become tighter. Managed care organizations as well as Medicare and Medicaid programs are demanding, and will continue to insist, that rehabilitation services be provided at the least expensive level of care. Rehabilitation nurses must participate in the planning process to provide quality care for less money by building creative staffing models and establishing innovative inpatient and outpatient programs.

Legislative involvement and client advocacy: Another challenge for rehabilitation nursing will be continued legislative involvement. To provide rehabilitation nurses with information on how to participate effectively in the legislative process, ARN encourages participation in the Nurse-in-Washington internship program, a 3-day seminar coordinated by NFSNO. ARN sponsors one member to attend each year through the Malcom Maloof Scholarship. Plans are under way as of this writing to offer an advanced internship on public policy. More rehabilitation nurses will need to increase their awareness of legislative issues; eventually, the specialty of rehabilitation nursing may need its own lobbyist.

Rehabilitation nursing must continue to advocate for the rights of people with disabilities, as it did with the Americans with Disabilities Act (ADA), and must promote the positive aspects of the ADA to the public. Similarly, rehabilitation nurses must continue to educate the public regarding prevention of disabilities and to continue activities such as advocating for helmet and seatbelt laws and teaching how to prevent spinal cord and brain injuries. They also should become more actively involved in areas such as prevention of AIDS, cancer, falls in the elderly, and other debilitating disease processes in the future.

Advanced technology: Rehabilitation nurses must be prepared to promote and use advanced technology as it becomes available both for clients and for use in the practice of nursing. Free time is less available today, and people want service that is timelier and faster. Time needs to be leveraged with technology so that more procedures can be done in less time (Burrus, 1992) without sacrificing quality.

Ethical issues: Rehabilitation units and hospitals will see ethical dilemmas increase in the future as a result of the Patient Self-Determination Act (see Chapter 30) and, possibly, of advances in technology. Issues such as whether tube feedings and ventilatory support should be continued will need to be thought out carefully. Members of rehabilitation nursing departments must discuss these issues to prepare for similar situations that could arise in their facilities. Frank Bowe (1992), author of "Handicapping America," wrote that in the future, genetic engineering may be used to correct a disability in a fetus. In such an event, additional ethical questions regarding rehabilitation care certainly will arise.

Innovative ideas often emerge as a result of challenges. Nurses need to be part of the solutions for the future and to accept leadership roles to ensure quality care for their patients. The field of rehabilitation nursing has been, and will continue to be, a very challenging and exciting specialty. As a team-oriented, dynamic, creative, and visionary group of professionals, rehabilitation nurses must be ready to meet any and all challenges the future may bring.

References

Bowe, F. (1992, August). Handicapping America. In A.Toppel (Chair), *A nation united: 25th anniversary celebration.* Symposium conducted at the meeting of the Commission on Accreditation of Rehabilitation Facilities in Washington, DC.

Burrus, D. (1992, August). Technological issues. In A. Toppel (Chair), *A nation united: 25th anniversary celebration.* Symposium conducted at the meeting of the Commission on Accreditation of Rehabilitation Facilities in Washington, DC.

Celtron, M. (1992, August). Future issues. In A. Toppel (Chair), *A nation united: 25th anniversary celebration.* Symposium conducted at the meeting of the Commission on Accreditation of Rehabilitation Facilities in Washington, DC.

Friedman, E. (1992, March). Managed health care: A closed door or a window of opportunity? In B. Desimone (Chair), *The Seventh Annual Casa Colina Case Management Conference for Catastrophic Injury.* Symposium conducted in Palm Springs, CA.

National Association of Rehabilitation Facilities & The American Hospital Association Section for Rehabilitation Hospitals and Programs. (1988). *Survey of rehabilitation awareness* [A Stanford Research Institute/Gallup market research study]. Unpublished study.

APPENDIX A

Patient and Family Guidelines for Selecting a Rehabilitation Facility

Note to healthcare professionals: It is common for families to believe that recovery will be completed in the acute care setting and the client will return directly to his or her home. Following are lists of questions and recommendations that could be offered to families to assist in the transition to a rehabilitation facility. Suggest that they take notes about all facilities and/or programs they have visited to aid in future comparison and decision making.

General guidelines

1. Visit all recommended programs and rehabilitation centers in the local area. Location should be just one of the many factors to consider in choosing a rehabilitation facility. It may be worth the effort to travel for specialized care. Consider the injury and anticipated length of stay.
2. Discuss payment. Some health insurance policies do not cover rehabilitation and/or management of chronic care unless it is performed in a hospital setting, and they set limits on the length of stay that is allowed.

Questions regarding the overall program

1. Has the disability in question been treated before in this program?
2. What are the admission criteria (e.g., evaluation procedures, costs, bed availability)?
3. How many individuals are currently receiving treatment here for the same disability?
4. What is the average length of stay?
5. What type of communication will occur with the referring facility and/or physician and the local physician who will assume care after discharge?
6. What effect will geographic distance have on the family's involvement in rehabilitation?

Questions regarding the program structure

1. Will rehabilitation (e.g., physical therapy or occupational therapy) be scheduled daily?
2. Are these team members full-time staff or consultants?
   - medical directors
   - physiatrists
   - neurologists
   - neuropsychologists
   - orthopedists
   - psychologists
   - rehabilitation nurses
   - physical therapists
   - occupational therapists
   - speech pathologists
   - recreational therapists
   - social workers

Questions regarding family involvement

1. If the family does not live nearby, what is the facility or program protocol for telephone contact?
2. How often will the family have conferences with the rehabilitation team?
3. What type of contact can the family expect with the attending physician?
4. What is the policy for home visits?
5. Are there educational and/or support groups within the facility?
6. Is individual counseling or family therapy, or both, available?

Questions regarding the medical aspects of rehabilitation

1. Is a physician available on site 24 hours daily?
2. How are emergency situations handled?
3. Is the facility prepared to handle the following:
   - X rays?
   - dental care?
   - routine laboratory work?
   - podiatry?
   - ophthalmology?
   - auditory testing?
4. What is the policy for the use of psychotropic drugs and/or physical restraints for management of behavior?

Questions regarding discharge planning

1. How does the facility assist the family with discharge?
2. Is there an established program of postdischarge follow-up?

Questions regarding the financial aspects of rehabilitation

1. What is the cost?
2. Will insurance cover all therapies, special equipment, and basic hygiene supplies?
3. How long will insurance benefits last?
4. What will happen if insurance coverage is denied?

Source Consulted

National Head Injury Foundation. (1992). *Selecting and monitoring head injury rehabilitation.* (Available from National Head Injury Foundation, 1776 Massachusetts Avenue NW, Suite 100, Washington, DC 20036)

APPENDIX **B**

Community Resources and Health-Related Organizations

This appendix contains a list of resources on many health-related topics. The list includes names, addresses, and telephone numbers that can be used to obtain further information. Information was confirmed at press time but is subject to change. This is not a complete listing; rather, it is meant to serve as a starting point.

Acquired Immune Deficiency Syndrome (AIDS)

Canadian AIDS Hotline/AIDS Clearinghouse
613/725-3769 (Ottawa)
416/392-AIDS (Toronto)

National AIDS Hotline
c/o American Social Health Association
PO Box 13827
Research Triangle Park, NC 27709
800/342-AIDS (2437), 800/342-7514

Architectural and Transportation Barriers

Overcoming Mobility Barriers International
1022 S. 41st Street
Omaha, NE 68105
402/342-5658

Arthritis

American Juvenile Arthritis Organization
1314 Spring Street NW
Atlanta, GA 30309
404/872-7100

Arthritis Foundation
1314 Spring Street NW
Atlanta, GA 30309
404/872-7100

National Osteoporosis Foundation
2100 M Street NW, Suite 602
Washington, DC 20037
202/223-2226

Blindness (*also see* Disability Services)

American Foundation for the Blind
15 W. 16th Street
New York, NY 10011
212/620-2000

Cancer

AMC Cancer Research Center
1600 Pierce Street
Denver, CO 80214
800/525-3777

American Cancer Society
1599 Clifford Road NE
Atlanta, GA 30329
800/227-2345

Cancer Information Service
(*This national number will direct callers to the hotline in the closest state.*)
c/o National Cancer Institute
9000 Rockville Pike, Building 31
Bethesda, MD 20892
800/4-CANCER (422-6237)

National Cancer Institute
Department of Health and Human Services
Public Inquiries Section
Office of Cancer Communications
Building 31, Room 10A-18
9000 Rockville Pike
Bethesda, MD 20892
301/496-5583

Oncology Nursing Society (*see* **Nursing Organizations**)

Children

American Juvenile Arthritis Organization (*see* **Arthritis**)

Boy Scouts of America
Scouting for the Handicapped Division
1325 Walnut Hill Lane
PO Box 152079
Irving, TX 75015-2079
214/580-2000

Child Help USA (for literature)
PO Box 630
Hollywood, CA 90028
800/422-4453

Children's Defense Fund
122 C Street NW, Suite 400
Washington, DC 20001
202/628-8789

Juvenile Diabetes Foundation (*see* **Diabetes**)

National Council on Child Abuse & Family Violence
1155 Connecticut Avenue NW, Suite 400
Washington, DC 20036
800/222-2000

National Information Center for Handicapped Children and Youth
PO Box 1492
Washington, DC 20013
800/999-5599 or 703/893-6061

National Resource Center on Child Abuse and Neglect
63 Inverness Drive East
Englewood, CO 80112
800/227-5242

Shriners Hospital Referral Line
PO Box 31356
Tampa, FL 33631-3356
800/237-5055

Spina Bifida Association of America
1700 Rockville Pike, Suite 540
Rockville, MD 20852
301/770-SBAA

Diabetes

Juvenile Diabetes Foundation (international hotline)
432 Park Avenue South
New York, NY 10016
800/223-1138

National Diabetes Information Clearinghouse
Box NDIC
9000 Rockville Pike
Bethesda, MD 20892
301/468-2162

Disability Services

American Health Care Association (*see* **Healthcare Facilities and Programs**)

Clearinghouse on Disability Information
U.S. Department of Education
Switzer Building, Room 3132
Washington, DC 20202
202/731-1241

Independent Living for the Handicapped
1301 Belmont Street NW
Washington, DC 20009
202/797-9803

Information Center for Individuals with Disabilities
Fort Point Place, First Floor
27-43 Wormwood Street
Boston, MA 02210-1606
617/727-5540

Library of Congress National Library Service for the Blind and Physically Handicapped
1291 Taylor Street NW
Washington, DC 20542
202/707-5100 or 800/424-9100 (TDD 202/707-0744)

Mainstream Inc.
1030 15th Street NW, Suite 1010
Washington, DC 20005
202/898-0202

National Council on Disability
800 Independence Avenue SW, Suite 808
Washington, DC 20591
202/267-3846 (TDD 202/267-3232)

National Easter Seal Society
70 E. Lake Street
Chicago, IL 60601
800/221-6827

National Foundation March of Dimes
1275 Mamaroneck Avenue
White Plains, NY 10605
914/428-7100

National Rehabilitation Information Center
8455 Colesville Road, Suite 935
Silver Springs, MD 20910-3319
800/346-2742 or 301/588-9284

President's Committee on Employment of the Handicapped
111 20th Street NW, Room 636
Washington, DC 20036
202/653-5044

Elderly (*also see* Arthritis, Incontinence, *and* Neuromuscular Disorders)

Alzheimer's Disease and Related Disorders Association
National Information Service
919 N. Michigan Avenue, Suite 1000
Chicago, IL 60611-1676
800/272-3900 or 312/335-8700

National Institute on Aging
National Institutes of Health
Federal Building, Room 6C12
Bethesda, MD 20892
301/496-1752

Farmers/Ranchers (services for disabled)

The AgrAbility Project
c/o National Easter Seal Society
1350 New York Avenue NW, Suite 915
Washington, DC 20005
202/347-3066
or
USDA Extension Service
Room 3346
South Building
Washington, DC 20250-0900
202/720-3920
or
Breaking New Ground Resource Center
Purdue University
1146 Agricultural Engineering Building
West Lafayette, IN 47907-1146
202/347-3066

Head Injury

National Head Injury Foundation
1776 Massachusetts Avenue NW, Suite 100
Washington, DC 20036
202/296-6443

Healthcare Facilities and Programs

American Health Care Association (information on facilities)
1202 L Street NW
Washington, DC 20005
202/842-4444

American Hospital Association
840 N. Lake Shore Drive
Chicago, IL 60611
312/280-6000

- American Hospital Publishing
  737 N. Michigan Avenue, Suite 600
  Chicago, IL 60611
  312/440-6800
- Section for Rehabilitation Hospitals and Programs
  840 N. Lake Shore Drive
  Chicago, IL 60611
  312/280-6671

Commission on Accreditation of Rehabilitation Facilities
101 N. Wilmot Road, Suite 500
Tucson, AZ 85711
602/748-1212

Council of Better Business Bureaus (home care/nursing home information)
4200 Wilson Boulevard, Suite 800
Arlington, VA 22203
703/276-0100

Joint Commission on Accreditation of Health Care Organizations
One Renaissance Boulevard
Oakbrook Terrace, IL 60181
708/916-5600

National Association of Rehabilitation Facilities
PO Box 17675
Washington, DC 20041-0675
800/368-3513 or 703/648-9300

National Consumers League (guides to life-care communities and long-term care)
815 15th Street, NW, Suite 516
Washington, DC 20005
202/639-8140

Healthcare-Related Federal Agencies

Agency for Health Care Policy and Research
Executive Office Center, Suite 501
2101 E. Jefferson Street
Rockville, MD 20892
301/495-3453

Consumer Information Center (for free and low-cost informational booklets)
PO Box 100
Pueblo, CO 81002

Food and Drug Administration
Office of Consumer Affairs, HFE-88
600 Fishers Lane
Rockville, MD 20857
301/443-3170

National Institute on Disability and Rehabilitation Research
U.S. Department of Education
400 Maryland Avenue SW, Room 3060
Washington, DC 20202
202/732-1134

Rehabilitation Services Administration
Department of Human Services
605 G Street NW, Room 101M
Washington, DC 20001
202/727-3211

U.S. Department of Health and Human Services
Office of Disease Prevention and Health Promotion
Room 2132, Switzer Building
330 C Street SW
Washington, DC 20201
202/205-8611

U.S. Public Health Service
200 Independence Avenue SW
Washington, DC 20201
202/245-7694

Hearing and Speech

American Speech-Language-Hearing Association
(*see* Rehabilitation Professionals)

Better Hearing Institute
PO Box 1840
Washington, DC 20013
800/EAR-WELL (327-9355)

National Association for Hearing and Speech Action Line
800/638-8255

Incontinence

Continence Restored, Inc.
407 Strawberry Hill
Stamford, CT 06905
212/879-3131 (day)
203/348-0601 (evening)

Help for Incontinent People (HIP)
PO Box 544
Union, SC 29379
803/579-7900

Neuromuscular Disorders

Amyotrophic Lateral Sclerosis Association
21021 Ventura Boulevard, Suite 321
Woodland Hills, CA 91364
818/990-2151

Epilepsy Foundation of America
4351 Garden City Drive
Landover, MD 20785
301/459-3700

Guillain-Barré Syndrome Foundation International
PO Box 262
Wynnewood, PA 19096
215/667-0131

Muscular Dystrophy Association
810 7th Avenue
New York, NY 10019
212/586-0808

Myasthenia Gravis Foundation, Inc.
53 W. Jackson Boulevard, Suite 660
Chicago, IL 60604
312/427-6252

National Ataxia Foundation
15500 Wayzata Boulevard, Suite 750
Wayzata, MN 55391
612/473-7666

National Multiple Sclerosis Society
205 E. 42nd Street
New York, NY 10017
800/624-8236

Parkinson's Disease Foundation
William Black Medical Research Building
Columbia Presbyterian Medical Center
650 W. 168th Street
New York, NY 10032
800/457-6676 or 212/923-4700

United Cerebral Palsy Foundation Associations
7 Penn Plaza, Suite 804
New York, NY 10001
212/268-6655

Nursing Organizations

American Association of Neuroscience Nurses
224 N. Des Plaines, Suite 601
Chicago, IL 60661
312/993-0043

American Association of Spinal Cord Injury Nurses
75-20 Astoria Boulevard
Jackson Heights, NY 11370-1177
718/803-3782

American Holistic Nurses' Association
4101 Lake Boone Trail, Suite 201
Raleigh, NC 27607
919/787-5181

American Nurses Association
600 Maryland Avenue SW, Suite 100 West
Washington, DC 20024-2571
202/554-4444

Association of Operating Room Nurses
10170 E. Mississippi Avenue
Denver, CO 80231
303/755-6300

Association of Rehabilitation Nurses (*see* Rehabilitation Professionals)

National Federation for Specialty Nursing Organizations
875 Kings Highway, Suite 200
West Deptford, NJ 08096
609/848-5932

National Nurses Society on Addictions
5700 Old Orchard Road, First Floor
Skokie, IL 60077-1057
708/966-5010

North American Nursing Diagnosis Association
1211 Locust Street
Philadelphia, PA 19107
800/647-9002

Nursing Organization Liaison Forum
600 Maryland Avenue SW, Suite 100 West
Washington, DC 20024-2571
202/554-4444

Oncology Nursing Society
501 Holiday Drive
Pittsburgh, PA 15220
412/921-7373

Respiratory Nursing Society
5700 Old Orchard Road, First Floor
Skokie, IL 60077-1057
708/966-8673

Rehabilitation Professionals

American Academy of Physical Medicine and Rehabilitation
122 S. Michigan Avenue, Suite 1300
Chicago, IL 60603-6107
312/922-9366

American Congress of Rehabilitation Medicine
5700 Old Orchard Road, First Floor
Skokie, IL 60077-1057
708/966-0095

American Occupational Therapy Association
1383 Piccard Drive, Suite 301
Rockville, MD 20850-4375
301/948-9626

American Physical Therapy Association
1111 N. Fairfax Street
Alexandria, VA 22314
703/684-2782

American Speech-Language-Hearing Association
(*also see* **Hearing and Speech**)
10801 Rockville Pike
Rockville, MD 20852
301/897-5700

Association of Rehabilitation Nurses
5700 Old Orchard Road, First Floor
Skokie, IL 60077-1057
708/966-3433

National Rehabilitation Association
633 S. Washington Street
Alexandria, VA 22314
703/836-7677

National Therapeutic Recreation Society
3101 Park Center Drive, 12th Floor
Alexandria, VA 22302
703/820-4940

Respiratory Disorders

American Lung Association
1740 Broadway
New York, NY 10019
212/315-8700

Asthma and Allergy Foundation of America
1717 Massachusetts Avenue, Suite 305
Washington, DC 20036
800/7-ASTHMA (727-8462) or 202/265-2065

Respiratory Nursing Society (*see* **Nursing Organizations)**

Sexuality

Sex Information and Education Council of the U.S.
130 W. 42nd Street, Suite 2500
New York, NY 10036
212/819-9770

Spinal Cord

American Association of Spinal Cord Injury Nurses
(*see* **Nursing Organizations)**

American Spinal Injury Association
250 E. Superior, Room 619
Chicago, IL 60611
312/908-3425

National Spinal Cord Injury Association
600 W. Cummings Park, Suite 2000
Woburn, MA 01801
617/935-2722

New England Paralyzed Veterans of America
1600 Providence Highway, Suite 101R
Walpole, MA 02081
508/660-1181

Paralyzed Veterans of America
801 18th Street NW
Washington, DC 20006
202/872-1300

Sports and Recreation

National Handicapped Sports and Recreation Association
4405 East-West Highway, Suite 603
Bethesda, MD 20814
301/652-7505

National parks
(Call specific park directly for complete information on access.)

Society for the Advancement of Travel for the Handicapped
347 Fifth Avenue, Suite 610
New York, NY 10016
212/447-7284

Special Olympics International
1350 New York Avenue NW, Suite 500
Washington, DC 20005
202/628-3630

Stroke

National Institute of Neurological and Communicative Disorders and Stroke
Building 31, Room 8A52
9000 Rockville Pike
Bethesda, MD 20892
301/496-9746

National Stroke Association
300 E. Hampden Avenue, Suite 240
Englewood, CO 80110-2654
303/762-9922

Stroke Clubs International
805 12th Street
Galveston, TX 77550
409/762-1022

Substance Abuse

Alcoholics Anonymous
Contact local chapters (which should be listed in local phone directories) directly.

MADD—Mothers Against Drunk Driving
National Headquarters
511 E. John Carpenter Highway
Irving, TX 75062
214/744-6233

National Clearinghouse for Alcohol and Drug Information
PO Box 2345
Rockville, MD 20852
800/729-6686 or 301/468-2600

National Nurses Society on Addictions
(*see* **Nursing Organizations**)

SADD—Students Against Driving Drunk
PO Box 800
Marlboro, MA 01752
508/481-3568
(SADD also has chapters in local high schools.)

Workers' Compensation Programs

Office of Workers' Compensation Programs
Office of the Director
Department of Labor, Room 5-3524
200 Constitution Avenue NW
Washington, DC 20210
202/219-7503

Private vocational rehabilitation services/state offices of vocational rehabilitation services
(See local telephone directory.)

Sources Consulted

Burek, D.M. (Ed.). (1992). *Encyclopedia of associations* (27th ed.). Detroit: Gale Research, Inc.

Chipps, E.M., Clanin, N.J., & Campbell, V.G. (1992). *Neurological disorders.* St. Louis: Mosby-Year Book, Inc.

Office of the Federal Register, National Archives and Records Administration. (1990). *U.S. Government Manual 1990-1991* (rev. ed.). Washington, DC: U.S. Government Printing Office.

Glossary of Terms

Below is a list of terms frequently used in rehabilitation. The glossary has been compiled as an easy-to-use reference for the practitioner. It is not an all-inclusive list, but it should offer helpful information.

abdominal massage—a method of helping to propel feces through the large intestine by stimulating the abdominal musculature

abulia—lack of spontaneity affecting all types of motor responses, including speech; occurs as a result of frontal lobe lesions

accessory muscles—neck muscles used as a secondary mechanism to assist breathing

advance directive—a written notification to one's physician and family outlining one's choice in regard to life-sustaining treatment under certain circumstances

affective domain—category of learning that deals with expression of feelings, attitudes, emotions, and values

agitation—excesses of behavior; often characterized by restlessness, inability to focus or maintain attention, irritability, and potential escalation to combativeness

agnosia—defect in the ability to recognize and interpret sensory stimuli appropriately

amnesia—a defect in memory; **anterograde amnesia** is loss of memory from a point of stress forward; **retrograde amnesia** is lack of awareness of events happening before the occurrence of a stressor

anal reflex—a reflex response of the anal sphincter that is elicited by a pinprick along both sides of the skin of the external anal sphincter; a visible contraction, also known as an *anal wink*, indicates that reflex-level function is present

anal wink—*see* **anal reflex**

androgogy—teaching of adults

ankylosis—fixation of a joint, usually resulting from destruction of articular cartilage

anosmia—absence of the sense of smell

anterior horn cell—cell in the ventral, or front, part of the spinal cord from which the lower motor neuron exits; the site of damage in poliomyelitis

aphasia—lack of speech; disordered language perception and expression

apraxia—inability to carry out voluntary movement in the absence of paralysis; results from dissociation of parts of the cerebrum, often as a result of parietal lobe lesions

astereognosis—inability to discriminate between objects based on their shapes, textures, weights, and sizes; inability to recognize an object by touch alone; occurs as a result of parietal lobe lesions

ataxia—movement that is irregular and jerky; commonly seen with cerebellar dysfunction

athetosis—involuntary, repetitive, gross movements; particularly affects posture

attention—the ability to respond to relevant information and to screen out information that is not important

autonomic dysreflexia—a potentially life-threatening condition occurring in persons with a spinal cord injury above T6, characterized by an unchecked sympathetic nervous system response to noxious stimuli below the level of injury; *also see* **autonomic nervous system**

autonomic nervous system—the portion of the nervous system concerned with control of involuntary bodily functions

Babinski reflex—a pathological reflex in adults occurring as a result of pyramidal tract damage; a positive Babinski reflex is seen when the toes of the foot dorsiflex and fan out after the sole of the foot is stroked

blanching—the whitening or loss of color in an area of skin that has experienced a decrease in blood supply

blood-brain barrier—a membrane that separates the brain from blood; occurs due to the thickening of basement membranes of cerebral vessels; prevents harmful substances from entering the brain and cerebrospinal fluid

bridging—a positioning technique used to elevate the hips and buttocks while patient is lying down; commonly used during dressing or to relieve skin pressure

Broca's aphasia—difficulty in speaking or inability to speak; also known as *expressive* or *nonfluent aphasia*

bulbar—refers to an area of the brainstem responsible for mechanisms involved in swallowing, coughing, speaking, chewing, and controlling facial expressions; bulbar dysfunction as a result of a brainstem lesion increases the patient's risk of aspiration

bulbocavernosus reflex—the response to stimulation of the bulbocavernosus muscle, a genital muscle found in both men and women, in which the muscle contracts around a finger in the rectum; stimulated in male patients by pressing on the dorsum of the penis and in female patients by pressing on the clitoris; a positive bulbocavernosus reflex indicates that the sacral segment reflexes are intact after spinal cord injury

clonus—repetitive, sustained stretch reflexes

cognitive domain—category of learning that deals with facts and concepts that involve an individual's intellectual abilities and problem-solving skills

confabulation—a method of verbally compensating for memory deficits by inventing details

confusion—the inability to recall minute-to-minute, hour-to-hour, or day-to-day events in life

conus medullaris—the conical portion of the lower spinal cord

corticospinal tract—a motor tract carrying messages from the cerebral cortex to various spinal segmental levels; the major voluntary motor tract; also known as the *pyramidal tract*

decerebrate posturing—abnormal extension of the arms and legs, seen as a result of brainstem damage or pressure

decorticate posturing—abnormal flexion of the arms and extension of the legs, seen as a result of brainstem damage or pressure

deglutition—the act of swallowing

detrusor muscle—the main muscle of the urinary bladder; composed of smooth muscle

detrusor sphincter dyssynergia—loss of coordination or synergy between the detrusor muscle of the urinary bladder and the external urinary sphincter; as a result of the dyssynergy, the detrusor muscle pushes down on a spastic or tightened urinary sphincter, creating undesirable high pressures in the bladder

diabetes insipidus—a condition resulting from lack of secretion of antidiuretic hormone (ADH) from the posterior pituitary gland; without the water-conserving function of ADH, the kidneys excrete large quantities of dilute urine; diabetes insipidus occurs frequently after cerebral injury, tumor, or surgery

digital stimulation—a technique used to stimulate a defecation reflex through the use of a gloved, lubricated index finger inserted in the rectum and rotated against the anal sphincter wall

disability—restriction in performing or lack of ability to perform an activity in the manner or range considered within normal limits

disinhibition—the inability to control verbalizations or behaviors in a socially appropriate way

durable medical equipment—nondisposable medical equipment expected to be used over a period of time (e.g., commode, hospital bed, elevated toilet seat)

durable power of attorney for health care (DPAHC)—authorizes a person to make medical decisions on behalf of another person should the latter become comatose or unable to act; usually becomes effective only with the incapacity of the granter

dysarthria—slurred speech due to weakness of the muscles of the face, neck, throat, and tongue

dysphagia—difficulty in swallowing

emotional lability—the inability to control emotion; generally seen as easily triggered bouts of crying or laughing even though the individual is not sad or happy

erythema—a form of macula with diffused redness over areas of skin (*see also* **nonblanchable erythema**)

experiential learning—learning by doing

expressive aphasia—*see* **Broca's aphasia**

extrapyramidal system—sensory and motor tracts of the brain and spinal cord outside the pyramidal tract

fasciculations—small, local contractions of muscles that are visible through the skin, caused by the spontaneous discharge of a number of fibers innervated by a single motor nerve filament

flaccidity—relaxed, flabby, or absent muscle tone that results from a lower motor neuron lesion in which the reflex arc is interrupted (*see also* **lower motor neuron** and **reflex arc**)

fluent aphasia—*see* **Wernicke's aphasia**

gait—manner in which locomotion is carried out; types of abnormal gaits include hemiplegic, ataxic, waddling, wide-based, and scissor

Glasgow Coma Scale—a neurological assessment scale that provides an objective and reliable tool for assessing and documenting a patient's level of consciousness

global aphasia—inability to speak and to comprehend words; also known as *mixed aphasia*

halo—a mechanical device attached to the skull of a person who has an unstable spine; the halo and attached thoracic body jacket provide vertebral stabilization, allowing the person to achieve some degree of mobility

handicap—disadvantage resulting from an impairment or disability that limits expected role fulfillment

hemiparesis—weakness of one side of the body

hemiplegia—paralysis of one side of the body

heterotopic ossification—formation of new bone at the joints following spinal cord injury or traumatic brain injury; a painful condition that can severely impair function by decreasing joint range of motion

Homan's sign—calf pain present during dorsiflexion of the foot; a reliable sign of potential deep vein thrombosis when accompanied by other symptoms such as pain, swelling, and warmth

homonymous hemianopsia—a visual defect affecting the temporal visual field of one eye and the nasal visual field of the opposite eye

horizontal gaze palsy—a condition in which the eye moves away from the side of a lesion; common with pontine lesions

hydrocephalus—an abnormal accumulation of cerebrospinal fluid resulting in enlargement of the cerebral ventricles

hyperphagia—inability to monitor food intake; desire to eat and drink excessively

hypertonia—increased muscle tone and increased resistance of joints to movement

hypotonia—decreased level of muscle tone; flaccid paralysis

impairment—loss or abnormality of psychological, physiological, or anatomic structure or function

impulsivity—the tendency to act without thinking

incidence—occurrence of a disease or disorder on an annual basis within a population (i.e., number of new cases per year)

incidental memory—the ability to spontaneously recall information not intentionally memorized (e.g., remembering where one put his or her keys upon arriving home)

independent living center—a group home for individuals with physical disabilities

intravesical pressure—a measurement of the volume of urine in the bladder; as the pressure rises, the bladder contains a larger volume

joint contracture—limitation of the range of motion in a joint as a result of tendon and muscle shortening

kinesis—muscular movement

learned helplessness—a psychological response to adverse situations from which there appear to be no escape or to tasks or problems that appear to have no solution

lingual—pertaining to the tongue musculature

locked-in syndrome—total paralysis of the body; the individual has an awareness of the environment but communication is limited to eye movement or eyelid blinking

locus of control—a person's belief regarding cause-and-effect relationships between his or her behaviors and their outcome

long-term memory—the storage and retrieval of past information about oneself and the outside world

lower motor neuron—connections between the spinal cord and the skeletal muscles; made up of the spinal nerves that innervate spinal muscles

Medicaid—a federally funded, state-administered program of medical assistance for people with low incomes

Medicare—a national health payment program for persons over 65 years of age

micturition—urination

milieu—an environment or setting (as in *treatment milieu*)

mixed aphasia—*see* **global aphasia**

muscle tone—the normal tension present in skeletal muscles that is needed to support and position parts of the body against gravity

myoclonus—sudden, brief jerking contraction involving a muscle or a muscle group

neglect—lack of awareness of a portion of the body

nociceptor—a nerve receptor carrying pain sensations

nonblanchable erythema—redness of skin surface that persists when pressure is applied

nonfluent aphasia—*see* **Broca's aphasia**

orientation—the ability to know about oneself (e.g., name, age, date of birth, home), the time (current day, month, and year), and facts about one's environment

orthostatic hypotension—a rapid drop in blood pressure when the erect position is assumed

orthosis—a device used to straighten and provide support to an extremity (the word is derived from the Greek *orthit*, meaning "straight"); orthoses are frequently named for the joints they support (e.g., an AFO is an ankle-foot orthosis, a KAFO is a knee-ankle-foot orthosis, and a WHO is a wrist-hand orthosis)

pedagogy—the teaching of children

perseveration—the persistence of a motor activity after the stimulus that prompted the activity has ceased

phantom sensation—the perception that pain exists in a removed body part; common after amputation of an extremity

poikilothermia—the tendency of an organism to assume the temperature of the surrounding environment; seen below the level of injury in spinal cord injured patients

posterior columns—sensory tracts located in the posterior portion of the spinal cord; posterior, or dorsal, columns convey messages regarding position, vibration, and touch sensation

posttraumatic amnesia—lack of memory of events since the occurrence of brain injury

premorbid—prior to the onset of disease or injury

pressure ulcer—any lesion caused by unrelieved pressure resulting in damage of underlying tissue; formerly called *decubitus*

prevalence—number of cases of a disease or disorder on any given day in the year

problem solving—the ability to consider a problem's important factors, recall them, organize them for analysis, and choose an appropriate solution from the possible alternatives

proprioception—awareness of position of body parts in space

psychomotor domain—category of learning dealing with tasks that are accomplished through physical or motor activities; also involves the ability to envision mentally how a skill is performed

pyramidal tract—*see* **corticospinal tract**

Rancho Los Amigos Levels of Cognitive Function Scale—a scale that objectively categorizes cognitive functioning and recovery following traumatic brain injury

range of motion—the extent of movement that each joint is intended to make

reactive hyperemia—reddening of the skin caused by blood rushing back into ischemic tissue

receptive aphasia—*see* **Wernicke's aphasia**

reflex arc—the neural pathway between the point of sensory stimulation and the responding muscle or gland; an involuntary response to a stimulus

reticulospinal tract—a motor tract carrying messages from the reticular formation of the brain to each segmental level of the spinal cord; one of the tracts of the extrapyramidal system (*see* **extrapyramidal system**)

saddle sensation—a sensation distribution in the saddle area of the perineum that is elicited by pinprick or light touch; the presence of sensation indicates intact sensory function at the sacral spinal cord segments

semantic memory—the process of understanding the context of written material

short-term memory—the recall of immediate or recent events

spasticity—undue resistance of muscles to passive lengthening

spinothalamic tract—a sensory tract that carries messages from each segmental level of the spinal cord to the thalamus

stigma—a negative stereotype that causes others to exercise discriminatory behavior toward a person based on a belief that the person is inferior

subluxation—a partial or complete dislocation

synergy—action of two or more agents or organs working with each other

syringomyelia—a progressive disorder of the spinal cord characterized by the formation of cavities; destruction of lateral and anterior gray matter in the spinal cord results in muscular atrophy and weakness

trigone muscle—an interlacing network of the smooth muscle forming the posterior base of the urinary bladder and continuing into the proximal urethra

unilateral neglect—inability to integrate sensory and perceptual stimuli from one side of the body or environment

upper motor neuron—nerve connections contained within the brain and spinal cord that carry messages from the brain to each segmental level of the spinal cord

vertigo—a neurological disorder characterized by a sensation of the head's spinning in space or the environment's spinning around the body

Wernicke's aphasia—difficulty comprehending sounds and speech; also known as *receptive* or *fluent aphasia*

white matter axons—myelinated fibers from nerve cell bodies that carry messages for nervous system activity

Acronyms

Below is a list of acronyms frequently used in the specialty practice of rehabilitation nursing. The list has been compiled as an easy-to-use reference for the practitioner. It is not an all-inclusive list, but it should offer helpful information.

ADA	Americans with Disabilities Act
ADH	antidiuretic hormone
ADLs	activities of daily living
AFDC	Aid to Families with Dependent Children
CARF	Commission on Accreditation of Rehabilitation Facilities
CSF	cerebrospinal fluid
DAI	diffuse axonal injury
DDST	Denver II Developmental Screening Test
DI	diabetes insipidus
DVT	deep vein thrombosis
FIM	Functional Independence Measure
GOAT	Galveston Orientation and Amnesia Test
HHA	household activities
HO	heterotopic ossification
ICP	intracranial pressure
ILC	independent living center
LMN	lower motor neuron
MMSE	Mini-Mental State Examination
NHIF	National Head Injury Foundation
OBRA	Omnibus Budget Reconciliation Act
OVR	Office of Vocational Rehabilitation
PECS	Patient Evaluation and Conference System
PEDI	Pediatric Evaluation of Disability Inventory
PTA	posttraumatic amnesia
QA	quality assessment
QI	quality improvement
RIND	reversible ischemic neurological deficit
SAH	subarachnoid hemorrhage
SIADH	syndrome of inappropriate antidiuretic hormone
SNF	skilled nursing facility
SSDI	Social Security Disability Insurance
SSI	Supplemental Security Income
TBI	traumatic brain injury
THR	total hip replacement
TIA	transient ischemic attack
TKR	total knee replacement
SCI	spinal cord injury
UMN	upper motor neuron
VNA	Visiting Nurses' Association
WMS-R	Wechsler Memory Scale–Revised

Index

T

U

V

W